Diabetes

A HANDBOOK FOR
THE PRIMARY HEALTHCARE TEAM

For Elsevier

Commissioning Editor: Mairi McCubbin
Development Editor: Helen Leng
Project Manager: Anne Dickie
Design Direction: Sarah Russell
Illustrator: Bruce Hogarth

Diabetes

A HANDBOOK FOR THE PRIMARY HEALTHCARE TEAM

Edited by

Joan R.S. McDowell

MN RGN SCM DN RNT
Head of Division of Nursing and Health Care
University of Glasgow
Glasgow, UK

David M. Matthews

BSc MBChB FRCP
Consultant Physician
Monklands Hospital
Airdrie, UK

Florence J. Brown

MPhil PGDip RGN RMN RHV
Diabetes Nurse Specialist
North Glasgow University Hospitals Division
Gartnavel General Hospital
Glasgow, UK

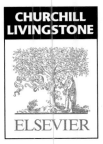

EDINBURGH   LONDON   NEW YORK   OXFORD   PHILADELPHIA   ST LOUIS   SYDNEY   TORONTO   2007

CHURCHILL
LIVINGSTONE
ELSEVIER

An imprint of Elsevier Limited

© Pearson Professional Limited 1996
© 2007, Elsevier Limited. All rights reserved.

First edition 1996
Second edition 2007

ISBN-13: 978 0443 101038

British Library Cataloguing in Publication Data
A catalogue record for this book is available from the British Library

Library of Congress Cataloging in Publication Data
A catalog record for this book is available from the Library of Congress

Note
Knowledge and best practice in this field are constantly changing. As new research and experience broaden our knowledge, changes in practice, treatment and drug therapy may become necessary or appropriate. Readers are advised to check the most current information provided (i) on procedures featured or (ii) by the manufacturer of each product to be administered, to verify the recommended dose or formula, the method and duration of administration, and contraindications. It is the responsibility of the practitioner, relying on their own experience and knowledge of the patient, to make diagnoses, to determine dosages and the best treatment for each individual patient, and to take all appropriate safety precautions. To the fullest extent of the law, neither the publisher nor the editors assume any liability for any injury and/or damage to persons or property arising out or related to any use of the material contained in this book.

The Publisher

ELSEVIER your source for books, journals and multimedia in the health sciences
www.elsevierhealth.com

Working together to grow libraries in developing countries
www.elsevier.com | www.bookaid.org | www.sabre.org

ELSEVIER   BOOK AID International   Sabre Foundation

The Publisher's policy is to use **paper manufactured from sustainable forests**

Printed in China

Contents

Contributors

Katharine D Barnard MSc BSc (Hons)
Health Psychologist
School of Psychology
University of Southampton, UK

3 Psychological care

Florence J Brown
MPhil PGDip RGN RMN RHV
Diabetes Nurse Specialist
North Glasgow University Hospitals
Division
Gartnavel General Hospital
Glasgow, UK

3 Psychological care
5 The person with type 1 diabetes
7 Monitoring diabetevii

David Chaney
MSc PGDip BNS DPSN RGN RNT
Lecturer in Nursing
University of Ulster at Magee
Derry, UK

11 Education for life

Vivien E Coates BA MPhil PhD RGN
Adv Dip FE (HE)
Professor of Nursing Research
Joint appointment: Altnagelvin
Hospitals HSS Trust & University
of Ulster,
Coleraine, UK

11 Education for life

Miles Fisher MD MBChB FRCP
Consultant Physician
Glasgow Royal Infirmary
Glasgow, UK

8 Cardiovascular risk reduction

Derek Gordon BSc (Hons) MD FRCP
Consultant Physician
Medical Directorate
Stobhill NHS Trust
Glasgow, UK

4 The person with type 2 diabetes
5 The person with type 1 diabetes
12 Improving care

June Gordon BSc SRD
Chronic Disease Management Dietician
Chronic Disease Management Team
Denburn Health Centre
Aberdeen, UK

6 Food for life

Eugene Hughes
MBBS DA DAC DRCOG MRCGP
Principal in General Practice
Ryde, Isle of Wight, UK

9 Microvascular disease

Ruth J D McArthur
BSc (Hons) RGN SCM GPN FPcert
STC/RCGP Dip Asthma
Practice Nurse/National Training
Co-ordinator
Education for Health
Mackintosh Practice
Hunter Health Centre
East Kilbride, UK

2 Diagnosis and screening for diabetes

Claire McDougall MBChB MRCP
Clinical Research Fellow
Division of Cardiovascular and
Medical Sciences
University of Glasgow
Glasgow, UK

8 Cardiovascular risk reduction

Joan R S McDowell
MN RGN SCM DN RNT
Head of Division of Nursing and
Health Care
University of Glasgow
Glasgow, UK

2 Diagnosis and screening for diabetes
7 Monitoring diabetes
12 Improving care

David M Matthews
BSc MBChB FRCP
Consultant Physician
Monklands Hospital
Airdrie, UK

1 What is diabetes?

T Chas Skinner BSc PhD
Associate Professor of Health Psychology
School of Psychology
University of Wollongong
Australia

3 Psychological care

Christine M Skinner BSc (Hons)
DPODM
Lecturer
Division of Podiatric Medicine and
Surgery
Glasgow Caledonian University,
Glasgow, UK

10 Foot care

Preface

This is a time of great change in the care of people with diabetes. Globally, we are facing an epidemic of type 2 diabetes with the associated burden on individuals and healthcare systems. Advances in science and technology mean that we can almost predict who will acquire diabetes and begin to consider preventive measures. Research has demonstrated the clinical benefits of normalising a blood glucose level, although this requires individuals with diabetes to lead and work in partnership with the healthcare team.

The care of people with diabetes requires a multiprofessional approach, with the diabetic individual at the centre. People living with diabetes are the experts in their own lives. The healthcare team works together with these people to support them as they adjust, cope and manage their condition in an effective way.

Coupled with this, national and international guidelines set the standards of care for people with diabetes. Within the past 10 years, there has been an increasing body of evidence to determine what care should be delivered, taking into consideration the individual aspects of people living with diabetes.

This book has, therefore, been written for healthcare professionals, caring for people with diabetes, who practice within a primary care setting. It has been written by members of the multidisciplinary team utilising the current evidence base. We trust that it will become a handbook for all professionals and a guide for their practice.

JMcD
DM
FB

What is diabetes?

David Matthews

DEFINITION

Diabetes mellitus is a chronic condition affecting around 171 million people worldwide; the World Health Organization (WHO) projects that this number will have more than doubled by 2030 (WHO 2005). The management of people with diabetes therefore poses a formidable challenge to the healthcare team, and to those in primary care in particular. Diabetes mellitus is a chronic condition characterised by hyperglycaemia due to deficiency or diminished effectiveness of insulin. This results in a disorder of carbohydrate metabolism; fat, protein and mineral metabolism can also be affected. Its importance as a disease is due to the irreversible tissue damage that results mainly from poor metabolic control. This irreversible tissue damage results in about 3.2 million deaths per annum from diabetes and in healthcare costs that range from 2.5 to 15% of overall budgets (WHO 2005). Diabetic retinopathy is the most common cause of blindness in persons aged less than 60 years in the UK and has an incidence of 50–65 per 100 000 of the diabetic population in Europe (Scottish Intercollegiate Guidelines Network (SIGN) 2001). One-third of people on programmes for the management of end-stage renal failure have diabetes. Having diabetes makes a person 2–3 times more likely to have a major vascular event such as myocardial infarction or stroke. Up to 15% of people with diabetes have a foot ulcer at some stage (Lancet 2005), with recurrence rates being greater than 50% after 3 years (Boulton et al 2005). Coupled with this, around 50% of people having amputations for non-traumatic reasons have diabetes. The resultant increased morbidity and mortality from diabetes is thus plain to see and explains why diabetes is a major consumer of healthcare resources world-wide.

CLASSIFICATION

Various classifications of diabetes were updated by the WHO in 1999 (Table 1.1). Type 2 diabetes is the most common, representing over 80% of all persons with diabetes; type 1 comprises most of the remaining 20%. Maturity onset diabetes of the young (MODY) and secondary diabetes are relatively uncommon and account for less than 5% of people. However, it is important to identify those individuals with secondary diabetes so that treatment can be directed to the underlying cause. Diabetes in association with other genetic syndromes is also very rare. In these instances, diabetes is another burden to be borne by these people.

TYPE 1 DIABETES MELLITUS

The hallmark of type 1 diabetes is a dependence on exogenously injected insulin to prevent ketosis and maintain life. Without injected insulin, people with type 1 diabetes die. This was the situation before the discovery of insulin in 1921. Some died very quickly over a matter of days. Others struggled along miserably for 3 or 4 years by eating almost starvation-type diets (Bliss 1983). In type 1 diabetes, therefore, there is an absolute deficiency of insulin.

Table 1.1
Classification of diabetes

Primary	
Type 1	
Type 2	
MODY, maturity onset diabetes of the young	
Secondary to other disorders	
1. Pancreatic disease	Chronic pancreatitis Haemochromatosis Pancreatectomy Carcinoma of pancreas Cystic fibrosis
2. Endocrine disease	Acromegaly Cushing's syndrome Phaeochromocytoma Gestational
3. Drugs	Thiazide diuretics Corticosteroids
Associated with genetic syndromes	
Friedreich's ataxia Muscular dystrophies Down's syndrome Diabetes insipidus, diabetes mellitus, optic atrophy and deafness (DIDMOAD)	

Case study 1.1

Joseph, a 10-year-old boy, is noticed leaving the classroom to go to the toilet more often than usual in the few days before he is taken seriously ill with a pyrexial illness and intermittent vomiting. His GP diagnoses a urinary tract infection and prescribes antibiotics. Over the next 48 hours, Joseph's condition deteriorates with continued vomiting and altered consciousness. When he proves unrousable, Joseph's parents take him to the local accident and emergency department where he is found to have diabetic ketoacidosis. Joseph is admitted to the children's ward where, after intravenous fluids and insulin and electrolyte replacement, he recovers.

Joseph's case is a fairly representative example of a person newly diagnosed with type 1 diabetes presenting in diabetic ketoacidotic coma (diabetic ketoacidosis is explained later in the chapter). Before the discovery of insulin, such a presentation was lethal. Joseph will be dependent on self-injected insulin for the rest of his life. Withdrawal of insulin would rapidly cause further ketoacidosis and he must be advised never to stop his insulin injections. Joseph and his family will require further support and education to give him the necessary skills for self-management (see Chapters 3, 5, 6, 7 and 11).

TYPE 2 DIABETES MELLITUS

Type 2 diabetes is the most common form of diabetes world wide and there is no requirement for insulin to prevent ketosis and preserve life. Many people with type 2 diabetes can be managed by dietary means alone (see Chapters 4 and 6). Sometimes, oral hypoglycaemic drugs are required in addition to diet. Most people are over the age of 30 years when diagnosed. The main associated feature is obesity and in such people the body tissues are relatively resistant to the effects of insulin, thus causing an elevation of blood glucose. By reducing body weight many people can make carbohydrate tolerance almost normal. The management of the person with type 2 diabetes is further expanded in Chapter 4.

There is a subgroup of people, however, who are not obese and who have a relative deficiency of insulin. These people cannot secrete enough insulin to cope with the carbohydrate load they consume. The pathological process in the cells of the islets of Langerhans in the pancreas is quite different from type 1 diabetes in that these individuals do not have autoimmune damage to the pancreas. However, they might eventually require insulin therapy, although they will not be classified as having true insulin dependence.

MATURITY ONSET DIABETES OF THE YOUNG

This is an inherited form of diabetes usually arising in a person's teenage years or in his or her early twenties and, although rare, affects about 1–2% of those with diabetes. It is passed down from one family member to another and each child has a 50% chance of inheriting the affected gene and a very high risk of developing diabetes (Shepherd 2003a).

People with MODY are usually managed with diet and/or sulphonylureas, regardless of age, for many years and ultimately will require insulin therapy. Insulin would also be required in special circumstances, such as pregnancy. Most people who have this form of diabetes have a multigenerational family history, with autosomal dominant inheritance and are usually not obese.

The molecular consequences are now well defined, with mutations in at least six genes. This means that diagnostic and predictive testing is now possible in 50–80% of families with MODY, which has implications for professional management (Shepherd 2003b). People with MODY have a mutation in the glucokinase gene, which results in mildly elevated fasting hyperglycaemia (> 5.5 mmol/L) (Barrow et al 2005). MODY 1 is due to a mutation in hepatocyte nuclear factor (HNF) 4α; MODY 2 is due to a mutation in the glycolytic enzyme glucokinase. Similarly, MODY 3 relates to HNF 1α, MODY 4 to insulin promoter factor 1, MODY 5 to HNF 1β and MODY 6 to neurogenic differentiation factor 1 (Fajans et al 2001). Genetic testing can define the subtype of diabetes as this has implications for different treatment options (Shepherd 2003a).

SECONDARY DIABETES

This type of diabetes is secondary to other disease processes that cause either pancreatic damage or production of hormones that antagonise the action of insulin (Box 1.1).

Pancreatic disease

The pancreas can be damaged as a result of frequent bouts of pancreatitis, which is often precipitated by alcohol abuse or the presence of gallstones in the common bile duct.

Box 1.1
Hormones that are antagonistic to the action of insulin

- Growth hormone
- Cortisol
- Glucagon
- Adrenaline
- Placental steroids
- Noradrenaline

The inherited condition of haemochromatosis causes iron to be deposited in the pancreas and this, in turn, causes pancreatic damage and diabetes. This condition is associated with gradual pigmentation of the skin, hence the common clinical name 'bronze diabetes'.

The presence of carcinoma within the pancreas can also cause destruction of normal insulin-secreting cells resulting in the development of diabetes. Pancreatic disorders causing diabetes usually require treatment with insulin.

Case study 1.2

Valentina is a 73-year-old woman who presents with a 9-kg weight loss associated with nausea, polydipsia, polyuria and vulvitis. Her random blood glucose is 19.7 mmol/L and she has 2% glycosuria. Valentina is diagnosed with diabetes and is treated with dietary measures and glipizide 2.5 mg to relieve her symptoms quickly. She returns to the GP surgery 3 weeks later. Her blood glucose has fallen to 9.1 mmol/L, she has no glycosuria, but her weight has fallen by a further 2 kg.

In Valentina's case, it is unusual to be nauseated with primary diabetes and weight loss should stop when the energy-losing glycosuria is abolished. Further investigation was thus necessary and she was found to have a carcinoma of the tail of her pancreas. Carcinoma of the pancreas can present as an apparent acute onset of diabetes and it is therefore important to think of secondary causes at the time of diagnosis, especially in elderly individuals with marked weight loss.

Endocrine disease

The secondary endocrine causes of diabetes involve excess endogenous production of hormones that are insulin antagonists (see Box 1.1):

- In acromegaly, growth hormone is secreted in excess by the pituitary gland.
- In Cushing's syndrome, the adrenal cortex makes excess cortisol due either to a primary tumour within the adrenal gland or to excess adrenocorticotrophic hormone (ACTH) production.
- In phaeochromocytoma there is excess secretion of adrenaline or noradrenaline by a tumour of the adrenal medulla or sympathetic plexus.

Hypertension, which is seen in acromegaly, Cushing's syndrome and phaeochromocytoma, commonly accompanies type 2 diabetes. When faced with an obese, hypertensive person with an elevated blood glucose it is important to consider the possibility of an underlying endocrine disorder before accepting a diagnosis of type 2 diabetes

The exceedingly rare glucagonoma results in diabetes because glucagon also antagonises insulin.

Gestational diabetes occurs in about 4% of women with normal pregnancies and is due to the insulin-antagonising effects of placental steroids and human placental lactogen. Gestational diabetes has been defined as carbohydrate intolerance of variable severity with onset during pregnancy, although there is no consensus about its diagnosis, treatment or management (SIGN 2001). Some women with gestational diabetes might need insulin treatment towards the end of pregnancy. Postnatally, the diabetes goes into remission but these women will enter the 'at risk' category for developing type 2 diabetes in later years (see Chapter 2).

Drug therapy

The thiazide diuretics, which are commonly used to treat essential hypertension, have a blood-glucose-raising effect by their inhibitory action on insulin secretion. Other drugs, such as corticosteroids (e.g. prednisolone), also make tissues relatively resistant to the effects of insulin and thus unmask diabetes.

GENETIC SYNDROMES

The genetic syndromes in Table 1.1 are rare but can be associated with diabetes mellitus, although the mechanisms are unknown. The syndrome comprising diabetes insipidus, diabetes mellitus, optic atrophy and deafness (DIDMOAD) is a well-recognised entity that can present with varying clinical features of the syndrome. Acanthosis nigricans, a rare skin condition sometimes associated with hirsutism and polycystic ovaries, is associated with a very insulin-resistant type of diabetes.

INCIDENCE AND PREVALENCE

The incidence of a disease is the number of new cases arising each year. The prevalence is the number of people with a disease in the population at any one time. The incidence of diabetes varies from country to country and area to area within countries (Hjelm et al 2003, Yach et al 2006). In the UK, the prevalence of diabetes is now around 3% and rising.

TYPE 1 DIABETES MELLITUS

The incidence varies between population groups and in the UK the cumulative risk of developing type 1 diabetes in persons aged under 20 is now 0.3–0.4%, with the peak between 10 and 14 years. This is increasing in all age groups being most marked in the 0–4 years.

TYPE 2 DIABETES MELLITUS

Accurate figures of the incidence of type 2 diabetes are difficult to establish, despite this being the more frequent type, because of inconsistent diagnostic criteria. The diagnosis of diabetes is addressed in Chapter 2.

The true prevalence is also difficult to determine accurately because of the relatively large population of people with type 2 diabetes who remain undiagnosed. There is, however, gathering evidence of a worldwide epidemic (Hjelm et al 2003). The prevalence of type 2 diabetes varies from country to country and population to population. A main feature is the low prevalence among Europeans who remain within Europe; there is a high prevalence among the Pima Indians, urban New Guineans and the Nauru (Diamond 2003, Knowler et al 1981, WHO 2005, Zimmet et al 1990). The population groups with the projected greatest increase are in Asia and Africa (Hjelm et al 2003).

Type 2 diabetes becomes more common with increasing age, with over 50% of people attending diabetes services in the UK aged over 60 years. There are now a growing number of younger people acquiring type 2 diabetes in the Western world, although it is still rare (Ehtisham et al 2004). The prevalence within the UK is only 2 in every million children. These young people tend to present later than young people with type 1 diabetes, are overweight, are usually female and a greater proportion are of ethnic minority origins. It is thought that this is due to more sedentary lifestyles and consuming more processed foods that are high in fat content.

AETIOLOGY OF DIABETES

TYPE 1 DIABETES

There is good evidence that type 1 diabetes is a T-cell-mediated autoimmune disorder and that affected persons are born with the tendency to destroy their own insulin-producing beta cells in the islets of Langerhans. There is evidence of familial clustering but there must also be some environmental trigger, as twin studies have shown that in only around 50% of identical twin pairs does the other twin develop diabetes (Devendra et al 2004).

Modern science is continually expanding our knowledge while exploring the basic genetic defect, the nature of the environmental agent and the immunopathological processes. It would appear that there is interplay between genetic susceptibility and environmental factors in the pathogenesis of type 1 diabetes (Devendra et al 2004).

Genetic predisposition

The risk of developing type 1 diabetes is mainly conferred by the inheritance of genes relating to the major histocompatibility complex (MHC) on chromosome 6. Gene mapping studies have shown that another important gene conferring susceptibility to diabetes is on chromosome 11, near the genes for insulin and insulin-like growth factor. In total, 20 independent chromosomal regions are associated with the genetic predisposition to type 1 diabetes (Atkinson & Eisenbarth 2001, Devendra et al 2004). Children are three times more likely to develop type 1 diabetes if their father has diabetes rather than their mother (Gale & Gillespie 2001).

The MHC was discovered when transplantation immunologists were trying to find out why recipients rejected donor organs. Sitting on the surface of all cells are protein molecules that allow the immune system to recognise cells as being 'self' or 'foreign'. These immune-system-recognition molecules, known as human leucocyte antigen (HLA), exist in two classes:

- Class I molecules are present on all nucleated cells and platelets. These proteins are recognised by specialised white blood cells known as CD8 (cytotoxic or suppressor) T lymphocytes. The main function of this type of T lymphocyte is to recognise antigens (e.g. a virus) but this requires the close association of the HLA class I molecule.
- Class II molecules of the HLA-D series (HLA-DP, DQ and DR) are present on other cells (but not platelets or nucleated cells) and present antigens to CD4 (helper or inducer) T lymphocytes. These T helper cells recognise antigens on macrophages and B lymphocytes. The complex interaction of these processes triggers activation and proliferation of T lymphocytes.

The main susceptibility genotypes for type 1 diabetes are HLA-DR3 and DR4 with the DQ2 and DQ8 the high-risk alleles (Gillespie et al 2004). The mode of action of these susceptibility genes is unclear. Human genome wide screens looking for areas that associate with the risk of type 1 diabetes have shown that the area upstream of the insulin gene on chromosome 11 is most likely to confer risk.

ENVIRONMENTAL FACTORS

Evidence for environmental factors having a role in aetiology of diabetes is emerging. Devendra et al (2004) summarise 16 studies that have investigated the impact of environmental factors on the development of type 1 diabetes. The overall conclusion appears to be that environmental factors alone do not cause type 1 diabetes. It is thought that the interaction between genetic disposition and environmental factors act as a trigger for an autoimmune process that results in type 1 diabetes (Bach 2005, Devendra et al 2004, Gillespie et al 2004).

The low concordance rate in monozygotic twins, the changes in the incidence of the disease in migrants from low-incidence to high-incidence regions and the increasing incidence in stable genetic populations do, however, suggest something. Cows' milk protein and Coxsackie virus B infection have been the most plausible postulates.

TYPE 1 DIABETES

PATHOGENESIS OF TYPE 1 DIABETES

Insulitis

Examination of the pancreases of people with long-standing type 1 diabetes has shown that there is destruction of the insulin-secreting beta cells while other cells are preserved. Even when pancreases of people newly diagnosed with diabetes are examined, most are deficient in beta cells. In other words, the destruction is highly selective to the beta cells.

In people newly diagnosed with diabetes there are large numbers of inflammatory cells including CD4 and CD8 T lymphocytes, B lymphocytes and others surrounding the beta cell (Atkinson & MacLaren 1994). This is referred to as insulitis. This inflammatory process is commonly associated with the presence of cytoplasmic antibodies in the peripheral blood. These circulating antibodies are more likely to be a marker of the insulitis rather than the cause. In people with type 1 diabetes, about 80% of the beta cells in the pancreas require to be destroyed by this autoimmune pathological process before the person presents with the more common symptoms of polyuria and polydipsia.

Circulating autoantibodies

Much has been learned about the natural history of type 1 diabetes by studying siblings of people with diabetes over a long period of time. A number of autoantibodies are specifically associated with type 1 diabetes (Kaufman 2003). Islet cell antibodies (ICA) are the most sensitive autoantibody marker of risk of future type 1 diabetes. Antibodies to other autoantigens, such as glutamic acid decarboxylase (GAD), IA-2 and IA-3 (phogrin), have also been found, although the role of these antibodies is unclear. Insulin autoantibodies (IAA) are directed against the insulin molecule but are indistinguishable from antibodies produced in response to exogenously injected insulin. IAA disappear with increasing ages of onset of type 1 diabetes so, if found, predict an early age of onset. GAD and ICA antibodies are more useful for predicting later-onset autoimmune diabetes. It is unlikely that these circulating antibodies contribute to the beta cell destruction as this is a predominantly T-cell-mediated phenomenon. The interaction between humoral and T-cell-mediated immunity in this situation remains unclear (Turner et al 1997).

Interestingly, in the UK Prospective Diabetes Study (UKPDS), ICA and GAD antibodies were measured in some 3672 people with typical type 2 diabetes, with 12% having at least one antibody (Turner et al 1997). This seemed to correlate with younger age, lower body mass index (BMI) and reduced beta cell function. This has led to the term latent autoimmune diabetes in adults (LADA) or slow onset type 1 diabetes (Davis et al 2005).

PREVENTION OF TYPE 1 DIABETES

Studies of the prevention of type 1 diabetes using a number of agents started late in the twentieth century but have proved uniformly disappointing (Devendra et al 2004, Diabetes Prevention Trial – Type 1 Diabetes Study Group 2002, European Nicotinamide Diabetes Intervention Trial (ENDIT) 2004). There is, however, some hope in preventing type 1 diabetes through preliminary work looking at interfering with the autoimmune processes by expanding specific cells or by blocking antibodies (von Boehmer 2004). This work is still at the early experimental stage.

TYPE 2 DIABETES

There is no evidence that type 2 diabetes is an autoimmune process. Twin studies have shown almost 90% concordance for type 2 diabetes. It is more common in certain racial groups, such as Pima Indians, and is much more likely to be a predominantly inherited condition. The precise genetic mechanisms have yet to be determined and, although it has a strong genetic component, only a small number of genes have been identified (Stumvoll et al 2005).

Many people with type 2 diabetes also have associated obesity. Despite the tendency to obesity being partly hereditary, its development is mainly related to environmental factors, such as the enormous availability of food in developed nations and the cultural factors that make food such an important factor in physical and psychological well-being. It has been shown that individuals from fairly primitive societies, where the incidence of diabetes is low, who then move to societies where food is too readily available, often progress to develop diabetes (Diamond 2003). Recent studies might provide a link between obesity and type 2 diabetes through the identification of key neural pathways that control glucose production from the liver (Seeley & Tschop 2006).

Insulin resistance is also associated with diabetes and is the best predictor of its development in the children of people with type 2 diabetes. The mechanism whereby this occurs is, as yet, unknown, although it is associated with a reduction in mitochondrial function in muscle and an increase in lipid content (Petersen et al 2004, Taylor 2004).

Past epidemiological research has shown that people who develop type 2 diabetes in later life were small babies at birth, suggesting that some intrauterine factor(s) might be important in determining susceptibility (Hales et al 1991, Hattersley & Tooke 1999).

Current research is challenging the main causes of diabetes and beginning to question if it is a disease of the central nervous system. This might especially be the case with type 2 diabetes (Elmquist & Marcus 2003, Obici et al 2003). In some ways, this serves to demonstrate the ongoing research into the cause of diabetes and the interplay between glucose regulation, food intake and the endocrine system.

PATHOGENESIS OF TYPE 2 DIABETES

There are three basic metabolic abnormalities in type 2 diabetes:

- insulin resistance
- impaired insulin secretion
- increased hepatic glucose production.

The sequence of events is shown in Fig. 1.1. The process from genetic disposition to the diagnosis of type 2 diabetes is progressive and will continue despite treatment.

Insulin resistance

The first step in developing type 2 diabetes is probably a defect in the action of insulin, resulting in impaired glucose uptake by the cells. To compensate for this, and to maintain normal blood glucose levels, there is a resulting increase in beta-cell insulin secretion with consequent hyperinsulinaemia (Fig. 1.1). This continues for a number of years, with insulin-secreting beta cells working very hard to maintain normal blood glucose (Kahn 1998, Taylor 2004).

As these overworked beta cells fail to keep pace with the insulin production required to maintain euglycaemia, impaired carbohydrate tolerance develops. Overt diabetes then follows, signalling that the beta cells are failing.

There is some evidence that this ineffectiveness of insulin action is inherited. The insulin receptor on the cell surface binds circulating insulin (Fig. 1.2). This receptor is made up of two extracellular alpha subunits. These bind insulin and are connected, through the cell membrane, to the intracellular milieu via two beta subunits. Binding of insulin to the alpha subunits results in the beta subunits triggering a cascade of metabolic events that involves the enzyme tyrosine kinase and culminates in the entry of glucose into the cell and subsequent metabolic processing. The entry of glucose is mediated by GLUT4, a cell membrane glucose transporter. Whereas abnormalities of this transporter might be expected to lead to type 2 diabetes, none has yet been identified.

Fig. 1.1
Sequence of events leading to type 2 diabetes.

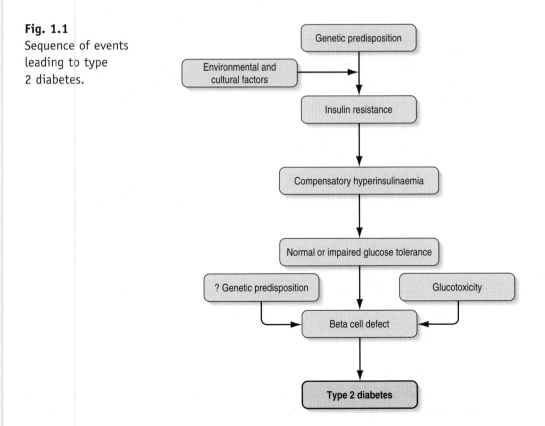

Fig. 1.2
The insulin receptor and
its actions.

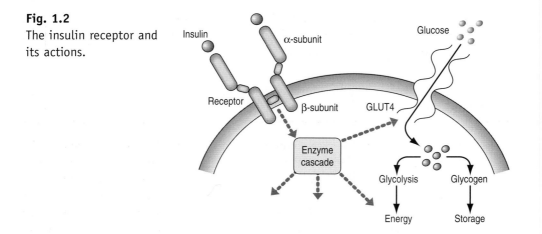

One of the important enzymes involved in the conversion of glucose into glycogen in muscle is glycogen synthase (GS), and abnormalities of this gene might also predispose to type 2 diabetes. Further potential genetic defects might exist in proteins or enzymes functioning after insulin/insulin receptor binding.

There is no doubt that the state of insulin resistance is fairly dynamic and that certain physiological states influence this. Weight gain is known to increase insulin resistance and regular exercise to decrease it. This explains why losing weight and exercise prescription are important measures in the treatment of type 2 diabetes (see Chapter 4). Ongoing research is attempting to understand the link between obesity-related chronic inflammation and insulin resistance (de Luca & Olefsky 2006).

Impaired insulin secretion

This is the definitive event in the transition from insulin resistance to the diabetic state. As the beta cells fail and insulin levels fall, blood glucose rises and the person progresses from an insulin-resistant state to developing symptomatic diabetes. Whether the decline in beta-cell function is genetically preprogrammed or, whether it is acquired, remains unclear.

In early type 2 diabetes, basal insulin levels are normal or even increased but appear inappropriately low for the raised blood glucose level. The immediate postprandial insulin response is impaired and, as blood glucose rises, this in turn leads to further impairment. It appears as if higher glucose levels blunt subsequent insulin secretion – this is termed glucotoxicity. This glucotoxicity probably explains why so many people with acute symptoms of hyperglycaemia can respond fairly dramatically to the immediate removal or reduction of simple sugars in their diet. The rapid fall in blood glucose induced by dietary measures restores insulin secretion, which in turn helps to reduce the blood glucose still further.

Increased hepatic glucose output

In the pathogenesis of type 2 diabetes, there is reduced muscle and adipose cell glucose uptake as well as excessive glucose output from the liver. The liver can generate glucose from fat and protein (gluconeogenesis) and this process is under the influence of insulin. The mechanisms involved are not well understood but reduced insulin in portal venous blood is important. The overall result is enhanced gluconeogenesis and hence hyperglycaemia.

INSULIN AND ITS ACTIONS

The hormone insulin is a 51-amino-acid peptide secreted by the beta cells of the islets of Langerhans. The insulin gene is situated on the short arm of chromosome 11 and controls the formation of a large insulin precursor molecule called pre-proinsulin. In the cytoplasm of the beta cell, preproinsulin is cleaved by enzymes to form proinsulin, which in turn is cleaved by a peptidase enzyme to form insulin and C-peptide. The insulin molecule (Fig. 1.3) consists of an A-chain (21 amino acids) and a B-chain (30 amino acids). Three disulphide bridges link the structure.

In people with diabetes the measurement of C-peptide (connecting-peptide) in plasma or urine allows the endogenous insulin-secretory status of the beta cells to be assessed. This is sometimes measured in people who are on insulin therapy to determine how much insulin their own pancreas is still producing.

The release of insulin from the beta cell can be stimulated by many factors, including glucose, amino acids and sulphonylureas. Glucose enters the beta cell and is probably metabolised there in order to stimulate insulin release.

Other agents can increase insulin release. These include the paracrine hormone, glucagon, which is released from the alpha cells, and another hormone, gastric inhibitory polypeptide (GIP), which stimulates insulin release. GIP is released when carbohydrate is eaten, which probably explains why ingested glucose is a much more potent stimulus of insulin release than intravenous glucose. This also accounts for the use of the oral glucose tolerance test, as opposed to the intravenous tolerance test, for diagnostic purposes in type 2 diabetes (see Chapter 2).

Glucose is normally absorbed from the small intestine and enters the portal vein. Most of the glucose then passes into the systemic circulation. The rise in blood glucose and GIP after a meal stimulates insulin release. Insulin then promotes glucose

Fig. 1.3
The structure of insulin

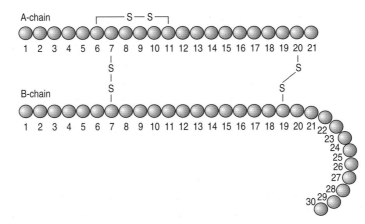

Fig. 1.4

The actions of insulin

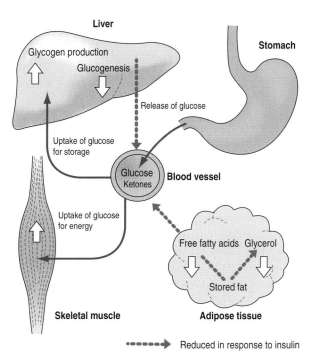

Reduced in response to insulin

uptake from the circulation into fat and muscle cells and enhances the production of glycogen in liver and muscle. It increases amino acid uptake and protein synthesis in the tissues as well as preventing protein breakdown (Fig. 1.4). The increased insulin also inhibits both the breakdown of protein to amino acids and triglycerides to free fatty acids and glycerol.

When insulin has done its work, driving the higher blood glucose out of the circulation into the tissues after a meal, its production wanes and the blood glucose levels are then maintained by the finely tuned liver production of glucose.

In the fasting state, insulin levels fall. The fall in insulin levels allows the breakdown of fat and proteins to occur. The fatty acids provide the main fuel for muscles, leaving glucose free to fuel the brain. The low continuing insulin concentrations are enough to limit ketone body formation and the normal buffering capacity of the blood prevents acidosis.

DIABETIC KETOACIDOSIS

In the pathological state of insulin deficiency there is an increased liver output of glucose from two sources. Glycogen is metabolised to glucose and glucose is also formed (gluconeogenesis) from a combination of the breakdown products of fatty acids and amino acids (see Fig. 1.4). In addition, the lack of insulin results in less glucose being taken up by the peripheral tissues such as muscle. Blood glucose thus rises, overcoming the renal threshold for glucose with resulting glycosuria. The resulting osmotic diuresis is responsible for the symptoms of polyuria, nocturia and polydipsia in uncontrolled diabetes.

In addition, fat and protein breakdown is quite unrestrained, with consequent weight loss. Fatty acid levels rise very high, which in turn causes the liver to increase the production of ketone bodies. Ketone levels eventually overwhelm the acid-buffering capacity of the blood and diabetic ketoacidosis (DKA) develops.

The combination of uncontrolled diabetes and acidosis with resultant circulatory collapse and clouded consciousness makes this a medical emergency that only intravenous fluids and insulin can reverse. Death can still occur from diabetic ketoacidosis, although this is now rare.

HYPEROSMOLAR NON-KETOTIC COMA

In a person presenting with hyperosmolar non-ketotic coma (HONK) there is a relative, rather than complete, lack of insulin. This differentiates it from diabetic ketoacidosis. Here, there is insufficient insulin production to prevent a rise in blood glucose yet there is just enough to prevent ketone body production. Hence ketonuria is not a feature.

Case study 1.3

> Mabel, a 75-year-old woman, lives alone. Her carer, who visits once per week, found her lying on the floor. Mabel was semiconscious and unable to give an account of what had happened to her. The previous week, her carer had found her rather tired and lethargic when she had called and, on reflection, states that Mabel might have been more thirsty than normal. Mabel is immediately admitted to hospital, where she is found to be mildly hypothermic and clinically dehydrated. Her feet are mottled in colour and her peripheral pulses are poor. Initial biochemistry confirms a dehydrated state with a urea 22.5 mmol/L and creatinine 200 micromol/L. Her blood glucose is found to be 52 mmol/L but there is no evidence of any ketonuria.

HONK usually occurs in people with type 2 diabetes and especially in people who are as yet undiagnosed, as in Mabel's situation, above. The elderly, who are at most risk of HONK, can become slowly unwell over a prolonged period as they fail to recognise the significance of their symptoms. This can result in the blood glucose rising to very high levels (often > 50 mmol/L), which causes a rise in plasma osmolality and results in severe dehydration. This is a medical emergency. Treatment is by slow intravenous fluids and insulin to gradually correct the blood glucose level and avoid the added complication of cerebral oedema. When restored to good health, the person is managed as an individual with type 2 diabetes. Long-term injected insulin is not usually required, suggesting that glucotoxicity might have played a role in the beta-cell failure.

A high mortality rate is associated with HONK, due to the fact that people can be comatose before they are discovered by relatives or friends. The dehydration reduces the circulation to the periphery and increases blood viscosity. Thrombosis of the arteries to the lower limbs and/or myocardial infarction is common and often contributes to the high mortality.

THE COUNTER-REGULATORY HORMONES

In both types of metabolic decompensation, DKA and HONK, it is important to recognise the actions of hormones that oppose the action of insulin (see Box 1.1).

Glucagon, adrenalin and noradrenaline modulate beta-cell insulin secretion. By increasing blood glucose levels they protect against hypoglycaemia and ensure fuel supplies to vital organs during stress. However, in the stressful situations of DKA or HONK, their actions are inappropriate and result in raising blood glucose to even greater levels.

THE CLINICAL DIFFERENCES BETWEEN TYPE 1 AND TYPE 2 DIABETES

AGE OF ONSET

People with newly diagnosed type 1 diabetes are usually children or young adults, although people with type 1 diabetes can be diagnosed at any age. Type 2 diabetes tends to present in people over the age of 30 years. However, increasing numbers of individuals are being identified at a younger age as the prevalence of obesity in younger people increases and as the public and healthcare professionals become more aware of type 2 diabetes.

GENDER

Type 1 diabetes is slightly more common in males, there being less sex bias than in type 2 diabetes.

PAST MEDICAL HISTORY

People with type 1 diabetes have usually been very healthy before the development of diabetes. It is very common, however, to find a history of hypertension and/or vascular disease in individuals who are diagnosed with type 2 diabetes.

FAMILY HISTORY

Sometimes, people presenting with type 1 diabetes have a family history of diabetes, but this is more common in individuals developing type 2 diabetes.

PRESENTATION

People with type 1 diabetes usually present with classic symptoms of polydipsia, polyuria, weight loss and tiredness. They might present with diabetic ketoacidosis.

People with type 2 diabetes can also present with classic symptoms but never develop ketoacidosis. They more often present with symptoms associated with mild elevation of blood and urinary glucose, namely balanitis or vulvitis, blurred vision or leg cramps. Type 2 diabetes is more commonly diagnosed by the finding of glycosuria or hyperglycaemia in the course of assessment of other medical conditions or during routine screening tests (see Chapter 2). It is not uncommon for people with type 2 diabetes to present with an established microvascular complication of diabetes, such as background retinopathy during routine eye screening, or with an infected neuropathic foot ulcer.

WEIGHT

People with type 1 diabetes have commonly lost weight at diagnosis, but not always. Many people with type 2 diabetes have coexistent obesity at diagnosis and it is not uncommon for some to claim recent great success in losing weight. This is, of course, due to the amount of energy lost in persisting glycosuria.

URINALYSIS

People who present with the classic symptoms of type 1 diabetes of polyuria and polydipsia will have glycosuria; ketonuria will be evident if presentation is with ketoacidosis. Most people with newly diagnosed type 1 diabetes will have significant ketonuria. Some people presenting with type 2 diabetes can have small or moderate amounts of ketonuria. If this occurs, it is usually because the person has reduced his/her calorie intake for whatever reason.

Sometimes, despite these clinical differences, it is difficult to tell whether people have type 1 or type 2 diabetes. This might not matter too much in the sense that initial treatments might not differ. However, it could be crucial in some individuals to know if they are likely to require insulin treatment because this might have serious implications in relation to employment, insurance and driving (see Chapter 11).

CONCLUSION

Diabetes mellitus is a chronic condition classified into two main types: type 1 and type 2. Type 1 diabetes is an autoimmune condition with a variable speed of onset. Type 2 diabetes is primarily an inherited disorder characterised by initial peripheral resistance to insulin with subsequent exhaustion of the pancreas's ability to secrete insulin.

Diabetes mellitus results in irreversible tissue damage and is a major source of morbidity and mortality within populations world wide.

REFERENCES

Atkinson MA, Eisenbarth GS 2001 Type 1 diabetes: new perspectives on disease pathogenesis and treatment. Lancet 358:221–229

Atkinson MA, MacLaren NK 1994 The pathogenesis of insulin dependent diabetes. New England Journal of Medicine 331:1428–1436

Bach JF 2005 A toll-like trigger for autoimmune disease. Nature Medicine 11(2):120–121

Barrow BA, Ellard S, Shepherd MH et al 2005 Patient recruitment strategy for family studies investigating novel genetic causes of maturity-onset diabetes of the young. European Diabetes Nursing 2(1):24–29

Bliss M 1983 The discovery of insulin. Paul Harris Publishing, Edinburgh

Boulton AJM, Vileikyte L, Ragnarson-Tennvall G, Apelqvist J 2005 The global burden of diabetic foot disease. Lancet 366:1719–1724

Davis TME, Wright AD, Mehta ZM et al 2005 Islet autoantibodies in clinically diagnosed type 2 diabetes: prevalence and relationship with metabolic control (UKPDS 70). Diabetologia 48:695–702

De Luca C, Olefsky JM 2006 Stressed out about obesity and insulin resistance. Nature Medicine 12(1):41–42

Devendra D, Liu E, Eisenbarth GS 2004 Type 1 diabetes: recent developments. British Medical Journal 328:750–754

Diabetes Prevention Trial – Type 1 Diabetes Study Group 2002 Effects of insulin in relatives of patients with type 1 diabetes mellitus. New England Journal of Medicine 346(22):1685–1691

Diamond J 2003 The double puzzle of diabetes. Nature 423:599–602

Ehtisham S, Hattersley AT, Dunger DB, Barrett TG 2004 First UK survey of paediatric type 2 diabetes and MODY. Archives of Disease in Childhood 89:526–529

Elmquist JK, Marcus JN 2003 Rethinking the central causes of diabetes. Nature Medicine 9(6):645–647

European Nicotinamide Diabetes Intervention Trial (ENDIT) 2004 A randomised controlled trial of intervention before the onset of type 1 diabetes. Lancet 363:925–931

Fajans SS, Bell GI, Polonsky KS 2001 Molecular mechanisms and clinical pathophysiology of maturity-onset diabetes of the young. New England Journal of Medicine 345:971–980

Gale EA, Gillespie KM 2001 Diabetes and gender. Diabetologia 44:3–15

Gillespie KM, Bain SC, Barnett AH et al 2004 The rising incidence of childhood type 1 diabetes and reduced contribution of high-risk HLA haplotypes. Lancet 364:1699–1700

Hales C, Barker DJP, Clark PMS et al 1991 Fetal and infant growth and impaired glucose tolerance at age 64 years. British Medical Journal 303:1019–1022

Hattersley AT, Tooke JE 1999 The fetal insulin hypothesis: an alternative explanation of the association of low birth weight with diabetes and vascular disease. Lancet 353:1789–1792

Hjelm K, Mufunda E, Nambozi G, Kemp J 2003 Preparing nurses to face the pandemic of diabetes mellitus: a literature review. Journal of Advanced Nursing 41(5):424–434

Kahn BB 1998 Type 2 diabetes: when insulin secretion fails to compensate for insulin resistance. Cell 92:593–596

Kaufman DL 2003 Murder mysteries in type 1 diabetes. Nature Medicine 9(2):161–162

Knowler WC, Pettit DJ, Bennett PH, Savage P I 1981 Diabetes incidence in Pima Indians: contributions of obesity and parental diabetes. American Journal of Epidemiology 113:144–156

Lancet 2005 Putting feet first in diabetes [editorial]. Lancet 366:1674

Obici S, Feng Z, Arduini A et al 2003 Inhibition of hypothalamic carnitine palmitoyltransferase-1 decreases food intake and glucose production. Nature Medicine 9:756–761

Petersen KF, Dufour S, Befroy D et al 2004 Impaired mitochondrial activity in the insulin-resistant offspring of patients with type 2 diabetes. New England Journal of Medicine 350:664–671

Scottish Intercollegiate Guidelines Network (SIGN) 2001 SIGN 55: management of diabetes. SIGN, Edinburgh

Seeley RJ, Tschop M 2006 How diabetes went to our heads. Nature Medicine 12(1):47–49

Shepherd M 2003a 'I'm amazed I've been able to come off injections': patients' perceptions of genetic testing in diabetes. Practical Diabetes International 20(9):338–343

Shepherd M 2003b Genetic testing in maturity onset diabetes of the young (MODY) – practical guidelines for professionals. Practical Diabetes International 20(3):108–110

Stumvoll M, Goldstein BJ, van Haeften TW 2005 Type 2 diabetes: principles of pathogenesis and therapy. Lancet 365:1333–1346

Taylor R 2004 Causation of type 2 diabetes – the Gordian knot unravels. New England Journal of Medicine 350(7):639–641

Turner R, Stratton I, Manley S et al 1997 UKPDS 2 Autoantibodies to islet-cell cytoplasm and glutamic acid decarboxylase for prediction of insulin requirement in type 2 diabetes. Lancet 350:1288–1293

Von Boehmer H 2004 Type 1 diabetes: focus on prevention. Nature Medicine 10(8):783–784

World Health Organization (WHO) 1999 Online. Available: www.who.int/mediacentre/factsheets/fs138/en/index.html

World Health Organization (WHO) 2005 Online. Available: www.who.int/dietphysicalactivity/publications/facts/diabetes/en/

Yach D, Stuckler D, Brownell KD 2006 Epidemiological and economic consequences of the global epidemic of obesity and diabetes. Nature Medicine 12(1):62–66

Zimmet P, Dowse G, Finch C et al 1990 The epidemiology and natural history of NIDDM-lessons to be learnt from the South Pacific. Diabetes/Metabolism Reviews 6:91–124

Diagnosis and screening for diabetes

Joan McDowell & Ruth McArthur

INTRODUCTION

It is known that there is a world epidemic of diabetes and projections have been made that there will be 2.9 million people with diabetes by the year 2010 (Amos et al 1997). As will be clear from Chapter 1, about 80% of these people will have type 2 diabetes, which presents a major challenge to any healthcare system.

Most healthcare professionals would have no difficulties in diagnosing diabetes in a person presenting with the classic symptoms of type 1 diabetes of polyuria, polydipsia, weight loss and tiredness. In such people, the diagnosis is easily confirmed by a clearly elevated blood glucose level confirmed by laboratory testing (Box 2.1) and appropriate treatment commenced. Similarly, it is easy to identify people who clearly do not have diabetes by finding a random plasma glucose below 5.5 mmol/L. Problems most frequently arise when a person is found to have glucose levels between 7.0 mmol/L and 11.1mmol/L and does not complain of any of the usual signs and symptoms of diabetes.

Diagnosing type 2 diabetes is often more problematic because the onset is very gradual and a person can have diabetes for many years before presenting with complications of the disease (Harris et al 1992, United Kingdom Prospective Study

Box 2.1
Diagnosing diabetes in the person with clinical symptoms

Diagnosing diabetes is clear where there are clinical symptoms and unequivocally elevated blood glucose. Patients with:

- symptoms and a random plasma glucose of 11.1 mol/L or above

or

- a fasting plasma glucose > 7.0 mol/L or above
  have diabetes as defined by the World Health Organization (WHO 1999).

Group (UKPDS) 1998). Hence the challenge to the healthcare team is to identify people with type 2 diabetes before they present with complications of the disease.

WHY IDENTIFY PEOPLE WITH TYPE 2 DIABETES?

Undiagnosed diabetes is not a benign condition. It carries with it costs to the individual – through the onset of complications – and costs to the healthcare system in the treatment of these. Therefore, to diagnose type 2 diabetes prior to complications arising seems a sensible way forward. Coupled with this, the costs of managing people with diabetes globally can be measured in clinical costs, indirect costs and the costs to carers on looking after people with diabetes (WHO 2004). Costs to the UK NHS vary between 8.7% of acute sector costs (Currie et al 1997) to 4.1% for type 2 diabetes alone (Williams et al 2001).

Although the prevalence of type 2 diabetes increases with age, it is now recognised in teenagers (Peters & Davidson 1992, Sinha et al 2002). The UKPDS (1998) found that up to 50% of people presented at diagnosis of diabetes with established complications, particularly retinopathy, indicating that they had diabetes for as long as 12 years. Diabetes remains the leading cause of blindness in working age adults, of end-stage renal disease and of non-traumatic lower extremity amputations; in addition it produces a 2- to 4-fold increase in cardiovascular risk. It is also recognised that mortality rates are higher in the population of people with diabetes whether diagnosed with diabetes or not than in the non-diabetic population (Jarrett & Shipley 1988). Hence the morbidity associated with type 2 diabetes is costly for the individuals concerned.

Case study 2.1

Fiona is a 55-year-old woman who attends the surgery for a routine hypertension review. Her body mass index is 20 (see Chapter 6) and her blood pressure is 130/80 mmHg; however, a routine urinalysis shows that she has glycosuria. With her consent, a random plasma glucose is taken, which is 13.0 mmol/L. On questioning, she admits to nocturia for a year, which she had attributed to her age and her daily fluid intake. She does not complain of thirst but does enjoy

Case study 2.1
Continued

drinking several cups of tea a day. She has had no weight loss within the previous year but admits to feeling tired. Further questioning elicits the fact that she had a 'touch of sugar' in her urine during her only pregnancy 30 years previously.

A careful history is taken to ascertain if Fiona is taking any drugs, e.g. corticosteroids or thiazide diuretics, which might reveal an underlying diabetic state. It is also important to enquire about family history, as a positive family history of type 2 diabetes predisposes her towards the same. On questioning, Fiona does not appear to have a family history of diabetes. Her only medication is her hypertensive therapy that she has taken for the preceding 2 years. Her history of gestational diabetes is not surprising as women who have had this are more likely to progress to type 2 diabetes in later life than those without gestational diabetes.

In pregnancy, the renal threshold for glucose is lowered, hence women will have glycosuria even though their blood glucose levels are normal. On questioning it would appear that Fiona's glycosuria had not been followed up during her pregnancy or postnatally. As the renal threshold for glucose rises with age, this means that there will be no glycosuria until the blood glucose level is significantly raised. As glycosuria acts as an osmotic diuretic, it is responsible for the more common symptoms of polyuria and polydipsia. Fiona's polyuria is due to her elevated blood glucose level, although her lack of polydipsia implies that she does not, as yet, have persistently elevated glucose levels.

A random plasma glucose equal to, or exceeding, 11.1 mmol/L is usually indicative of diabetes but a diagnosis should not be made on the basis of only one abnormal finding in the absence of clinical symptoms (WHO 1999). Fiona will be informed that she has diabetes if she has one additional glucose test on another day with a value in the diabetic range (Box 2.2). It is strongly recommended that only plasma venous samples are used to diagnose diabetes (Table 2.1).

Box 2.2
Criteria for diagnosing diabetes in the person without clinical symptoms

A person who is found to have an elevated blood glucose but who does not present with clinical symptoms needs to have two biochemical results on two separate days above the stated range before the diagnosis of diabetes can be made. Results must be one of the following:

- A random venous plasma glucose at any time of day regardless of last food intake that is $\geq$ 11.1 mmol/L
- A fasting plasma glucose $\geq$ 7.0 mmol/L
- A 2 hour plasma glucose $\geq$ 11.1 mmol/L at 2 hours after 75 g glucose in an oral glucose tolerance test

Table 2.1 The diagnosis of diabetes after an oral glucose tolerance test (OGTT). Diabetes mellitus is present if the blood glucose result is greater than the levels indicated below 2 hours after 75 g glucose load

Patient state	Glucose concentration (mmol/L)			
	Whole blood		Plasma	
	Venous	Capillary	Venous	Capillary
Fasting	> 6.7	> 6.7	> 7.8	> 7.8
2 hours after 75 g glucose load	> 10.0	> 11.1	> 11.1	> 12.1

Fiona's case study is not uncharacteristic, as people usually present in primary care with other associated medical conditions. The primary healthcare team (PHCT) should be alert to the possibility of undiagnosed diabetes hindering a person's anticipated recovery, e.g. the slow-to-heal leg ulcer. Likewise, members of the PHCT attending people with a sore toe, vaginal or penile thrush, blurred vision, boils and carbuncles or complaints of weight loss must be proactive in their role to assist in the early detection of diabetes. The PHCT should be aware of the risk factors for developing type 2 diabetes that are frequently associated with undiagnosed diabetes (Box 2.3). These risk factors are only pertinent to the person with type 2 diabetes.

Case study 2.2

Kahlil is a 42-year-old business man who has attended his general practitioner for a medical examination for his health insurance. A random blood glucose is 11.5 mmol/L and, as both his parents have type 2 diabetes and the family are of Asian origin, Kahlil is at high risk of developing type 2 diabetes. His body mass index is 27 and he admits that his working day is mainly sedentary; he takes little exercise and frequently has business lunches during the week.

Box 2.3
Risk factors for developing type 2 diabetes

- Family history of type 2 diabetes
- Obesity, with a body mass index in excess of 25
- Increasing age over 40 years
- Hypertension or significant hyperlipidaemia
- Black and ethnic minorities
- Gestational diabetes
- Any woman with a history of delivering babies weighing over 4 kg
- Women with polycystic ovary syndrome who are obese
- People known to have impaired fasting glycaemia
- People known to have impaired glucose tolerance
- Hypertension or hyperlipidaemia

In Kahlil's situation, it is important to determine whether he is developing diabetes or not. Although there are several lifestyle changes that he could make, it is first important to establish a diagnosis. Kahlil would therefore be invited to attend for an oral glucose tolerance test.

THE ORAL GLUCOSE TOLERANCE TEST

The oral glucose tolerance test (OGTT) remains the definitive standard for diagnosing diabetes despite the concerns expressed regarding its poor reproducibility and the fact that it is subject to a wide variety of influences (Yudkin et al 1990). The OGTT is still recommended if there is any doubt about the diagnosis (Vaccaro et al 1999, WHO 1999). As a test, however, it is time consuming for the person, can be rather unpleasant and can be quite inconvenient for both people and staff.

It should be remembered that the OGTT is conducted only where there is an equivocal blood glucose result in the absence of any symptoms. It is usually performed within general practice; those hospitals involved in administering the test do so on an outpatient basis. Educating the person before the test is essential as several factors can influence its reproducibility (Box 2.4). This is usually done by nursing staff and can be reinforced by literature. It is important that the person knows who to contact with any queries regarding the test as it can be seen that many factors can influence the result.

PROCEDURE

The OGTT should be postponed if the person is unwell or has had a prolonged period of bed rest before the test. The person should take his or her normal diet for 3 days before the test; it is important that diet is not altered prior to the OGTT. The person should fast overnight for 10–16 hours prior to the test, although water may be drunk. The OGTT should be performed in the morning and the person advised not to smoke the night before the OGTT, immediately prior to or during the test. The healthcare professional responsible for the OGTT should record any factor that might influence the interpretation of the results (Box 2.4).

Box 2.4
Factors that influence the oral glucose tolerance test

- Prolonged bed rest
- Restricting diet prior to the test
- The length of time in a true fast prior to the test
- Any intercurrent illness
- Medication that the person may be taking
- Smoking prior to or during the test

A sample for blood glucose estimation is taken when the person is fasting. The person is advised to drink 75 g glucose diluted in warm water. This is usually palatable in the form of Lucozade, although people are referred to criteria produced by the GlaxoSmithKline Group as the varying formulations means different volumes are required to acquire 75 g. The person should drink this within 5 minutes. A further blood glucose estimation is then taken 2 hours after the glucose load.

After the test, a return appointment should be made to discuss the results and the person goes home. No particular aftercare is required and the person should be advised to live their life as normal until the return visit.

INTERPRETING THE RESULTS

The WHO criteria for diagnosing diabetes were developed over many years and included research carried out both in the UK and in the USA (WHO 1999). These studies found that people who had a glucose level ≥ 11.1 mmol/L 2 hours after a glucose challenge were at greatest risk of developing microvascular complications of diabetes, primarily retinopathy (Harris 1993), whereas both fasting and postprandial glucose are associated with an increased risk of cardiovascular disease. The criteria used for diagnosing diabetes are outlined in Table 2.1.

Kahlil (in case study 2.2) will not have diabetes if none of his glucose samples exceeds the levels in Table 2.1. He would, however, be advised about his food intake and encouraged to undertake a weight-reduction programme. He would also be advised about taking some exercise to help with his weight management. Due to his family history, his obesity and his ethnic origins, he would be advised to have a screening test for diabetes every 3 years.

Another scenario is where only one of Kahlil's results is abnormal. Take, for example, a fasting plasma glucose of 6.0 mmol/L but a 2-hour plasma glucose of 12.1 mmol/L. The second result is clearly within the diabetic range, but Kahlil does not have clinical symptoms of diabetes. In this instance it is recommended that a second result is acquired on another day and both results would be compared. The second result could be obtained from a random sample or repeat OGTT.

Alternatively, Kahlil's fasting plasma glucose could be normal or elevated but his 2-hour plasma glucose normal. This is not within the diabetic range but is clearly an elevated result. Kahlil would therefore have impaired glucose tolerance that is discussed below.

It is important when interpreting any glucose results that the person reading them knows whether the sample is on whole blood or plasma, venous or capillary, and interprets the results accordingly (Table 2.2). Within the PHCT it is usual for venous plasma samples to be collected.

In some PHCTs there is a move towards taking a fasting blood glucose instead of undertaking a full OGTT. Although this is not diagnostic, for people who are asymptomatic it can be used as a screening test for diabetes and will be discussed under that heading. The use of fasting glucose levels alone to diagnose diabetes does not appear to identify subjects at increased risk of death due to hyperglycaemia (DECODE Study Group 1999).

Table 2.2
Comparative figures of plasma glucose versus whole blood glucose

Venous plasma glucose	Whole blood glucose
7.0 mmol/n	6.1 mmol/L
7.8 mmol/n	6.7 mmol/L
11.1 mmol/n	10 mmol/L

IMPAIRED GLUCOSE TOLERANCE AND IMPAIRED FASTING GLUCOSE

DIAGNOSIS AND PREVALENCE

Both these definitions have been clarified under the new classifications system (Box 2.5). The diagnosis of impaired glucose tolerance (IGT) is made only following an OGTT. IGT is typified by hyperglycaemia and insulin resistance.

The prevalence of IGT is between 13% and 40%, depending on studies and population groups (Tringham & Davies 2002). Studies undertaken on multiethnic populations state that between 7% and 72% of the population progress to type 2 diabetes within 5–10 years (Tringham & Davies 2002, Wylie et al 2002), demonstrating that the state of IGT is unstable. The numbers who revert to normal glucose tolerance vary considerably between 28% and 67% (Yudkin et al 1990).

The recognition of IFG identifies people who have a higher-than-normal fasting glucose that is below the diagnostic level for diabetes.

In a study of 167 children and adolescents whose body mass index was above the upper 95% confidence limit for their age, Sinha et al (2002) reported that 25% had IGT and 4% of the adolescents had unsuspected type 2 diabetes. These markedly obese young people were insulin resistant. This study is important in that it documents a strong relationship between childhood obesity and diabetes, with its attendant cardiovascular risks. With the increasing incidence of type 2 diabetes in young people, there is a need for public health efforts to prevent diabetes by encouraging healthier lifestyles in early life.

Box 2.5
Diagnosis of impaired glucose tolerance and impaired fasting glycaemia

The diagnosis of impaired glucose tolerance after an OGTT

People have impaired glucose tolerance (IGT) if their results lie within this range:
- Fasting plasma glucose < 7.0 mmol/L and OGTT 2-hour value ≥ 7.8 mmol/L but < 11.1 mmol/L

The diagnosis of impaired fasting glycaemia

People have impaired fasting glycaemia (IFG) if their results lie within this range:
- Fasting plasma glucose ≥ 6.1 mmol/L but < 7.0 mmol/L

Case study 2.3

Gregor is a 59-year-old man who is admitted to hospital with chest pain. This pain is later confirmed as a reflux oesophagitis. Routine blood tests show that he has a fasting plasma glucose of 6.5 mmol/L. Gregor works as a lorry driver. He is diagnosed with impaired fasting glycaemia.

Clinical implications

Gregor has been diagnosed as having IFG. Both IGT and IFT carry important clinical implications. IGT carries an increased risk of macrovascular disease and mortality (DECODE Study Group 1999, Jarrett & Shipley 1988). As with type 2 diabetes, people often present with cardiovascular disease before the diagnosis of IFG is made, as in Gregor's situation.

A person who is identified as having IGT should be screened for other risk factors, e.g. smoking, obesity, lack of exercise, hypertension and hyperlipidaemia and, thereafter, encouraged to make the necessary lifestyle changes. It is recommended that people with IGT are screened every 3 years for diabetes (Paterson 1993).

There is also evidence that IFG is associated with progression to type 2 diabetes (Vaccaro et al 1999), although evidence in relation to its increased risk of cardiovascular disease is as yet uncertain (Tringham & Davies 2002). Anyone found to have IFG should have an OGTT to exclude the diagnosis of diabetes, hence Gregor's management would include undertaking an OGTT.

It would appear that there is poor awareness of the clinical significance and management of people with IGT within a primary care setting (Wylie et al 2002). As primary care is the preferred place for screening and diagnosing of diabetes, it is clear that the PHCT need more guidance not only diagnosing these entities but also appreciating the clinical significance of the same and possible prevention strategies.

PREVENTION STUDIES

Several studies have been undertaken on people who have been identified with IGT to determine if there are any interventions that would prevent the progression to type 2 diabetes (Tringham & Davies 2002). Such studies have employed different research methodologies and interventions. Interventions have included lifestyle changes, incorporating exercise regimes, dietary modification and – as a preventive measure – the utilisation of oral medications normally used to treat diabetes. There have been various outcomes to these studies. Some have demonstrated a 58% reduction in progression to diabetes (Pan et al 1997, Tuomilehto et al 2001) with statistical significance for clinical practice demonstrating that progression to diabetes can be delayed by intensive lifestyle changes and by using metformin or acarbose.

PSYCHOLOGICAL ASPECTS OF DIAGNOSIS OF TYPE 2 DIABETES

People react to the diagnosis of type 2 diabetes in a variety of ways (Lawton et al 2005, Peel et al 2004). There is the perception that type 2 diabetes is not considered serious if the diagnosis is made in primary care without referral to secondary care. People whose diabetes is picked up because of other factors, like Kahlil in case study 2.2, sometimes struggle to conceptualise their illness because they have never felt ill nor experienced any of the side effects of diabetes (Lawton et al 2005). Such individuals do not perceive their lack of adherence to prescribed treatment management as a problem, because they do not actually perceive that they are ill. One study (Lawton et al 2005) demonstrated that people's perceptions of diabetes were influenced mainly by whether it was their GP or a hospital consultant who informed them of the diagnosis, and whether this took place in primary or secondary care. People can also interpret their lack of referral to secondary care as reflecting the fact that diabetes is not a serious disease and hence, where there is predominantly primary-led care, it is important that individuals are informed about the seriousness of the disease.

Peel et al (2004) found that people arrived at their own diagnosis of diabetes using one of three routes. The first route was where the person suspected that they had diabetes either from prior knowledge from a family member or else through reading about the symptoms on posters, etc. This would be the situation with Kahlil (case study 2.2), both of whose parents had type 2 diabetes and hence, were diabetes to be confirmed, he would almost expect this. The second group identified were those who arrived at their diagnosis through an 'illness' route. Fiona, in case study 2.1 epitomises this. People experience some symptoms of hyperglycaemia, have some sort of contact with health professionals and, when a diagnosis is made, there is a feeling of amazement and a sense of relief. The third route was the 'routine' route. Here, people were diagnosed with diabetes secondary to other health-related issues like Kahlil (case study 2.2) and Gregor (case study 2.3). These people described a wide range of emotional responses to the diagnosis of diabetes. People diagnosed with type 2 diabetes secondary to other health-related issues pose particular challenges to the healthcare team because they have not actually felt ill and hence might not accept the diagnosis or the proposed treatment. It is therefore essential that it is impressed on such people that diabetes is a serious, life-threatening disease even though their initial management might not appear to reflect this.

SCREENING PROGRAMMES FOR DIABETES

How does one detect the large number of people with undiagnosed diabetes? Perhaps the answer is in screening programmes, although there is some debate around these (Engelgau et al 2000, WHO 2003). The concept of screening is not

Box 2.7
Guidelines for interpreting the result after screening for diabetes using the modified OGTT (Paterson 1993)

■ Capillary plasma > 8.8 mmol/L or capillary whole blood > 8.0 mmol/L or venous plasma > 8.0 mmol/L is a positive screening test.

ADVICE FOR THE PERSON AFTER A SCREENING TEST

It is recommended that those with a positive screening test or equivocal result require a formal diagnosis to be made in line with the WHO criterion detailed above using a full OGTT (Paterson 1993). Individuals should be advised that the test has indicated that there is a possible rise in their blood glucose and that this should be investigated further. They should be instructed to make an appointment to attend their GP's surgery at their earliest convenience and not to alter their diet in the meantime.

The effects on the person of the possibility of diabetes should not be underestimated. Members of the PHCT must be prepared to counsel such people to help alleviate their anxieties before a definite diagnosis is made. Screening for diabetes might result in people who feel well being told that, in fact, they are ill. This can have implications for their employment prospects, life insurance, driving licence and so on. It is imperative that appropriate advice and counselling is offered to the person being screened at this stressful time. It is further recommended that those with a negative screening test and no risk factors for diabetes should be rescreened every 5 years. Those who have risk factors should be screened every 3 years (Paterson 1993), although it would appear that there is no optimal period for screening (Engelgau et al 2000). However, within the PHCT these recommendations might be considered impossible and hence a decision might be made to develop a team policy to target certain age groups or ethnic minority groups for screening. The frequency of this screening programme will depend on resources within the PHCT.

In Gregor's situation (case study 2.3), his impaired glucose tolerance was not detected until he presented with another condition. As Gregor does not meet any of the high-risk criteria, he would not be included in any targeted screening programme. Opportunistic screening might detect diabetes; however, increasing public awareness of diabetes could achieve a similar outcome.

PUBLIC AWARENESS OF DIABETES

As diabetes is difficult to diagnose in the absence of clinical symptoms, problematic to screen for, yet has debilitating long-term effects on individuals, perhaps increasing public awareness of the disease could increase the number of people presenting earlier to their GP.

Diabetes UK launched its 'Missing million' campaign (Diabetes UK 2000) by suggesting that there might be one million people in the UK with undiagnosed diabetes who require treatment. More recently, some pharmaceutical retailers within the UK have advertised on local television that they will offer a blood glucose test to anyone who requests it.

One study attempted to determine the impact of posters on the knowledge of the public on the symptoms of diabetes (Singh et al 1994). The posters chosen were predominantly in written form and aimed to educate on the symptoms of diabetes; they had a positive tone. It was hoped that this would avoid causing anxiety, which could result in people not seeking help should they have the symptoms. The hypothesis that increasing the general public's knowledge about the symptoms of diabetes would lead to the early diagnosis of type 2 diabetes was supported (Singh et al 1994). Hence it does compare competitively with other conventional screening methods.

CONCLUSION

Diabetes has high morbidity and mortality rates. Particular concern is expressed regarding the diagnosing of those people who are as yet unaware that they have the disease. This is because they often present when they already have complications of the disease and early detection of diabetes might assist in the prevention of diabetic complications. The obesity epidemic is further increasing the number of people developing type 2 diabetes at an even earlier age.

Various tests are available to diagnose diabetes, to screen for diabetes and to monitor diabetes (see Chapter 7). It is important that the correct test is used for the correct purpose to facilitate the correct interpretation of the results.

All members of the PHCT have a role to play in the diagnosing of diabetes. Being alert to the possibility of diabetes and adopting the appropriate methods of screening or diagnosing diabetes can identify the newly diagnosed person before the symptoms or complications are evident.

Increasing the knowledge of the general public regarding the symptoms of diabetes through poster campaigns is an effective way to persuade people to self-select for further investigation for diabetes.

REFERENCES

Amos AF, McCarty DJ, Zimmet P 1997 The rising global burden of diabetes and its complications. Diabetic Medicine 14:S7–S85

Bandolier 2005 Finding type 2 diabetics in primary care. Online. Available: www.jr2.ox.ac.uk/bandolier/band128/b128-4.html

Currie CJ, Kraus D, Morgan CL et al 1997 NHS acute sector expenditure for diabetes: the present, future and excess in-patient cost of care. Diabetic Medicine 14:686–692

If the person with diabetes expresses a lack of confidence about a behaviour change, it is possible to explore the nature of the lack of confidence by using open questions. Such as:

> *What do you see as the difficulties in giving up cigarettes?*

The person with diabetes might then embark on his or her experiences around, for example, peer pressure to smoke and the sense of needing cigarettes to reduce stress. It might then be possible for the person to identify an achievable goal and plan in detail how to achieve that goal. This will enhance the person's sense of self-efficacy. Goals and action planning are discussed further on in this chapter.

LOCUS OF CONTROL

According to the Health Locus of Control Model, people demonstrate internal locus of control when they believe that they have responsibility for their own health. Having an external locus of control means that health is seen as the responsibility of others, that what happens is a result of influences beyond our control (Wallston et al 1976). Peyrot and Rubin (1994) have investigated the locus of control construct further in the context of diabetes. Having noted that studies examining the relationship between locus of control and health outcomes had mixed results, they designed a diabetes-specific locus-of-control instrument that enabled them to identify and explain these paradoxical differences. Their results showed that internal locus of control had two components that can predict opposing outcomes in terms of self-management. The first component, autonomy, is linked with successful self-care that reinforces competence and becomes self-perpetuating. The second component is self-blame, which is related to negative outcomes. Peyrot and Rubin (1994) also sought to clarify conflicting reports about health outcomes and external locus of control. Again two dimensions were implicated in opposing health outcomes. They found that so-called healthy outcomes (e.g. glycaemic control within normal or near-normal limits) were associated with the dimension of 'powerful others'. They found that 'chance' locus of control (where people believe that things that happen to them are as a result of chance) resulted in suboptimal health outcomes.

HEALTH BELIEFS

Four important belief factors constitute Becker's (1974) Health Belief Model, which determines whether or not an individual will follow a recommended treatment plan. These beliefs involve perceptions of:

1. The severity of the disorder: the more severe the perceived consequences, the more likely the person is to actively take care of his or her diabetes.
2. Vulnerability to the disorder: there is a difference between the degree of susceptibility felt by people with type 1 diabetes and people with type 2 diabetes. According to the Health Belief Model, the more susceptible a person feels, the more likely he or she is to actively self-manage the diabetes.
3. The benefits of treatment: in diabetes, those who understand and see the benefits of self-management are more likely to perform self-care behaviours than those who don't see the benefits.
4. The barriers to treatment: there are many costs to diabetes self-management, for example dietary restriction and fear of hypoglycaemia, and individuals need to believe that the benefits outweigh the costs.

Becker later described these health beliefs in relation to diabetes self-management (Becker & Janz 1985). A person's readiness to follow the treatment regimen is highly dependent on two aspects: (1) the perceived desirability of avoiding the symptoms and the complications of the disorder; (2) the belief that the health actions necessary will be effective but not too costly when compared to other valued aspects of the individual's lifestyle.

Understanding health beliefs, the issues of self-responsibility and making choices are components in psychological care and in the concept of empowerment.

> *Question 'How can I actually motivate a person with diabetes to take responsibility for his or her diabetes?'*

The reality is that people with diabetes already have, and take, responsibility for making countless decisions regarding self-management every day. Clinicians often believe the person with diabetes 'is not motivated' if his or her decisions are at odds with clinician recommendations. In their book *Health behaviour change: a guide for practitioners*, Rollnick et al (1999) describe motivation as being the individual's 'expressed degree of readiness to change' (p 23).

Readiness to change is a component of motivational interviewing, which also includes consideration of the individual's confidence and how important the change is to the person. In motivational interviewing the role of the clinician is to understand the reasons for the decisions taken and to elicit barriers to particular decisions. If barriers exist, it might be possible to work collaboratively to find strategies. A common example would be the individual who chose hyperglycaemia in order to avoid hypoglycaemia. Once recognised as a barrier, it might be possible, through negotiation, to look at options that would enable more stable blood glucose levels while still avoiding hypoglycaemia. Conversely, there might be no realistic alternatives and the person with diabetes is making an informed choice.

A number of issues are associated with the psychology of diabetes; these are covered below.

STRESS AND DIABETES

MAJOR LIFE EVENTS AND DAILY HASSLES

Everyone experiences major life events from time to time. Life events can be graded according to how disruptive to one's life they are (Holmes & Rahe 1967). Death of a spouse, divorce and redundancy come near the top of the list for causing most disruption and stress (Box 3.1). Marriage and moving house come somewhere in the middle, whereas holidays and Christmas come closer to the bottom. Alternatively, the accumulation of minor routine aspects of daily living – 'daily hassles' – can result in the person feeling stressed. These daily hassles might or might not be directly connected with living with diabetes (Polonsky 2002). Experiencing a major life event and/or daily hassles will produce a certain degree of stress, which interferes with diabetes both physiologically and behaviourally (Riazi et al 2004).

What is stress?

It has been suggested that 'the essence of stress is the feeling of doubt about being able to cope...' (Lancet 1994). The reasons why people feel they can or cannot cope are varied. Whereas some people can cope with very major problems, others are unable to cope with seemingly minor difficulties.

Box 3.1
Life events in decreasing order of severity (Holmes & Rahe 1967)

- Death of a partner
- Separation or divorce
- Death of close family member or friend
- Personal injury or illness
- Marriage
- Dismissal from job
- Marital reconciliation
- Retirement
- Change in health of family member
- Pregnancy
- Sex difficulties
- New baby
- Changes at work
- Change in financial situation
- Son or daughter leaving home
- Outstanding personal achievement
- Starting or leaving school
- Trouble with boss
- Moving house
- Change in school
- Going on holiday
- Christmas

People who experience sustained stress can develop symptoms such as depression, agitation, apparently irrational anger, lethargy, anxiety, feeling muddled and irritability. Chronically tensed muscles can lead to general aches and pains, including headaches, and there might be other symptoms, such as indigestion, palpitations, diarrhoea, skin problems and loss of sex drive.

During times of stress, people find that their diabetes becomes more difficult to control. Most people find that their blood glucose seems to rise during stress, but others find that they alternate between hypoglycaemia and hyperglycaemia. This occurs for two reasons. First, the physiological response to stress produces several stress hormones, including adrenaline. These hormones work in opposition to the action of insulin and usually cause the blood glucose to rise. Less commonly, some people become hypoglycaemic in response to stress, but this mechanism is less well understood (Riazi et al 2004).

Second, people who are experiencing stress try to find ways of alleviating the symptoms and blocking out the problems causing that stress. This response is usually behavioural. Some people eat more than usual or turn to more highly refined carbohydrate foods such as chocolate. Others drink more alcohol than usual, whereas smokers tend to smoke more cigarettes. Some find that they lose their appetite when they are under stress, which might be another reason for hypoglycaemia at that time. All of these responses can interfere with diabetic control.

GRIEF AND DIABETES

It is usual for people to experience a sense of loss in response to many situations, including a death, the break-up of a relationship, redundancy or retirement. Even the diagnosis of diabetes or diabetic complications can involve grieving for the loss of health and lifestyle.

Grieving is well described as a staged process of coming to terms with the new situation. People experience a variety of reactions including denial, anger, bargaining, isolation and depression prior to acceptance (Kubler Ross 1990). This process is normal and the timeframe varies from person to person. Case study 3.1 demonstrates how grief, due to bereavement, can affect a person's blood glucose control.

Case study 3.1

Claudette is in her late forties. She came to see the nurse because she knew her diabetes was 'out of control'. She wasn't eating well and she was either hypoglycaemic because she hadn't eaten enough or feeling tired and thirsty because she had eaten too much of the 'wrong' foods. When asked if anything else was going on in her life to cause her to overeat, she burst into tears and cried vigorously about the death of her father.

Case study 3.1
Continued

Initially, it was thought that Claudette's father had died within the last few days, but it transpired that he had died 9 months before. It was obvious that she had not made any progress in grieving for her father. On further questioning the reason became obvious. Claudette's father had lived with her for 9 years. During that time she and her husband had never had a holiday and they had finally decided to spend a week away on their own. Claudette's father went to stay with his other daughter but within 24 hours he had died suddenly and unexpectedly. This resulted in Claudette being consumed with guilt, believing that, if she had been less selfish about going on holiday, her father would still be alive.

COPING WITH DIABETES

People have different ways of coping with the difficulties they experience. Unconscious strategies such as denial, obsessional behaviour and projection are employed to lessen the impact of living with diabetes.

DENIAL

It is a normal and protective response for some people to use 'switching off' or denial as a way of coping. Denial can be present at diagnosis and remain for several years afterwards, however, it can also cause the person to be 'switched off' from good self-care practices, especially in type 1 diabetes (Lo et al 2001). For example:

> *I really don't think the diabetes is a problem. I have never felt better. I wonder if the doctor has made a mistake – I mean, I don't do as they ask me to do, and I am neither up nor down – what's the point in going to the clinic?*

OBSESSIONAL BEHAVIOUR

Some people who experience a great deal of anxiety in relation to their diabetes find that they feel more in control if they are very precise about their self-care practices. They might monitor their blood and urine more frequently than necessary and document everything they have eaten. They are particularly aware of calorie and carbohydrate exchanges and try to make sense of differences in glycaemic levels in terms of their energy expenditure, diet, stress levels, etc. This level of self-care activity is only of concern if it intensifies and becomes the main feature of the individual's daily life. If this has happened then these behaviours suggest that the person might not have come to terms with the diagnosis:

> *The doctor said that I could cut down my blood testing to two days a week instead of testing every day and he asked me to stop urine testing altogether. But I don't want to reduce my testing. I always like to know what is going on. I feel much safer if I am testing every day.*

PROJECTION

Although the clinician encourages the person with diabetes to take responsibility for his or her diabetes, the person believes that what happens to the diabetes – good or bad – is as a result of outside influences. The person places (projects) the responsibility of his or her diabetes onto others – doctors, nurses, dieticians, family and/or friends:

> *I said to the doctor that the diet the dietician has given me is completely unacceptable. I can't be eating one thing and my family eating another. The dietician said that I should give my family the same diet as me, she said it was healthy for all of us, but I told her that the family wouldn't put up with that...anyway, it is far too expensive.*

Projecting responsibility onto others demonstrates an external locus of control.

DEPRESSION AND DIABETES

Depression is common – both in people with diabetes and in those who do not have the condition. However, research has shown that it is more common in people with diabetes. In the general population 5–8% of people will be experiencing a major depressive episode at any point in time; this figure rises to 15–20% for people with diabetes, two to three times that of the general population (Anderson et al 2001, Gavard et al 1993, Lustman et al 1997). In two UK studies, just under 38% of people with diabetes attending outpatients reported moderate to severe levels of anxiety or depression, with no apparent differences in levels of depression in type 1 and type 2 diabetes.

Meta-analyses link depression in diabetes with hyperglycaemia (Lustman et al 2000) and with an increased risk for complications (de Groot et al 2000). People at elevated risk for depression can be identified through their medical history and clinical presentation, and by asking depression-specific questions or through use of depression screening tools. People with a history of depression, anxiety disorder, mental health treatment, substance abuse or smoking are at heightened risk for depression, as are women and those with a family history of depression or mental health treatment. People who have multiple complications are more likely to be depressed, especially when those complications include neuropathy, impotence, or cardiovascular disease (de Berardis et al 2003, de Groot et al 2001).

EFFECTS OF DEPRESSION

Apart from depression being a serious condition that can have a substantial effect on people's quality of life, it affects diabetes in several ways. When depressed, individuals lack the motivation for self-management, which leads to poor dietary care, lack of physical activity and infrequent monitoring, which in turn can lead to further feelings of failure and hopelessness. This is frequently managed by comfort eating or drinking and, for those who smoke, increased smoking. This is often referred to as the indirect effect of depression on diabetes, but there is also thought to be a direct effect. That is, depression is associated with increased levels of the hormone cortisol, which acts in a number of ways (stimulating glucose release from the liver and blocking the action of insulin) to increase circulating blood glucose levels. For these reasons, depression in people with diabetes is predictive of poorer metabolic control, earlier onset of complications and more rapid progression of diabetes; it is particularly predictive of the onset of coronary heart disease.

INSULIN INJECTION PHOBIA

Injection phobia, although a common phrase, is actually very rare. Being anxious at the thought of injecting oneself is a normal emotional response. Recent evidence suggests that true injection phobia is only likely to occur in people who have had or who currently have a genuine phobia, for example, agoraphobia.

EMOTIONS

The diagnosis of diabetes generates a wide range of emotions, from utter shock and disbelief through to relatively calm acceptance of the news. The way in which a healthcare professional breaks the news can have a substantial impact on the short- and long-term process of adjusting to living with diabetes. Diabetes carries with it a level of emotional weight or burden. People with diabetes will demonstrate different emotional responses as they adjust to the impact of diabetes on their lives. The burden of diabetes will increase and decrease according to perceived difficulty and hardship. The emotional burden of diabetes can be measured by a recently developed instrument know as the Diabetes Distress Scale (DDS) (Polonsky et al 2005). It should be noted, however, that not all of the emotional consequences of diabetes are negative.

EATING DISORDERS

Research indicates that the emphasis placed on dietary control in the management of type 1 diabetes can place a person with diabetes at an increased risk of some disturbance in eating behaviour. The true prevalence of eating disorders among people with diabetes is unknown, partly because it is difficult to distinguish between a focus on food and the body that is a necessary part of life with diabetes and the abnormal concerns and behaviour that are used to diagnose eating disorder (Hall 1997). Recent research suggests that between one-third and one-half of all young women with type 1 diabetes engage in insulin purging, i.e. deliberately taking less insulin than they need for good glycaemic control, in order to control their weight (Rydall et al 1997). This causes blood glucose levels to remain high, fat storage to be inhibited and excess glucose to pass from the blood and be excreted in the urine. Many individuals with type 1 diabetes and disordered eating believe this behaviour to be easier and less unpleasant than vomiting. In people with type 2 diabetes, binge eating is relatively common, with estimates of disordered eating in this population ranging from 5 to 25% (Crow et al 2001, Hepertz et al 2000, Kenardy et al 2001, Mannucci et al 2002).

SECTION TWO: THE CHANGING PHILOSOPHY OF DIABETES CARE

Education is a major aspect of diabetes care and so it is important to consider some of the psychological elements of learning and behaviour change. Traditionally, diabetes education was seen as an information-giving exercise (see Chapter 11). The assumption was that once information had been provided, good self-care practices would follow. For example, someone might be asked to perform blood glucose monitoring but seems not to be doing so. One approach would be to assume that, for some reason, the person had not understood either the procedure or the importance of doing the procedure. The demonstration of the procedure could be repeated and the individual encouraged to practise that skill. The importance of blood glucose monitoring on a regular basis would be re-emphasised. This method is known as the 'compliance or traditional medical model approach' (Anderson & Funnell 2005).

However, there could be other reasons for a person with diabetes not testing for blood glucose. For example:

> *I can't bring myself to test my blood. Every time I think about it I feel angry about it and about having diabetes. Why me? I don't need this. I've got enough on my plate; I'm not going to do it.*

Here the person might be ignoring blood testing because he or she has not yet accepted the diabetes. Blood glucose monitoring is a physical reminder of the diabetes. The person might be denying the diabetes (as a way of coping) and blood glucose monitoring acts as an emotionally painful reminder of the anger about having a life-long disease and all that this entails.

In the last 15 years there has been a change from what was seen as a compliance-based approach to diabetes education, where the role of the educator was to teach the facts and skills of diabetes self-management and the person with diabetes was expected to 'toe the line'. There is now a more empowering person-centred approach, whereby a respectful and balanced collaborative partnership between the educator and person with diabetes is taken as the starting point. The partnership acknowledges the clinician's expertise in terms of knowledge and experience of working with others who have diabetes, *and* the expertise of the person with diabetes in terms of the rich and unique biopsychosocial elements that make up that person and how he or she lives his or her life. These elements include the person's beliefs and values about life in general and life with diabetes. An example of this might be:

> *Being able to drive is the most important thing for me [value]...Driving is an essential element of my work and I need to work to pay the bills. I can't risk hypoglycaemia so I choose to run my blood glucose levels a bit higher even though I know I am increasing my risk of complications.*

Another person might look at things differently:

> *My health is the most important thing to me...I don't want to get complications [value]. I drive as part of my work but I am worried about hypoglycaemia so I find that if I test my blood glucose before each drive and make sure I eat regularly – and for me that means snacks in between meals – then I feel I am as safe as anyone else [belief].*

Understanding a person's values and beliefs, and acknowledging that they might be different from your own, is a first step to effective psychological and educational care. These differences, however, can be uncomfortable for healthcare practitioners. In case study 3.2, Reuben demonstrates how his values affect his beliefs.

Case study 3.2

> Reuben is an intelligent, articulate 49-year-old sales manager who has had type 1 diabetes for 30 years. He has most of the diabetic complications, including diabetic nephropathy (which required a kidney transplant 2 years previously), retinopathy and neuropathy. His blood glucose levels remain consistently high, although having developed complications he might be expected to be highly motivated to improve his diabetic control, not least to protect his new kidney. The specialist nurse assumed that this was the case. Several education sessions failed to persuade Reuben to adjust his insulin. When he is eventually asked at what levels he prefers his blood glucose to be, he explains that he would rather risk further deterioration in his complications than risk hypoglycaemia. For Reuben, hypoglycaemia was an experience akin to a nightmare:

> *I know that I am putting myself at risk in terms of worsening eye and kidney disease but I cannot put myself at risk of hypoglycaemia, I would never be able to relax. I don't get the warnings anymore, I would have to stop driving and then I would lose my job and maybe my home as a result. I know you regularly check the progress of my complications and so I have decided that this is how I must live my life.*

> *Question 'How can I avoid feeling angry when people with diabetes do not comply?'*

Clinicians spend years acquiring their expertise in their chosen subject. Additionally, they see what happens to people with diabetes after years of suboptimal glycaemic control in terms of serious microvascular and macrovascular complications. There is no doubt that there is often conflict between what the clinician might want for a person with diabetes and what any individual with diabetes wants for him- or herself. Rather than feeling effective as a clinician one might feel a degree of inadequacy if a person with diabetes is making choices that could be considered detrimental to long-term health. This situation can result in the healthcare professional feeling angry and this might, unwittingly, be communicated to the person with diabetes.

Reflecting on your own beliefs and values in relation to helping people with diabetes can help you understand the nature of your anger. To be effective as a person-centred practitioner you need to communicate genuineness, empathy and unconditional positive regard. If you are person-centred then you will have certain beliefs about the human race and one of those beliefs is that people do the best for themselves given their internal and external circumstances. This understanding is crucial in underpinning good psychological and educational practice because it acknowledges that, despite a person's best efforts, there are barriers to optimal self-management. The role of the clinician in a collaborative relationship is to use one's communication/counselling skills to broach barriers to optimal self-care. Ultimately, however, the choices are with the person with diabetes and, in an empowering relationship, the clinician will respectfully accept the decisions that person makes. That doesn't mean to say that decisions about self-care cannot be discussed and modified sometime in the future; barriers can be revisited.

> *Question 'What evidence is there that psychological care makes a difference and is it only a psychological difference or does it also make a difference to HbA1c?'*

A study by Michie et al (2003) demonstrated that facilitating people to take action can result in significant behaviour change. This study noted that physical and psychological outcomes of patient-centred care are often inconsistent. Following a review of the person-centred literature in the context of those with chronic disease, it was identified that patient-centredness can be defined in two distinctive ways and has two distinctive outcomes. A total of 30 studies were examined: 20 took the perspective of the individual and 10 'sought to activate' the person with diabetes. The studies taking the latter approach were more consistently associated with good physical outcomes. Based on an examination of the studies, Michie et al (2003) describe taking the perspective of the individual with diabetes as the 'first ingredient' and activating the person's self-management as the 'second ingredient'.

There might be times in the diabetes consultation when the first ingredient – taking the person's perspective – is more appropriate, for example, when an individual has received news regarding diabetes diagnosis, diagnosis of complications or there is some other aspect of life for which the person with diabetes might need emotional space in which to adjust.

In the UK, most diabetes education, management and support is done in the context of 1 : 1 consultations with different clinicians, each of whom will offer education as part of the consultation process. Evidence suggests that these consultations are didactic in nature and promote a compliance-based model of consultation (Parkin & Skinner 2003, Pill et al 1998). Conversely, investigation of the diabetes literature intimates that patient self-efficacy and self-management improve when consultations with primary care physicians involve agreement about the content of the consultation (Heisler et al 2003, Williams et al 1998). However, the Heisler study tended to highlight the negative effects of consultations where there was disagreement between physicians and people with diabetes on treatment goals and strategies.

> *Question 'Is person-centredness not just about being nice?'*

Whereas a person-centred approach is seen by some as a passive activity (Michie et al 2003), Brown (1996) suggests that it is often seen as 'being nice' while still expecting compliance. To be person-centred, however, requires the practitioner to be aware of his or her guiding philosophy of practice and to have certain qualities and skills to communicate that philosophy. These are described below.

Person-centredness is a philosophy of counselling and of education developed by the American psychologist Carl Rogers. His basic premise (Rogers 1978) was that the individual:

> *...is basically a trustworthy organism, capable of evaluating the outer and inner situation, understanding him- or herself in its context, making constructive choices as to the next steps, and acting on those choices.*

Rogers' philosophy was that the person, not the problem, was the focus in counselling and education. Some beliefs held by person-centred practitioners include:

- That human nature is essentially constructive.
- That people do their best to grow and to preserve themselves given their internal and external circumstances.
- That it is important to reject the pursuit of authority or control over others and seek to share power (Bozarth & Temaner Brodley 1986).

SECTION THREE: WHAT IS COUNSELLING AND HOW CAN IT HELP?

So what can the professional do? What is counselling and how can it help?

In some ways it is easier to say what counselling is not. Counselling is not about giving advice, it is not about solving people's emotional problems, nor is it about stopping people's distress.

The following definition of counselling might help to clarify the philosophy of what counselling is:

> *Counselling is a process through which one person helps another by purposeful conversation in an understanding atmosphere. It aims to establish a helping relationship, in which the one counselled can express his thoughts and feelings in such a way as to clarify his own situation, come to terms with some new experience, and see his difficulty more objectively and so face his problems with less anxiety and tension. Its basic purpose is to assist the individual to make his own decision from the choices available to him. (Royal College of Nursing Working Party 1978)*

Let us analyse the definition in a bit more detail by looking at the definition more closely.

A PURPOSEFUL CONVERSATION

Counselling, or a consultation, is sometimes regarded as a 'chat' about psychosocial issues. What can often happen is that the 'chat' or 'counselling' consists of a number of closed questions that the clinician might think are relevant but which do not allow the person with diabetes to elaborate or to express new material.

Counselling is a precise way of communicating with someone. Many counselling skills can be used to facilitate a person-centred approach in the consultation; some of these are described later in the chapter.

REFLECTING FEELINGS

Feelings can be reflected back to the client when the clinician is trying to understand the client's emotional experiences. To reflect feelings, the clinician must not only recognise and correctly label the feeling but also interpret the level of intensity. As a result, the person with diabetes sees that his or her feelings are accepted and are receiving attention. The person might then feel able to disclose further feelings and to become more aware of them. Sometimes people have mixed feelings, which can inhibit them from getting a clear picture:

> Person with diabetes: 'Diabetes has been the worst thing that has happened to me.'
> Clinician (not getting it quite right): 'So you've been a bit upset about this?'

An alternative and more appropriate response would be:

> Clinician: 'It sounds as if you have been devastated by what has happened.'

People show their feelings in different ways: verbally, non-verbally or a combination of both. An individual's non-verbal communication can be acknowledged by verbal response, for instance:

The person with diabetes drums his fingers on the table and appears 'jumpy'.

> Clinician: 'You seem quite agitated about this?'

SUMMARISATION

The key purpose of summarisation is to help the person with diabetes draw together the thoughts and feelings that he or she has communicated. When the clinician uses summarisation, the individual's verbal and non-verbal statements will be attended to. This is particularly useful during a consultation if the clinician becomes unclear about what is being communicated. Summarising either part way through, or at the end, can clarify thoughts and feelings for both the person and the clinician. As with other skills, summarising should be done tentatively. Clarifying a problem or difficulty can lead to the person with diabetes gaining insight and making progress.

> Clinician: 'I wonder if I could recap the last 10 minutes or so. You started off by saying that everything was "in a mess" and this included your marriage, your job and your diabetes. You decided to concentrate on talking about your diabetes and we would set aside another time to discuss your work and your marriage. In the last few weeks since you

were diagnosed with diabetes you have been finding it difficult to stick to your diet and this is partly because you feel rebellious but also angry, as you believe that having diabetes has affected the way other people think of you, and this includes your husband and your colleagues at work. Is there anything that you would like to change or add?'

THE QUALITIES OF A COUNSELLOR

The core qualities of the person-centred approach have been adopted by most counselling disciplines as being central to the healing process of clients and are seen to be therapeutic. The core qualities are:

- genuineness
- empathy
- acceptance.

These conditions or qualities are expressed through the use of communication skills above.

GENUINENESS

This quality is also known as 'realness' or 'congruence'. The genuine practitioner communicates a set of attitudes and counsellor behaviours (Egan 1998). The genuine practitioner will be him- or herself in interactions with others whilst maintaining professional boundaries. He or she will not need to hide behind a uniform or to have a different persona when with the person with diabetes. Two ways to communicate genuineness are not to overemphasise the 'helping' role and to avoid defensiveness when faced with challenging behaviour (Egan 1998).

EMPATHY

To be empathic means to truly comprehend another person's experience by paying careful attention to the individual's story, observing verbal and non-verbal content and reflecting back. True empathy comes from exploring, using the skills above, the nature of the person's experience. Being empathic requires 100% attention and so the listener's own agenda is set aside as he or she listens empathically (Egan 1998).

ACCEPTANCE

This is also known as being non-judgemental or having unconditional positive regard. The accepting practitioner values and has a deep regard for the humanity of the person with diabetes. This regard goes beyond, and is unaffected by, the behaviours of the person, which might otherwise be seen as negative, destructive or self-defeating (Mearns & Thorne 1999).

Whereas the counselling process serves to increase self-esteem and enables the person with diabetes to think in a more positive way about him- or herself, the following questions can help clinicians to think about issues that occur when working with people with diabetes:

> *Question 'Empowerment seems to be important in the political health agenda in the UK but is it not just a byword for people to be able to do what they want?'*

It is right that some people are concerned that empowerment is synonymous with patient choice and that patient choice means passivity on the part of the clinician.

There are three key principles of the empowerment approach to diabetes care. First, the reality is that more than 98% of care is provided by the person with diabetes; therefore, that person is the locus of control and decision-maker in the daily treatment of his/her diabetes. Second, the primary aim of the healthcare team is to provide on-going diabetes expertise, education and psychosocial support so that the person with diabetes can make informed decisions about his or her daily diabetes self-care. Finally, people with diabetes are more likely to make and maintain behaviour changes if those changes are personally meaningful and freely chosen (Anderson 1995).

The empowerment approach acknowledges the person with diabetes as expert and at the same time provides knowledge and encourages motivation for self-care. An empowerment approach also acknowledges that people with diabetes have to make choices and ensures that these choices are informed ones. Moreover, it allows for consideration of the emotional context of living with, and caring for, diabetes and provides a forum for support of that care. Research shows that using the empowerment approach in consultations (including listening/taking note of opinions, acknowledgement of emotional context, joint decision making and motivating) is related to improvements in self-care and glycaemic control (Anderson 1995, Kyngas et al 1998, Street et al 1993, Williams et al 1998; all cited in Skinner & Cradock 2000).

Funnell et al (1991) stated that for people with diabetes to be self-empowered they require:

> *...the knowledge, skills, attitudes and self-awareness to influence their own behaviour and that of others in order to improve the quality of their lives.*

The concept suggests that people should be enabled to assume more control over those aspects of their lives that affect their health. Individuals are expected to participate actively in health care and decision making.

To facilitate self-empowerment, health professionals *also* need self-awareness and skills in terms of their own attitude and approach towards people with diabetes. Anderson & Funnell (2005) compare the traditional medical model style of diabetes consultation with a person-centred empowering model style of consultation (Table 3.1). Changing from the traditional medical style to the person-centred empowering way of consulting can be achieved by the use of communication skills in the consultation, for example using open questioning. Having a structure to the consultation allows the clinician and the person with diabetes to identify issues, to learn what is important (values), to look at options, to decide on goals and to commit to actioning choices. This empowerment model of consultation also tests whether the options are realistic and invites the person with diabetes to consider what support he or she needs to achieve his or her identified goals. The aim of an empowering style of consultation is to assist the individual to problem solve.

Table 3.1
Traditional medical model versus empowering person-centred model

Traditional medical model	Empowering person-centred model
Diabetes is a physical illness	Diabetes is a biopsychosocial condition
Relationship of provider and patient is authoritarian, based on provider expertise	Relationship of professional and patient is democratic and based on shared expertise
Problems and learning needs are usually identified by professional	Problems and learning needs are usually identified by the patient
Professional is viewed as problem solver and caregiver, i.e. the professional is responsible for diagnosis and treatment	Patient is viewed as a problem solver and caregiver, i.e. professional acts as a resource and both share responsibility for treatment and outcome
Goal is compliance with recommendations	Goal is to be enable patients to make informed choices
Behavioural strategies are used to increase compliance with recommended treatment. A lack of compliance is viewed as a failure of patient and provider	Behavioural strategies are used to help patients change behaviours of their choosing A lack of goal achievement is used as feedback to modify goals and strategies
Behaviour changes are externally motivated	Behaviour changes are internally motivated
Patient is powerless, professional is powerful	Patient and professional are powerful

From Anderson & Funnell 2005.

CHRONIC DISEASE MODEL OF SELF-MANAGEMENT

PROBLEM SOLVING

Self-management is enhanced if people with diabetes have the confidence to work things out from themselves. This confidence can be nurtured by facilitating the setting of individually identified goals and talking through how best to implement the chosen goal, taking into account internal and external barriers. The goals are usually short-term, specific and realistic. They are not all-or-nothing goals, i.e. 'I will lose 4 stones', where failure is highly likely to induce negative feelings in the individual around confidence and competence. Instead, a more realistic short-term weight loss should be agreed, such as 'In the next 4 weeks I will lose 7 lbs.' The person with diabetes should have an opportunity to review and modify his or her goals depending on outcome. Clinicians should communicate clearly that they are inviting the person with diabetes to be his or her own expert (Lorig 2002).

Lorig (2003) goes on to describe four ways in which self-efficacy can be enhanced:

1. Skills mastery: confidence is gained through experience of doing things. Goal setting and action planning will enhance this process. It is for this reason that goal setting or action planning is part of all good self-management programmes. The presence or absence of goal setting was a key issue separating successful from unsuccessful education in asthma education (Bodenheimer et al 2002).
2. Modelling also enhances self-efficacy. Learning from others who have the same condition with similar experiences is far more powerful than learning from health care professionals who do not have the experience of living with the condition.
3. Reinterpretation of symptoms contributes towards self-efficacy. This is an area where it is important to understand the beliefs of the person with diabetes. For example the person with diabetes may believe that treatment is the responsibility of the clinician and not be aware that lifestyle changes can have a significant effect on symptoms and on outcomes.
4. Social persuasion supports confidence. Support for the individual with diabetes from one's health professionals, friends, family and community are all-important, particularly peer support from others who have similar experiences.

Ideally, the goal(s) you agree with a person needs to be SMART:

- **S**pecific
- **M**easurable
- **A**ction-orientated
- **R**ealistic
- **T**ime limited.

Case study 3.3

Bill is 45 years old and has type 2 diabetes. Following a structured diabetes education programme, where he was invited to consider what goal he would work on to improve his health, Bill decided that he wanted to lose weight. (Result goal). One way to do this would be to be more

Case study 3.3
Continued

physically active (Treatment goal). Bill was asked to think about what activity might be most suitable for him. He used to play football but as he works erratic hours it would be difficult to make a regular commitment. He needed to do something that he enjoyed and could do on his own. He decided that brisk walking would suit his lifestyle (behaviour/action). Bill was asked to think through in detail how he would make a commitment to achieving his goal (action plan). Bill decided that he would walk on three days a week and specified the days and times: Tuesday and Friday evenings, after his meal and Sunday mornings, after breakfast. He planned a route that he would walk and estimated that this would take him about 40 minutes. He decided to ask his wife to join him as he knew that she was also keen to lose weight and they could encourage and support each other (evidence shows that social support helps people achieve behaviour change). When asked how confident he was that he could achieve this on a scale of 1-10 (1 being not at all confident and 10 being very confident) he scored himself at 8 out of 10. If he scored himself at less than 7 then he would be less likely to achieve his goal.

Recent research shows that if individuals actually plan how they will enact or implement their generalised intention, there is a substantial increase in the likelihood that they will follow through on their intentions. Therefore, by helping people set goals that are specific, measurable, realistic and time-limited actions, they are being encouraged to develop an implementation intention. It is important that these SMART goals are behaviours.

For example, setting weight loss or lower blood glucose values as goals will not work; people with diabetes do not have complete control over these outcomes because they are influenced by their medication regimens, stress responses, etc.

In addition, goals must be specific, so, for example 'eating less fat' is not specific enough. It is essential that we support people with diabetes in detailing *how, when* and *where* they are going to achieve their goals.

Once the goals are established, it is important to help the individual plan, and identify anything that might get in the way. If the person is to commit to action, he or she will drive the planning process.

> Question *'I have read lots about different psychological theories and their impact on self-management but when I sit down with someone where do I start?'*

Much is written about the different effects of psychological theories such as health beliefs, self-efficacy, locus of control and quality of life and it can feel somewhat like a melting pot. A number of possible interventions could be usefully applied if only you could remember what they were and integrate them cleverly into your consultation. Unfortunately, this smacks of the sticking-plaster scenario. From the physical standpoint, a person with diabetes is not a collection of organs with an abnormal blood glucose; similarly, the person with diabetes is not a collection of psychological theories needing to be fixed. How can psychological theory help us? The evidence tells us that self-efficacy is important, as is good quality of life. Social support is also important and having certain health beliefs and a particular locus of control can also effect self-management positively or negatively.

QUALITY OF LIFE

In Funnell et al's (1991) definition of empowerment, quality of life is specifically cited as an optimal outcome. Defining quality of life, however, can be a somewhat treacherous area. The term 'quality of life' means different things to different people. At one level the term has become an advertiser's cliché, at another it can be the main outcome of a scientific study. A bibliographic study of quality of life as reported in randomised controlled trials demonstrated that in many studies, quality of life was either poorly defined or not defined at all (Sanders et al 1998). This was partly attributed to the complex nature of the construct. This is highlighted by the multitude of instruments, both generic and disease specific, measuring quality of life.

Quality of life is a multidimensional construct containing several domains broadly covering emotional and physical well-being, social support, role functioning and treatment satisfaction with diabetes. Self-management decisions are often driven by quality of life issues. The comment below reveals quality of life issues in the psychological and physical domains. The person here has chosen to feel psychologically and physically well whilst acknowledging the long-term effects of his decision.

> *I'd rather not live as long than live the way you've got to live to keep them (blood glucose results) low. You're just miserable all day, you don't feel right. You can't live like that for the rest of your life...I just try and live a normal life and I keep my sugars a bit higher...I know it's not good for me in the long run but you still feel alright. If you are running too low then you are like an old man going about. That's not for me.*

> *Question 'I worry that if I discuss feelings with a person with diabetes I might open a can of worms. Could I do any damage by doing this?'*

Clinicians worry that by acknowledging that a person with diabetes has feelings they open up a can of worms or a floodgate of emotions that overwhelm the person with diabetes and/or the clinician and somehow 'damage' the person with diabetes. It *is* possible during a consultation that a masked depression or other psychological illness might be revealed; however, this will not have been *caused* by its acknowledgement. It is important that appropriate treatment is received. If the clinician finds him- or herself in an emotionally difficult situation beyond his or her abilities then it is important to refer the patient on to a colleague or specialist services if these are available. Listening to someone who is troubled is the first step to healing and the only time that a consultation is unlikely to be therapeutic is if the presenting problem is similar to an unresolved problem within the clinician, i.e. unresolved grief or experience of similar major life events that are still fresh for both the clinician and the individual.

Awareness of local psychological and psychiatric services is important; most major towns and cities have such services and many general practices in the UK employ counselling services. Most reputable counselling services will have British Association of Counselling and Psychotherapy approval. Some services will charge a fee but this is often tailored to suit the client concerned.

> *Question 'So is it better to use a clinical psychologist attached to a diabetes unit to see people referred by members of the team or to 'upskill' the team to address psychological issues themselves?'*

Both of these options have advantages and disadvantages. A clinical psychologist has the benefit of specialist expertise; however, delays in appointment availability can hinder progress. Also, referral to a clinical psychologist can be daunting for the individual with diabetes. 'Upskilling' the team to address psychological issues has the advantage of dealing with issues as they arise in consultations. However, the team cannot be expected to have the expertise held by a clinical psychologist.

> *Question 'This is all very well but do I have the time?'*

Psychological care can feel time-consuming, especially if emotional problems are detected. The use of listening skills will allow the person with diabetes to identify and address what is important. Conversely, not to use these skills may mean that clinicians are addressing their own agendas and are not meeting the needs of the person with diabetes (Parkin & Skinner 2003).

CONCLUSION

Psychological care of people with diabetes is an essential part of overall diabetes care. All clinicians involved in such care need to acknowledge and address the influences of psychosocial factors on people's lives, their self-management, diabetic control, long-term health and quality of life. The primary healthcare team is in a position to view diabetes in a person-centred way rather than a disease-centred way and can enhance the delivery of psychological care by the use of communication skills that acknowledge the needs of each individual and assist in promoting self-management.

It is important that clinicians seeking to improve both metabolic control and psychological well-being of people with diabetes acknowledge the daily demands placed on people with diabetes and offer appropriate advice and support. Suboptimal self-care can contribute to elevated blood glucose levels and/or hypoglycaemia, with increased risk of long-term diabetes complications and worsened quality of life.

Diagnosing psychological disorders in people with diabetes requires special care, as the signs and symptoms of most common disorders can overlap with diabetes symptoms. Clinicians should retain a willingness to refer for appropriate investigation and treatment by a psychologist or other mental health specialists ideally within the diabetes care team.

REFERENCES

Anderson RM 1995 Patient empowerment and the traditional medical model. A case of irreconcilable differences? Diabetes Care 18(3):412–415

Anderson RM, Funnell MM 2005 The art of empowerment. Stories and strategies for diabetes educators, 2nd edn. American Diabetes Association Alexandria, VA.

Anderson RM, Funnell MM, Fitzgerald JT, Marrero DG 2000 The diabetes empowerment scale: a measure of psychosocial self-efficacy. Diabetes Care 23(6):739–743

Anderson RJ, Freedland KE, Clouse RE, Lustman PJ 2001 The prevalence of comorbid depression in adults with diabetes – a meta-analysis. Diabetes Care 24(6):1069–1078

Anderson RM, Fitzgerald JT, Gruppen LD et al 2003 The diabetes empowerment scale – short form (DES-SF) Diabetes Care 26(5):1641–1642

Bandura A 1977 Self efficacy: towards a unifying theory of behaviour change. Psychological Review 84:191–215

Becker MH 1974 The health belief model and personal health behaviour. Health Education Monographs 2:324–473

Becker MH, Janz NK 1985 The health belief model applied to understanding diabetes regimen compliance. Diabetes Educator 11(1):41–47

Bodenheimer T, Lorig K, Holman H, Grumbach K 2002 Patient self-management of chronic disease in primary care. Journal of the American Medical Association 288(19):2469–2475

Bozarth J, Temaner Brodley B 1986 The Core Values and Theory of the Person-Centred Approach. Paper prepared for the First Annual Meeting of the Association for the Development of the Person-Centred Approach, Chicago

Brown F 1996 A hard lesson in psychological care: being nice is not enough [leader]. Practical Diabetes International 13(5):143

Crow S, Kendall D, Praus B, Thuras P 2001 Binge eating and other psychopathology in patients with type II diabetes mellitus. International Journal of Eating Disorders 30:222–226

de Berardis G, Pellegrini F, Franciosi M et al 2003 Identifying patients with type 2 diabetes with higher likelihood of erectile dysfunction: the role of the interaction between clinical and psychological factors. Journal of Urology 169:422–428

de Groot M, Anderson RJ, Freedland KE et al 2000 Association of diabetes complications and depression in type 1 and type 2 diabetes: a meta-analysis [abstract]. Diabetes 49:A63

de Groot M, Anderson R, Freedland KE et al 2001 Association of depression and diabetes complications: a meta-analysis. Psychosomatic Medicine 63:619–630

Donnan PT, MacDonald TM, Morris AD 2002 Adherence to prescribed oral hypoglycaemic medication in a population of patients with type 2 diabetes: a retrospective cohort study. Diabetic Medicine 19(4):279–284

Egan G 1998 The skilled helper. A problem-management approach to helping. 6th edn. Brooks/Coles Publishing Company, Pacific Grove, CA

Evans JM, Newton RW, Ruta DA et al 1999 Frequency of blood glucose monitoring in relation to glycaemic control: observational study with diabetes database. British Medical Journal 319(7202):83–86

Funnell MM, Anderson RM, Arnold MS et al 1991 Empowerment: an idea whose time has come in diabetes education. The Diabetes Educator 17:37–41

Gavard JA, Lustman PJ, Clouse RE 1993 Prevalence of depression in adults with diabetes: an epidemiological evaluation. Diabetes Care 16:1167–1178

Hall RCW 1997 Bulimia nervosa and diabetes mellitus. Seminars in Clinical Neuropsychiatry 2:24–30

Heisler M, Vijan S, Anderson RM et al 2003 When do patients and their physicians agree on diabetes treatment goals and strategies, and what difference does it make? Journal of General Internal Medicine 18(11):893–902

Hepertz S, Albus C, Lichtblau K et al 2000 Relationship of weight and eating disorders in type 2 diabetic patients: a multicenter study. International Journal of Eating Disorders 28:68–77

Holmes TH, Rahe RH 1967 The social readjustment rating scale. Journal of Psychosomatic Research 11:213

Kenardy J, Mensch M, Bown K et al 2001 Disordered eating behaviours in women with type 2 diabetes mellitus. Eating Behaviours 2:183–192

Kubler Ross E 1990 On death and dying. Routledge, London

Kyngas H, Hentinen M, Barlow JH 1998 Adolescents' perceptions of physicians, nurses, parents and friends: help or hindrance in compliance with diabetes self-care? Journal of Advanced Nursing 27:760–769

Lancet 1994 Essence of stress [editorial]. Lancet 344:8939:1713–1714

Lo R, MacLean D 2001 The dynamics of coping and adapting to the impact when diagnosed with diabetes. Australian Journal of Advanced Nursing 19(2):26–32

Lorig K 2002 Partnerships between expert patients and physicians. Lancet 359(9309): 814–815

Lorig K 2003 Self-management education: more than a nice extra. Medical Care 41(6):699–701

Lustman PJ, Griffith LS, Clouse RE et al 1997 Effects of nortriptyline on depression and glucose regulation in diabetes: results of a double-blind, placebo-controlled trial. Psychosomatic Medicine 59:241–250

Lustman PJ, Anderson RJ, Freedland KE et al 2000 Depression and poor glycemic control: a meta-analytic review of the literature. Diabetes Care 23:434–442

Mannucci E, Tesi F, Rica V et al 2002 Eating behavior in obese patients with and without type 2 diabetes mellitus. International Journal of Obesity-related Metabolic Disorders 26:848–853

Mearns D, Thorne B 1999 Person-centred counselling in action, 2nd edn. Sage Publications, London

Michie S, Miles J, Weinman J 2003 Patient-centredness in chronic illness: what is it and does it matter? Patient Education and Counseling 51(3):197–206

Morris AD, Boyle DI, McMahon AD et al 1997 Adherence to insulin treatment, glycaemic control, and ketoacidosis in insulin-dependent diabetes mellitus. The DARTS/MEMO

Collaboration. Diabetes Audit and Research in Tayside Scotland. Medicines Monitoring Unit. Lancet 350(9090):1505–1510

Parkin T, Skinner TC 2003 Discrepancies between patient and professional's recall and perception of an outpatient consultation. Diabetic Medicine 20(11):909–914

Peyrot M, Rubin RR 1994 Structures and correlates of diabetes-specific locus of control. Diabetes Care 17(9):994–1001

Pill R, Stott NC, Rollnick SR, Rees M 1998 A randomized controlled trial of an intervention designed to improve the care given in general practice to type II diabetic patients: patient outcomes and professional ability to change behaviour. Family Practice 15(3):229–235

Polonsky WH 1999 Diabetes burnout: what to do when you can't take it anymore. American Diabetes Association, Alexandria, VA.

Polonsky WH 2002 Emotional and quality-of-life aspects of diabetes management. Current Diabetes Reports 2(2):153–159

Polonsky WH, Fisher L, Earles J et al 2005 Assessing psychosocial distress in diabetes: development of the diabetes distress scale. Diabetes Care 28(3):626–631

Riazi A, Pickup J, Bradley C 2004. Daily stress and glycaemic control in type 1 diabetes: individual differences in magnitude, direction and timing of stress-reactivity. Diabetes Research and Clinical Practice 66:237–244

Rogers C 1978 Carl Rogers on personal power. Constable, London, p 15

Rogers C 1980 A way of being. Houghton Mifflin, Boston, MA

Rollnick S, Mason P, Butler C 1999 Health behaviour change: a guide for practitioners. Churchill Livingstone, Edinburgh

Royal College of Nursing Working Party 1978 Counselling in nursing. Royal College of Nursing, London, p 14

Rydall AC, Rodin GM, Olmsted MP et al 1997 Disordered eating behavior and microvascular complications in young women with insulin-dependent diabetes mellitus. New England Journal of Medicine 336:1849–1854

Sanders C, Egger M, Donovan J et al 1998 Reporting on quality of life in randomised controlled trials: bibliographic study. British Medical Journal 317:1191–1194

Skinner, TC, Cradock S 2000 Empowerment: what about the evidence? Practical Diabetes International 17(3):91–95

Street RL, Piziak VK, Herzog J et al 1993 Provider–patient communication and metabolic control. Diabetes Care 16:714–721

Wallston BS, Wallston KA, Kaplan GD, Maides SA 1976 Development and validation of the health locus of control (HLC) scale. Journal of Consulting and Clinical Psychology 44:580–585

Williams GC, Freedman ZR, Deci EL 1998 Supporting autonomy to motivate patients with diabetes for glucose control. Diabetes Care 21(10):1644–1651

The person with type 2 diabetes

Derek Gordon

A WORLDWIDE EPIDEMIC

Type 2 diabetes has reached epidemic proportions both in developing countries and in the developed world. It is estimated that throughout the world there are currently 150 million people with diabetes, and that number will double by 2025. Globally, 97% of these people will have type 2 diabetes, although in the industrialised countries this figure falls to 90%.

In the UK, it is estimated there will be 2.88 million people with type 2 diabetes by 2010. Data from eight European countries indicate that the mean cost per patient with diabetes is US$2928 annually (1999 values), and the proportion of healthcare spending on diabetes ranges from 1.6% to 6.6%, depending on the country.

Changes in human lifestyle over the past century have precipitated this dramatic increase in the incidence of diabetes. Increasing prosperity, ready access to food – much of which is now ready-made, convenience food – and a more sedentary way of life have resulted in an explosion in the incidence of obesity. The Nurses' Health Study found that in 91% of people with type 2 diabetes the condition could be attributed to a body mass index (BMI) > 23, lack of exercise, unhealthy diet, smoking and abstinence from alcohol (Hu et al 2001).

Obesity is associated with increased resistance to insulin action and the development of type 2 diabetes. Insulin resistance also increases with age and an ageing population has also contributed to the numbers of people with diabetes.

THE METABOLIC SYNDROME

It is now recognised that insulin resistance is associated with a cluster of factors known as the 'metabolic syndrome'. Overall obesity, and in particular central obesity, dyslipidaemia [characterised by elevated levels of triglycerides and low levels of high-density lipoprotein (HDL) cholesterol], hyperglycaemia and hypertension are common traits that, when they occur together, constitute the metabolic syndrome. The metabolic syndrome is very common, affecting about 24% of US adults between the ages of 20 and 70 years. People with the syndrome are about twice as likely to develop coronary heart disease as people without it.

It should, therefore, be recognised that type 2 diabetes is usually part of a more complex metabolic disorder and that treatment of the blood glucose levels should not be undertaken in isolation. It is important to tackle all aspects of the metabolic syndrome, that is, obesity, dyslipidaemia and hypertension. This chapter deals with the management of diabetes control; Chapter 8 covers the management of other cardiovascular risk factors.

THE PREDIABETIC STATE

The development of diabetes takes many years. The earliest feature in most people is the development of insulin resistance. The pancreas can initially compensate by producing more insulin and blood glucose levels can be maintained within normal limits. Eventually, however, the pancreas can no longer produce sufficient insulin to overcome the worsening insulin resistance and blood glucose levels begin to rise. At this stage people will have impaired glucose tolerance. Eventually the pancreatic beta cells begin to fail and insulin levels fall. This results in higher blood glucose concentrations and the development of diabetes.

THE SPECTRUM OF TYPE 2 DIABETES

Type 2 diabetes is therefore the result of both insulin resistance and insulin lack, hence people with type 2 diabetes form a classic spectrum of disease. At one end of the spectrum are obese people who have predominantly insulin resistance, at the opposite end are non-obese individuals with predominant insulin insufficiency.

WHY TREAT TYPE 2 DIABETES?

There are several reasons for treating the blood glucose concentrations in diabetes. Hyperglycaemia is associated with symptoms of lethargy, thirst and frequency of urination, including nocturia. Poorly controlled diabetes can lead to vaginal or penile thrush. Treatment of diabetes can relieve the symptoms of hyperglycaemia.

It had also been assumed for many years that control of blood glucose levels would prevent some of the complications of diabetes. This was demonstrated, for people with type 2 diabetes, when the results of the UK Prospective Diabetes Study (UKPDS 1998a, 1998b) were published.

UK PROSPECTIVE DIABETES STUDY

The UK Prospective Diabetes Study (UKPDS) was a large, multicentre, clinical trial that started in 1977 and reported its final results in 1998. The aims of the study were to identify whether, in people with type 2 diabetes, tight metabolic control reduced the macrovascular and microvascular complications and whether any particular form of therapy was best in achieving tight control. In addition, the study aimed to demonstrate whether tight control of blood pressure prevented macro- and microvascular complications. The blood pressure control part of the study will not be discussed in this chapter.

During the course of the study, several UKPDS reports were published that revealed aspects of the epidemiology and natural history of type 2 diabetes. The study followed 3867 people with newly diagnosed type 2 diabetes. Individuals were randomly assigned to conventional treatment (the aim of which was to maintain fasting blood glucose at < 15 mmol/L) or intensive treatment (the aim of which was to achieve fasting blood glucose levels < 6 mmol/L).

People were allocated to treatment by diet, a sulphonylurea or insulin therapy. In addition, a small subgroup of obese individuals was allocated to initial treatment with metformin.

Results of the UKPDS

The study demonstrated that in both the conventional and intensive treatment groups, there was a steady increase in fasting blood glucose and glycated haemoglobin (HbA1c) over the period of the study. Type 2 diabetes is therefore a progressive disease associated with worsening metabolic control over a number of years (Fig. 4.1). This implies that metabolic control can be maintained in type 2 diabetes only by progressive increases in doses of medications and the utilisation of multiple therapies, including insulin. The different treatment modalities showed little difference on their effect on fasting blood glucose or HbA1c. Only people treated with chlorpropamide had significantly improved metabolic control when compared with other sulphonylureas or insulin.

The intensively treated group showed an 11% reduction in HbA1c when compared to the conventional group (HbA1c 7.0% compared to 7.9%). For every 1% increment in HbA1c the study demonstrated a:

- 21% increased risk of any diabetes-related endpoint
- 21% increased risk of any diabetes-related death
- 14% increased risk of a myocardial infarction (MI)
- 37% increased risk of any microvascular complication.

Fig. 4.1

HbA1c rises with time in both the conventional and the intensively treated groups of patients with type 2 diabetes. Reprinted from UKPDS (1998a), with permission from Elsevier.

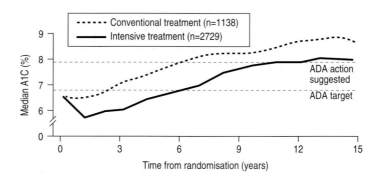

Furthermore, the UKPDS (1998a) demonstrated that benefits could be achieved by reducing HbA1c results no matter how low they were to start with; in other words the lower the HbA1c the better. Microvascular risk became low when HbA1c reached levels of 7–8% whereas macrovascular risk continued to fall, down to HbA1c levels of 6–7%.

The difference in HbA1c results between the conventional and intensive treatment groups was associated with a significantly reduced frequency of microvascular endpoints; the reduction in diabetes-related mortality or macrovascular endpoints did not quite reach statistical significance. However, the group of obese people who were treated intensively with metformin showed a significant reduction in cardiovascular risk.

Metformin was the only treatment that was not associated with weight gain and raised circulating concentrations of plasma insulin. Sulphonylureas and insulin treatments were associated with increased plasma insulin concentrations and insulin resistance, and this might therefore have accounted for their poorer influence on long-term cardiovascular morbidity.

SELF-MONITORING IN TYPE 2 DIABETES

There is no evidence that blood or urine testing improves HbA1c, body weight or the incidence of hypoglycaemic events in people with type 2 diabetes. The National Institute for Health and Clinical Excellence (NICE) does not recommend the use of self-monitoring as a stand-alone intervention in people with type 2 diabetes (NICE 2004). Rather, it recommends that self-monitoring be taught only if the purpose or need for it is clear and agreed with the individual with diabetes.

Self-monitoring can be useful in the period immediately after diagnosis, when people can learn the effects of various foodstuffs on their blood or urine glucose levels. This can sometimes be effective in encouraging alterations to diet. It can be useful to teach self-monitoring to people in whom oral hypoglycaemic agents are failing; this can act as an incentive to improve control. Also, if they subsequently require insulin treatment they will already have mastered the technique prior to starting insulin. No doubt there are other situations when self-monitoring can be useful. However, prolonged self-monitoring with no clear purpose is an expensive practice that may not be beneficial. See Chapter 7 for further elaboration.

NON-DRUG TREATMENT OF TYPE 2 DIABETES

DIET

Dietary review is fundamental to the management of the person with type 2 diabetes. The basic tenets of dietary management should therefore be known to the primary healthcare team so that preliminary advice can be given in the community at the time of diagnosis (see Chapter 6). However, few doctors or nurses have adequate training to provide complete dietary advice and all newly diagnosed people should receive advice from a dietician.

Well over 50% of all newly diagnosed people with type 2 diabetes are overweight (BMI 25–30 kg/m^2) or obese (BMI > 30 kg/m^2). The cornerstone to their diet is an individualised reduced-calorie diet (see Chapter 6). Eating less reduces energy intake and allows weight reduction. Weight reduction will improve insulin resistance and allow the person to utilise his or her own insulin production more effectively.

When diet succeeds, the benefits are evident. Blood glucose, lipids and blood pressure fall. However, the response to diet is often disappointing. Most diabetic clinics in general practice or hospital lack the resources required to allow frequent dietary review and people often lack motivation or find it impossible to alter deeply ingrained eating habits. The UKPDS found that only 16% of newly diagnosed people with type 2 diabetes achieved near-normal fasting blood glucose concentrations after 3 months of dieting. Those people with the highest fasting blood glucose levels at the time of diagnosis were least likely to achieve good diabetic control by diet alone (UKPDS 1990).

EXERCISE

Several studies have demonstrated the benefit of lifestyle intervention on the development and management of diabetes. Modest weight loss and increased physical activity have been shown to cause substantial reduction in the risk of developing type 2 diabetes (Helmrich et al 1991, Manson et al 1991). For each 500-kcal increment in weekly energy expenditure, the risk of developing type 2 diabetes can be reduced by 6%.

Decreased cardiac risk

Exercise confers the well-established benefit of improved insulin sensitivity for people with or without diabetes. As with weight loss, improved insulin sensitivity is associated with reduction in blood pressure and improvement in lipid profiles, thus reducing cardiovascular risk. Improved fitness and exercise are associated with a reduction in coronary disease in the general population, but evidence for such a decrease among people with diabetes has not appeared.

Weight loss

The addition of exercise training to a conventional diet has been shown to be beneficial (Blonk 1994) with people showing greater weight loss and improved HbA1c. However, weight loss tends to be modest in most people and only a minority maintain their weight loss over a 3-year period (Stevens et al 2001).

Improved glucose utilisation

Increased insulin sensitivity allows glucose to enter muscle cells more efficiently both acutely and chronically with exercise. Improvements in glucose tolerance testing have been shown in type 2 diabetes after as little as 1 week of aerobic training. Increased insulin sensitivity begins to decline however, in as little as 1 or 2 days without exercise.

Exercise can therefore improve diabetic control and allow lower doses of oral hypoglycaemic drugs or insulin. However, the exercise must be maintained and this requires both self-motivation by the individuals and continuing encouragement by their families, friends and health carers. The optimal methods for maintaining motivation are still to be identified.

Case study 4.1

Bernard is a 52-year-old taxi driver who was recently diagnosed as having type 2 diabetes when he attended his GP complaining of tiredness and thirst. A random blood glucose was found to be 23 mmol/L. He has been overweight for many years and currently weighs 107 kg (BMI 34 kg/m^2). When working, he eats erratically from cheap hot-food stalls. He smokes 30 cigarettes per day and never takes any exercise. His GP estimates his weekly alcohol intake at approximately 28 units. His mother and two brothers have type 2 diabetes.

The finding of a random blood glucose above 11.1 mmol/L in a person with osmotic symptoms confirms diabetes. Bernard's elevated blood glucose might be the cause of his lethargy. In addition to his diabetes, his unhealthy lifestyle will further increase his risk of vascular catastrophe in the future unless he makes major alterations to the way he lives.

Bernard's case history is fairly typical of the person with type 2 diabetes. There is a strong family history of diabetes and he has the associated risk factor of being overweight. He is likely to have other features of the metabolic syndrome; namely hypertension and hyperlipidaemia. His initial management will involve appropriate changes to his lifestyle including diet and exercise.

Diet should include calorie restriction to promote weight loss. If he is found to be hypertensive, Bernard would be advised to restrict his intake of salt to around 3 g/day. This can usually be achieved by limiting the use of salt to cooking and by not adding salt at the table. A suitable low-fat diet should be recommended if his total cholesterol and triglyceride levels are raised.

As Bernard has a sedentary lifestyle, he should be encouraged to increase his exercise activity. It is recommended that all individuals (including those with diabetes) undertake aerobic physical activity on a minimum of 3 days per week with sessions lasting 20–60 minutes. However, our 52-year-old taxi driver might have to start with low intensity exercise for shorter periods of time. In some areas of the UK, general practitioners can prescribe an exercise programme at a local gym. It is important to undertake a pre-exercise assessment of people with diabetes prior to entry into any such programme. Watch for signs and symptoms of peripheral vascular disease, such as intermittent claudication, cold feet, decreased or absent peripheral pulses. Diminished light touch, pin-prick or vibration sense might signal a peripheral neuropathy. Such people might be at risk of foot ulceration if asked to undertake exercise. Eyes should be examined to identify new vessel formation (see Chapter 9).

A history of postural hypotension, hypoglycaemia unawareness, gustatory sweating or impotence might signal the presence of autonomic neuropathy which, if present, could make exercise dangerous because of risks to the heart.

An exercise stress test is recommended for people at risk of heart disease who anticipate engaging in moderate to intense exercise. Among people with diabetes who are considered at risk are those who are older than 35 years, who have had type 2 diabetes for longer than 10 years and those who have had type 1 diabetes for longer than 15 years.

Case study 4.1
Continued

> Despite adherence to a restricted-calorie diet for 6 months and some increase in his exercise activities, Bernard continues to complain of thirst and frequency of urination during the night. His weight has fallen by 4 kg but his HbA1c remains elevated at 9.2%. His GP decides to start him on metformin.

PHARMACOLOGICAL TREATMENT OF TYPE 2 DIABETES

METFORMIN: A BIGUANIDE

In medieval times, the plant, *Galega officialis,* (goat's rue or French lilac) was used as a traditional remedy for diabetes in Southern and Eastern Europe. The plant was subsequently shown to be rich in guanidine and in 1918 guanidine was shown to have mild hypoglycaemic effects. However, guanidine was too toxic for clinical use and in the 1950s the biguanide, metformin, was derived and introduced into clinical practice.

Modes of action

Metformin lowers blood glucose concentrations by several mechanisms. Its most important effect is to enhance insulin sensitivity in peripheral tissues, in particular the liver and skeletal muscles. By improving insulin action on the liver, metformin inhibits glucose production and release. It also stimulates insulin uptake by skeletal muscle. It might have direct or indirect effects on reducing appetite (Bailey 1992).

The UKPDS included a subgroup of overweight people who were allocated to treatment with metformin, sulphonylureas (chlorpropamide or glibenclamide) or insulin therapy. Only metformin therapy was associated with improved insulin sensitivity and reduced circulating concentrations of insulin.

Reduced insulin resistance would be expected to improve cardiovascular risk and, indeed, the UKPDS showed that metformin had the greatest effects on any diabetes-related end point, on overall mortality due to any cause and also on the incidence of stroke. The UKPDS also reported that, in overweight people, metformin was not associated with weight gain and produced fewer hypoglycaemic attacks than sulphonylureas or insulin therapy (UKPDS 1998b). It is therefore recommended that metformin is used as first-line treatment in overweight people if lifestyle changes fail to improve diabetic control.

Metformin is likely to reduce blood glucose concentrations by 2–3 mmol/L when prescribed for people in whom diet has failed. This is a comparable blood glucose lowering effect to sulphonylureas. About 30% of people so treated will achieve good diabetic control. However, in a further 5–10% of people per year, metformin treatment will fail to achieve adequate control.

Prescribing metformin

Metformin is available in the UK as 500- and 850-mg tablets. The drug should be taken with meals and the dose increased gradually to lessen side effects. A typical starting dose would be 850 mg once daily or 500 mg once or twice daily. The dosage can be increased in a stepwise fashion over a period of several weeks to prevent adverse drug effects. Garber et al (1997) showed that metformin lowered HbA1c and fasting blood glucose in a dose-related manner, up to 2000 mg per day. Beyond this dosage there is little therapeutic gain but a much higher incidence of side effects.

Side effects of metformin

The most common side effects of metformin are gastrointestinal in origin. About 20% of people experience diarrhoea, flatulence or abdominal pain, whereas others complain of a metallic taste, nausea or anorexia. Although a reduction in appetite might be desirable in the overweight person, for the sake of compliance any nausea or anorexia must be considered seriously. These disturbances are generally transient and can be minimised by starting treatment at a low dosage and taking the drug with food.

Metformin can cause the blood lactate levels to rise. However, if it is prescribed taking into account recognised contraindications, there is no increased risk of serious lactic acidosis or increased levels of lactate compared to other antihyperglycaemic agents (Aguilar et al 1992). Metformin is normally excreted through the kidneys and is contraindicated in people with impaired renal function (e.g. serum creatinine > 130 micromol/L) as this can result in accumulation of the drug in the body, enhancing its effect on lactate production. Liver disease is also a contraindication, because adequate hepatic function is required to metabolise the increased lactic acid. People with cardiac failure perfuse their tissues poorly and the resulting tissue hypoxia causes lactic acid production. It is therefore unwise to prescribe metformin for such individuals. Metformin should be temporarily withdrawn in people undergoing surgery or radiology procedures requiring injection of contrast.

Case study 4.2

Annie is a 62-year-old housewife who has had type 2 diabetes for 10 years and was initially managed on diet alone. After 3 years her metabolic control deteriorated and as she was obese (BMI 31 kg/m^2), metformin was started at an initial dose of 500 mg daily. Gradually, over a number of years, the dose was increased to 1 g twice daily. Over the past 3 months Annie has developed thirst and she has begun to monitor her urine for glycosuria. This has shown persistently elevated results. She denies any recent change to her diet. A clinic HbA1c result is 9.5%, confirming recent poor control.

Before making additions to Annie's current therapy, it is important to determine if she is actually taking her current prescribed medication. Further dietary assessment should also be undertaken to determine her understanding, identify any necessary changes to be made and to assess her motivation and adherence.

One of the most important findings of the UKPDS was the demonstration that type 2 diabetes is a progressive condition. All modalities of therapy were associated with a relentless rise in HbA1c with duration of disease (see Fig. 4.1). This results in the need for increasing doses of medication and the introduction of multiple therapies to maintain diabetic control. UKPDS (1990) suggested that 3 years after diagnosis approximately half of people controlled on diet alone were failing in their control and required more than one glucose-lowering drug. After 9 years this increased to 75% of people requiring multiple therapies to achieve HbA1c levels averaging 7.0%. Following the failure of metformin to control Annie's diabetes, the introduction of an insulin secretogogue is recommended (NICE 2004).

INSULIN SECRETOGOGUES

The sulphonylureas

Sulphonylureas have been used to treat type 2 diabetes for more than 50 years. In recent years, understanding of their mode of action has developed. Sulphonylureas bind to cell membrane receptors on the beta cell. This causes the potassium channel across the membrane to close and the membrane to depolarise. In turn, this causes calcium influx and insulin granule release into the extracellular medium. Therefore the effect of sulphonylureas is limited to people with preserved pancreatic cell function. The pancreas can only be squeezed to produce more insulin if there are functioning beta cells there to be squeezed!

It is generally recommended that sulphonylureas are ingested about 30 minutes before meals as this will stimulate insulin production to coincide with the time of eating. This in turn has been shown to reduce the postprandial rise in blood glucose (Melander et al 1989). Most drugs in this group are given twice daily when used at higher doses. The maximum therapeutic effect of most sulphonylureas is achieved at relatively low doses. This is likely to be due to cell receptors for the drug becoming saturated at low doses and further increases in drug dose have no additional effects. A person who shows poor glycaemic control on a dose of gliclazide 160 mg daily or glibenclamide or glipizide 10 mg daily is unlikely to respond optimally to higher doses and a decision to start additional therapy should not be delayed unnecessarily.

Which agent to use?   There are very few studies of the older sulphonylureas such as tolbutamide. For the more recently introduced sulphonylureas there is little evidence that one compound is more effective than another and little to be gained by changing from one agent to another (Gordon 1996).

Nevertheless, there are important differences between the sulphonylureas, in particular their duration of effect (Table 4.1). The shorter-acting sulphonylureas require more frequent dosing, with consequent influence on concordance with treatment (see below). The longer-acting sulphonylureas – glibenclamide and chlorpropamide – are associated with a higher incidence of severe hypoglycaemic attacks (Gordon 1996).

Glimepiride is the most recently introduced sulphonylurea and can be prescribed as a once-daily preparation even at higher dosage (Sonnenberg et al 1997). The starting dose is usually 1 mg daily and this can be increased in 1-mg steps every 1–2 weeks to the usual maximum dose of 6 mg. Glimepiride has been shown to be less likely to cause symptomatic hypoglycaemia than glibenclamide (Dills & Schneider 1996).

Table 4.1

The sulphonylureas

Drug	Effect duration (hours)	Daily dose (mg)
tolbutamide	6–10	500–2000
gliquidone	6–18	15–180
gliclazide	12–20	40–320
glipizide	6–16	2.5–20
glimepiride	12– > 24	1–6
glibenclamide	12– > 24	2.5–20
chlorpropamide	24–72	100–500

Side effects of sulphonylureas   These agents tend to cause weight gain and should only be used in obese patients when dietary restriction and metformin therapy have proved inadequate in controlling blood glucose levels.

The most important side effect with sulphonylureas is the development of serious and prolonged hypoglycaemia. For this reason, any person who becomes hypoglycaemic due to a sulphonylurea should be admitted to hospital for at least 24 hours for observation. The elderly are most at risk, probably because of coexisting vascular disease of the brain and heart. Almost all causes of prolonged hypoglycaemia have involved people over the age of 70 years (Ferner & Neil 1988). Of those admitted to hospital, 10% will die and 3% will be left with permanent brain damage. The longer-acting sulphonylureas should be avoided in the elderly.

The short-acting tolbutamide can be used in renal impairment, as can gliquidone and gliclazide, which are mainly metabolised and inactivated by the liver. However, care should be taken to monitor blood glucose levels regularly in order to avoid hypoglycaemia.

Sulphonylurea failure   As type 2 diabetes progresses, beta-cell function deteriorates further and the ability of the sulphonylureas to stimulate insulin secretion also deteriorates. Indeed, by 'flogging a dying horse' it is possible that the sulphonylureas might actually hasten the demise of the beta cell. Harrower and Wong (1990) reported 5-year failure rates for gliclazide at 7%, glibenclamide 17.9% and glipizide 25.6%.

SHORT-ACTING INSULIN SECRETOGOGUES

The glinides (meglitinides and D-phenylalanine derivatives)

Glinides, such as repaglinide and nateglinide, are recently introduced insulin secretogogues. Like the sulphonylureas, they bind to the sulphonylurea receptor on the surface of the beta cell. The binding, however, occurs at a different position on the sulphonylurea receptor. Nevertheless, their action is similar to that of the sulphonylureas, causing closure of the transmembrane, potassium channel and subsequent release of insulin from the beta cell.

These drugs are short acting and should be taken before main meals. Their function is mainly to reduce postprandial rises in blood glucose. There is some evidence to support the hypothesis that rapid rises in blood glucose levels are particularly important in the development of diabetic complications. Therefore, drugs that can reduce postprandial glucose excursions might be important in reducing the morbidity and mortality associated with diabetes. However, this theory is at present unproven and controversial.

Repaglinide   Repaglinide is the first meglitinide to become available for clinical use. It is taken before meals at doses of 0.5–4 mg. Studies have shown that repaglinide as monotherapy or in combination with other hypoglycaemic agents such as metformin or rosiglitazone (see below) achieves good metabolic control similar to that achieved by glibenclamide regimens. Repaglinide is associated with

mum dose is 200 mg thrice daily. The tablets should be chewed with the first mouthful of food or swallowed immediately before food.

Acarbose does not cause hypoglycaemia itself but, when used in combination with insulin or insulin secretogogues, hypoglycaemia can occur. People should be warned that they need to carry glucose and *not* sucrose with them to treat hypoglycaemic episodes. This is because acarbose interferes with sucrose absorption from the gut.

Several studies have shown that acarbose can reduce postprandial hyperglycaemia (Lindstrom et al 2000, Scorpiglione et al 1999) as well as HbA1c levels by generally small amounts (Chan et al 1998, Holman et al 1999, Scott et al 1999).

However, acarbose is poorly tolerated and there is a high incidence of gastrointestinal side effects, mainly flatulence, abdominal pain and diarrhoea. Several studies have demonstrated high drop-out rates because of side effects (Chan et al 1998, Holman et al 1999) and these findings have led NICE (2004) to recommend that acarbose should probably only be considered for people who cannot tolerate other oral glucose-lowering therapies.

CONCORDANCE

NICE (2004) defines concordance as being:

> *... concerned with the extent to which an individual's behaviour, in terms of lifestyle practices and medication taking, coincides with medical or health advice.*

In the management of diabetes, the emphasis is on individual empowerment and partnership between people and healthcare professionals. The term 'concordance' recognises this more equitable relationship and is now the preferred expression, as opposed to either compliance or adherence.

The Diabetes Audit and Research Tayside Study

The Diabetes Audit and Research in Tayside Scotland (DARTS) programme has added substantially to our understanding of concordance with drug therapy for people with type 2 diabetes. Using information obtained from dispensed prescription data from community pharmacies, Donnan and colleagues (2002) were able to derive adherence indices for individuals taking sulphonylureas or metformin as monotherapy. Adequate adherence was defined as the amount of drug dispensed being ≥ 90% of individuals' requirements. The authors were able to show that adequate adherence was found in only one in three people with type 2 diabetes receiving a single oral hypoglycaemic agent. Adherence was poorer with an increasing daily number of tablets for both sulphonylurea and metformin, with only one in four people remaining adherent when treatment involved more than once daily dosing. Adherence also fell as the number of co-medications rose. Poorer adherence was also associated with more socially deprived groups.

As explained elsewhere, type 2 diabetes often requires multiple therapies to control blood glucose. In addition, multiple risk-factor interventions are required to control blood pressure, hyperlipidaemia and cardiovascular risk. It is, therefore, highly likely that the person with longstanding type 2 diabetes will be on multiple medications.

The data from the DARTS project (Donnan et al 2002) have encouraged pharmaceutical companies to develop long-standing, once-a-day preparations and combination drugs to improve concordance by individuals with diabetes.

MODIFIED-RELEASE MEDICATIONS

Diamicron MR is a slow-release preparation of gliclazide. It is prescribed as a once-daily medication and it is hoped that this will improve concordance. Preliminary studies with Diamicron MR have shown that HbA1c can be improved following conversion from conventional gliclazide to the long-acting preparation. Diamicron MR is also associated with a decreased incidence of hypoglycaemic events.

A slow-release preparation of metformin, Glucophage SR is available and may be associated with fewer gastorintestinal side effects.

COMBINATION DRUGS

Avandamet is currently available in the UK. This drug is a combination of metformin and rosiglitazone and is available in a number of dose variations. Combination treatments are expected to improve concordance for people with type 2 diabetes who are on multiple drug regimens.

Similarly Competact is a combination of metformin and pioglitazone which has recently gained marketing authorisation in Europe.

ANTI-OBESITY DRUGS

Anti-obesity drugs should be used only as part of a comprehensive weight-management programme, with frequently reinforced guidance on diet, exercise and healthy living. These agents should only be considered when people have a BMI > 30 kg/m^2 and when at least 3 months of lifestyle intervention has failed to induce weight loss. In the presence of comorbidity such as diabetes, coronary heart disease, hypertension or obstructive sleep apnoea, anti-obesity drugs can be used for individuals with BMI > 28 kg/m^2. Drug treatment should be withdrawn if weight loss is insignificant (< 5% initial body weight after 3 months) or if there is weight gain at any time while receiving drug treatment.

Orlistat

Orlistat is a pancreatic lipase inhibitor. Lipases are required to break down fats before they can be absorbed from the gastrointestinal tract. Weight loss therefore occurs by reducing the absorption of fat from the diet by about 30%. Orlistat is licensed for use in the UK in conjunction with a mildly hypocaloric diet in those with BMI of > 30 kg/m^2. It can also be used in those with a BMI of 28 kg/m^2 or greater and associated risk factors such as diabetes. Treatment should only be started if a low-fat diet has previously produced a weight loss of 2.5 kg over a period of four consecutive weeks. Orlistat is prescribed at a dose of 120 mg before, during or up to 1 hour after main meals.

Several studies have shown that orlistat in conjunction with a hypocalorific diet causes increased weight loss, when compared with placebo, in obese people with type 2 diabetes treated by diet alone, metformin, sulphonylureas or insulin. This effect is seen in studies lasting as long as 1 year (Greenway 1999, Halpern et al 2003 Hanefeld & Sachse 2002). Similarly, these studies have demonstrated that people treated with orlistat have significant improvements in HbA1c, fasting glucose and postprandial glucose levels.

Orlistat and dyslipidaemia   There is now a significant body of evidence that demonstrates the effect of orlistat on lipid profiles. Orlistat has been shown to cause significant reductions in total cholesterol, low-density lipoprotein (LDL) cholesterol and fasting free fatty acids. The reduction in circulating free fatty acids was associated with a reduction in insulin resistance (Kelley et al 2002, 2004).

Orlistat and blood pressure   Orlistat has also been shown to produce modest reductions in systolic blood pressure in people with type 2 diabetes when compared to placebo (Miles et al 2002, Tong et al 2002). This contrasts with sibutramine (see below) and might prove to be of clinical significance.

Orlistat and the prevention of diabetes   The XENDOS study (Torgeson et al 2004) has reported results that show that the modest weight loss achieved with orlistat in people with impaired glucose tolerance can delay the development of diabetes over a 4-year period.

Sibutramine

Sibutramine is a centrally acting drug that prolongs the action of the neurotransmitters serotonin and noradrenaline by blocking their reuptake at nerve endings. This results in the induction of premature satiety and the maintenance of thermogenic energy expenditure. Sibutramine therefore helps to prevent the reduction in energy expenditure that normally occurs during dieting.

Several studies have demonstrated the ability of sibutramine to improve both weight loss and diabetic control in overweight and obese people with type 2 diabetes (Finer et al 2000, Fujioka et al 2000, Serrano-Rios et al 2002). The improvement in glycaemic control was generally commensurate with the amount of weight loss. In general, reductions in HbA1c were < 0.5% but could be > 1% for people achieving substantial weight loss.

The ability of sibutramine to maintain weight loss has been demonstrated in several trials. For example, a multicentre French trial started individuals on a very low calorie diet for 1 month before randomising people to sibutramine or placebo. After 12 months the sibutramine group had lost a further 5 kg whereas the placebo group had regained 0.5 kg (Apfelbaum et al 1999).

Sibutramine and dyslipidaemia Sibutramine treatment has been shown to improve the typical pattern of dyslipidaemia seen in obese people or those with diabetes (i.e. raised triglycerides and low HDL cholesterol). The reduction in triglycerides and the increase in HDL cholesterol achieved by sibutramine is in excess of that seen by equivalent weight reduction by diet alone (Dujovne et al 2001).

Sibutramine and blood pressure Sibutramine can cause small increases in blood pressure and heart rate, probably by means of its central, inhibitory action on noradrenaline reuptake. This drug is therefore contraindicated in people with uncontrolled hypertension. However, if blood pressure is well controlled, studies have shown no detrimental cardiovascular effects (Faria et al 2002, Hazenburg 2000, McMahon et al 2000, Sharma 2001). However, NICE guidelines (2004) suggest that the detrimental effect of sibutramine on blood pressure negates the beneficial effects of weight loss on cardiovascular outcomes.

Rimonabant is a selective cannabinoid type 1 receptor blocker which has recently been introduced. In combination with an energy-restricted diet and exercise this can reduce bodyweight and HbA1c in obese persons with type 2 diabetes inadequately controlled on metformin or sulphonylurea (Scheen et al 2006).

LONG-TERM SAFETY

Dexfenfluramine (a stimulator of serotonin release) and phentermine (a stimulator of noradrenaline release) have been withdrawn from clinical use because of serious side effects; in particular cardiac valve disease and pulmonary hypertension. These complications have not been identified in people on sibutramine treatment.

INSULIN THERAPY

Case study 4.4

Margaret is a 68-year-old woman who has had type 2 diabetes for 5 years. She was treated initially by diet alone and subsequently with a sulphonylurea. Her control has never been good and 6 months ago metformin was introduced. She has never been overweight and she has lost 4 kg in weight over the past 6 months. She is symptomatic, with polydipsia and nocturia. The need for insulin therapy has been discussed with her on several occasions but she is reluctant to consider this option.

The thin person with type 2 diabetes who is symptomatic and losing weight has reached the point where the pancreatic beta cells have failed and the person is insulin deficient. Insulin therapy will correct the insulin deficiency and reduce blood glucose concentrations. This in turn will reduce the toxic effects of chronically high glucose levels on the beta cells and endogenous insulin secretion may improve.

Many people have a deep-seated fear of self-injection and are understandably reluctant to consider insulin treatment. It can be explained that insulin will be given for a trial period and can subsequently be withdrawn if the person so wishes. This often reassures the individual, who feels that the introduction of insulin treatment is a 'life sentence'. Most people requiring insulin therapy are tired and lethargic, although they might not appreciate the significance of these symptoms, attributing them to old age. It is important to point out to the doubting person that insulin therapy can give them a new lease of life. Most people started on insulin treatment feel a lot better: their symptoms of polydipsia and polyuria recede, they regain lost weight and they generally feel more energetic. Most people 'never look back' after starting insulin therapy and do not contemplate reverting to oral treatments.

INSULIN TREATMENT IN THE ELDERLY

It should be remembered that starting elderly people on insulin treatment can have far-reaching consequences. Many elderly people are unable to learn the technique of self-injection. There can be several reasons for this: failing eyesight, poor muscle coordination due to cerebrovascular disease or degenerative diseases, arthritis or the inability to grasp new concepts may limit the ability of the individual to undertake self injection. Under these circumstances, the person becomes dependent on a relative or healthcare worker for insulin treatment. A previously independent person can therefore be rendered dependent on others. This loss of independence can be associated with a reduction in self-esteem and the development of depression.

Case study 4.5

Jean, who is also 68 years old, has had type 2 diabetes for 6 years. She weighs 117 kg and has been unable to lose weight on diet or metformin treatment. Gliclazide was introduced about 1 year ago. This improved metabolic control initially but resulted in weight gain of nearly 6.5 kg over a 6-month period. The dose of gliclazide has been increased to maximum without further benefit and Jean's blood glucose levels at the clinic are usually greater than 17 mmol/L. Jean is troubled by recurrent carbuncles and recurrent vaginal thrush.

Jean is markedly obese and likely to be insulin resistant. Attempts to achieve control of blood glucose can result in massive doses of insulin being prescribed. This in turn can result in further weight gain. However, the UKPDS has demonstrated the benefit of insulin therapy in preventing long-term complications, despite weight gain. Every effort should be made to encourage weight loss by dieting and exercise, and the use of an anti-obesity drug may be justified. Improved metabolic control in Jean's situation will reduce the incidence of repeated skin and vaginal infections.

INSULIN PROTOCOLS

Until recently, most general practitioners in the UK referred individuals requiring insulin therapy to the local hospital diabetic clinic. Increasingly, however, insulin therapy is being instigated in the community. The principles of insulin therapy in type 2 diabetes will be briefly described here and the reader is referred to Chapter 5, where the subject is dealt with in greater depth.

The UKPDS used once-daily ultralente insulin or isophane insulin, which reflected common practice during the 1970s and 1980s. During that era, oral hypoglycaemic agents were withdrawn and replaced by insulin treatment. Once-daily insulin injections would be particularly suitable for elderly people who might require community nursing assistance with injections. However, for the majority of individuals the aim is to achieve optimum metabolic control, and such regimens are rarely adequate. An early study suggested that if once-daily isophane insulin was used, there was some evidence that better overall control of the diabetes could be achieved if the insulin was given at bedtime rather than before breakfast (Seigler et al 1992). However, as bedtime insulin can be associated with nocturnal hypoglycaemia, this form of therapy has been discouraged. When once-daily insulin injections failed to adequately control hyperglycaemia, the person was normally switched to twice-daily or multiple injection regimens. New insulin analogues available nowadays mean that night-time injections are again feasible (see Chapter 5).

INSULIN AND ORAL HYPOGLYCAEMIC AGENT COMBINATIONS

Sulphonylurea plus insulin

Increasingly, the trend in recent years has been to continue sulphonylurea and/or metformin treatment while introducing insulin therapy. The launch of insulin glargine has encouraged this trend and studies have shown that bedtime insulin glargine in combination with oral therapy can achieve tight diabetic control while causing significantly less nocturnal hypoglycaemia than isophane insulins (Riddle et al 2003).

Combination sulphonylurea and insulin therapy can be effective in people with a partial beta-cell response to sulphonylureas. As the sulphonylureas stimulate endogenous insulin secretion, lower insulin doses might be expected to be effective. The combination of an oral agent with a single daily insulin injection can make the introduction of insulin more acceptable to the individual person.

This combination has been the subject of several studies and a meta-analysis of 16 studies has shown that the combination of sulphonylurea plus insulin improves glycaemic control with reduced insulin requirements and with no adverse effect on weight (Johnson et al 1996). Combination therapy was associated with a 1.1% reduction in HbA1c as compared to 0.25% reduction with insulin monotherapy.

Metformin plus insulin

For the obese person with insulin resistance, a combination of metformin and insulin seems logical. Metformin improves the action of insulin on peripheral tissues and one would expect it to reduce the requirement for high doses of insulin in this type of individual. The addition of metformin to insulin therapy might also be expected to reduce or prevent the inevitable weight gain which occurs in obese people with type 2 diabetes following the introduction of insulin therapy.

Metformin plus insulin therapy has been associated with an insulin sparing effect of between 15–32% in people with type 2 diabetes (Buse 2000). This combination has been shown to reduce HbA1c to a greater extent than insulin alone, while using a lower dose of insulin.

If combination treatment with oral agents and insulin fails to control blood glucose levels, people can be changed onto twice-daily insulin regimens. Fixed mixtures of short-acting and isophane insulins are probably the simplest insulins to use in this group of people.

Thiazolidinedione therapy is contraindicated for people on insulin treatment. Thiazolidinediones should therefore be withdrawn before the introduction of insulin treatment.

Case study 4.6

Beatrice is a 67-year-old woman who was admitted to hospital 7 months ago having sustained a dense right hemiplegia and aphasia. On admission to hospital a random blood glucose was measured at 17 mmol/L and, in accordance with the protocol for acute treatment of stroke, she was started on an insulin infusion to control her hyperglycaemia. Initially, Beatrice required nasogastric feeding and intravenous insulin was continued. When she was again able to swallow and eat, the insulin was changed to twice-daily injections of a fixed insulin mixture. She had a prolonged period of rehabilitation but remained chair-bound and profoundly dysphasic.

On discharge from hospital, Beatrice's insulin requirements were 28 units per day. However, over the next few weeks, she had several hypoglycaemic episodes and the insulin was gradually reduced to 12 units per day. It was therefore decided to stop insulin treatment and she was converted to gliclazide 80 mg twice daily. The dose of gliclazide was, however, reduced first to 80 mg once daily and then 40 mg daily. Diabetic control remained tight and the oral agent was also stopped. Months later, Beatrice's blood glucose remains in the range 4.0–8.0 mmol/L on diet alone.

Beatrice's case illustrates that treatment with insulin or oral hypoglycaemic drugs is not always permanent. In the acute situation such as Beatrice's stroke, her newly diagnosed diabetes might well require insulin treatment initially. The acute stress of her cerebrovascular accident was sufficient to cause an increase in insulin resistance and resulted in blood glucose levels rising. Any significant medical or surgical emergencies can result in such a rise in blood glucose and these changes can persist for several weeks.

Similarly, the introduction of medications such as steroids can result in deterioration in glycaemic control and the need to increase glucose lowering therapy. On cessation of steroid treatment, the insulin or oral agent might need to be reduced in dosage or withdrawn.

DRUGS OF THE FUTURE

DUAL PPARα AND PPARγ RECEPTOR AGONISTS

Current PPARγ receptor agonists exhibit only mild lipid-lowering effects in addition to their insulin-sensitising action. Fibrates are PPARα receptor agonists and have been used for many years as lipid-lowering agents. They reduce plasma triglycerides and raise HDL cholesterol while reducing LDL cholesterol. By combining the therapeutic effects of PPARα and γ receptor agonists, the major metabolic disorders of type 2 diabetes, hyperglycaemia, insulin resistance and dyslipidaemia can be addressed simultaneously.

Aside from improving dyslipidaemia, cardiovascular risks can be further modified by dual activation of PPARα and γ receptors, as this has been shown to exert direct antiatherogenic effects (Jackson et al 1999, Marx et al 1999). In addition, this dual activation has been shown in animal models to reduce the undesirable weight gain associated with TZD therapy (Chaput et al 2000, Guerre-Millo et al 2000). By simultaneously stimulating both PPARα and γ, the propensity for adipogenesis resulting from PPARγ activation might be offset by the propensity of PPARα activation to stimulate lipid catabolism.

Muraglitazar

Muraglitazar is a novel non-TZD dual PPARα and γ agonist. This drug, along with other dual PPARα and γ agonists is currently under development.

The amylin story

Amylin is a pancreatic hormone that is co-localised with insulin in the beta cells and co-secreted with insulin in response to meals. Postprandial insulin and amylin responses become markedly reduced as beta-cell function deteriorates with advancing type 2 diabetes.

Modes of action   Following its release from the pancreas, amylin acts on the brain. It binds to specific sites, including the area postrema. Signals sent via the vagus nerve then result in the slowing of gastric emptying. Amylin also acts centrally as an appetite suppressant (Young et al 2000). In addition, amylin suppresses nutrient-stimulated secretion of glucagon (Gedulin et al 1997). This hormone is responsible for stimulating postprandial release of glucose from the liver.

Thus amylin contributes to normal glucose homeostasis through actions that limit nutrient influx during the postprandial period.

Pramlintide

Pramlintide is a synthetic analogue of human amylin and has similar biological actions. Studies with pramlintide are now well advanced. Current regimens of insulin therapy in type 2 diabetes are associated with excessive weight gain, failure to adequately control postprandial glycaemic excursions and an increased risk of hypoglycaemia. Studies of pramlintide in both type 1 and type 2 diabetes have shown beneficial effects when it is co-injected with insulin (Thompson et al 1997, 1998). These studies have demonstrated that the addition of pramlintide to insulin can result in improved glycaemic control without the need to increase insulin doses and in association with significant weight loss. The improvement in glycaemic control with pramlintide was not associated with an increased incidence of severe hypoglycaemia. Pramlintide therefore appears to go some way to counter the detrimental effects of insulin treatment in type 2 diabetes. It is likely that this compound will come to the market in the near future.

The incretin story

It has long been recognised that orally administered glucose provokes greater stimulation of insulin release than similar amounts infused intravenously. Hence, it has been postulated that oral nutrient ingestion must stimulate gut-derived signals that are potent stimulators of insulin release (incretins). The neurotransmitter substances glucagon-like peptide-1 (GLP-1) and glucose-dependent insulinotropic peptide (GIP) have been identified as the most important peptides for the majority of nutrient-stimulated insulin secretion.

Unlike the potent glucose-lowering actions of GIP in normal rodents, exogenous administration of GIP is less effective in diabetic rodents. It is, therefore, unlikely to be of clinical benefit for people with type 2 diabetes. However, GLP-1 appears to be equipotent in diabetic and non-diabetic animals. GLP-1 has been shown to have additional glucose-lowering properties. These include inhibition of glucagon secretion, inhibition of gastric emptying and reduction of food intake.

GLP-1 is metabolised very rapidly by the enzyme dipeptidyl peptidase IV (DPP-IV). Because of this, the effects of a single injection of GLP-1 are short-lasting and continuous intravenous infusions are required for sustained effects. In order to overcome this problem, degradation-resistant GLP-1 analogues with longer duration of action have been developed.

Exendin-4 (exenatide)

Exendin-4 is a naturally occurring GLP-1 receptor agonist isolated from the salivary gland venom of the lizard *Heloderma suspectum*. Exendin-4 is highly resistant to the proteolytic activity of DPP IV and exhibits a longer duration of action.

Exendin-4, now renamed exenatide, must be given by twice-daily subcutaneous injections. It is currently being evaluated for treatment of type 2 diabetes in combination with metformin, sulphonylureas or both (Fineman et al 2003).

Liraglutide is a fatty-acid-linked DPP-IV-resistant GLP-1 analogue that is given once daily and is also undergoing clinical trials for treatment of type 2 diabetes. A further GLP-1 analogue currently named CJC-1131 and with a half-life of 10 days is undergoing preliminary studies in humans (Baggio & Drucker 2004).

DPP IV inhibitors

An alternative therapeutic approach to prolong the action of GLP-1 is to inhibit the enzyme DDP IV. Several DDP IV inhibitors (LAF-237, MK-0431 and P93/01) are currently undergoing clinical trials. These drugs have the advantage over GLP-1 analogues that they can be administered orally.

MEDICATIONS ALTERING GLUCOSE TOLERANCE AND DRUG INTERACTIONS

Individuals with type 2 diabetes are likely to be middle aged or elderly and might have other medical conditions that need to be treated simultaneously. As stated elsewhere, type 2 diabetes is associated with hypertension, hyperlipidaemia and vascular disease. Polypharmacy is the norm for these people, who may often be taking medications that interfere with their diabetes (Table 4.2).

HYPERGLYCAEMIC EFFECTS

Diuretics

Thiazide diuretics such as bendroflumethiazide are known to increase blood glucose levels by causing increased resistance to the action of insulin on peripheral tissues. Thiazides are often included in 'combination pills' such as Tenoretic and Capozide. The loop diuretics, furosemide and bumetanide, also have mild effects on glucose tolerance.

Table 4.2
Drugs influencing glycaemic control

Hypoglycaemic effects	hyperglycaemic effects
alcohol	corticosteroids
monoamine oxidase inhibitors	thiazide and loop diuretics
fibrates	chlorpromazine
miconazole	chronic alcohol
salicylates	oral contraceptives
cimetidine, ranitidine	anabolic steroids

Beta-blockers

The beta-blockers are now less commonly used as first-line therapy for hypertension. They remain useful drugs, however, in people who also have angina. These drugs also impair glucose tolerance and might worsen diabetic control.

Oestrogen

Oestrogen-containing preparations or drugs with oestrogen-like actions can increase blood glucose levels. Although oral contraceptive agents are not often used in this age group, hormone replacement therapy *is* used and must be introduced with care in the older female with type 2 diabetes lest diabetic control deteriorates. The anti-oestrogen, tamoxifen, has oestrogenic effects and can worsen glucose tolerance. This medication is commonly used in older persons with breast malignancy.

Steroids

Corticosteroids antagonise the action of insulin and therefore medications, such as prednisolone, used for the treatment of asthma or for immunosuppression will result in raising blood glucose concentrations. Anabolic steroids are used in some people with malignancy and are also used illegally for body building. They will also cause blood glucose levels to rise.

Adrenaline

Adrenaline is another hormone that can counter the action of insulin and it is important to remember that adrenaline or adrenaline-like compounds (phenylpropanolamine and ephedrine) are frequently found in decongestants and cold remedies.

Atypical antipsychotics

Over the past 10 years, the atypical (also known as novel or second-generation) antipsychotic drugs have increasingly been used to treat schizophrenia and related disorders in which psychosis is a prominent feature. The *British National Formulary* currently lists amisulpride, clozapine, olanzapine, quetiapine, risperidone, aripiprazole, sertindole and zotepine as atypical antipsychotics.

Recently, evidence has been mounting to suggest that atypical antipsychotic drugs are associated with adverse metabolic effects, including weight gain, new-onset diabetes (both type 2 and diabetic ketoacidosis) and hypertriglyceridaemia. (Koller et al 2001, Newcomer et al 2002). These drugs have also been noted to exacerbate pre-existing diabetes.

The mechanism by which atypical antipsychotic drugs affect glucose metabolism remains unclear but it is likely that multiple factors are involved. These drugs can cause weight gain, with an associated increase in insulin resistance. However, it is likely that these drugs have an adverse effect on insulin sensitivity independent of their tendency to cause weight gain. It is therefore recommended that fasting glucose, HbA1c and lipids are monitored at least 6-monthly in people taking atypical antipsychotics, and more often in those at greater risk of diabetes.

HYPOGLYCAEMIC EFFECTS

A variety of drugs can have hypoglycaemic effects (Table 4.3). Aspirin and other non-steroidal anti-inflammatory agents have a mild blood-glucose-lowering effect. Similarly, alcohol can cause hypoglycaemia, particularly if a person is taking insulin or on sulphonylurea treatment. Alcohol acts on the liver and reduces the ability of the liver to produce glucose. Hence alcohol will enhance the hypoglycaemic effects of insulin or oral hypoglycaemic agents.

Drug interactions with sulphonylureas

Drugs that bind to proteins in the blood can displace the sulphonylureas from their binding sites and release the more active drug into the circulation, thus causing hypoglycaemia. The sulphonamide antibiotics and trimethoprim are examples of drugs that compete with the sulphonylureas for their protein binding sites. Other antibiotics, such as chloramphenicol and the 4-quinolones, can also enhance the hypoglycaemic action of the sulphonylureas. Rifampicin, however, is an antibiotic that accelerates the metabolism of the sulphonylureas and therefore reduces their therapeutic effect.

Drug interactions with meglitinides

A potentially dangerous interaction between repaglinide and gemfibrozil has been identified. Gemfibrozil markedly increases the systemic exposure to repaglinide and this combination of drugs should be avoided. A similar interaction occurs between repaglinide and clarithromycin and this may require a reduction in the dose of repaglinide.

Table 4.3 also lists medications that alter the hypoglycaemic effects of the above agents. The reader is also referred to the *British National Formulary* for a more extensive list of interactions.

Table 4.3
Drug interactions with oral hypoglycaemic agents

Sulphonylureas	meglitinides	metformin	glitizones
sulphonamides*	gemfibrozil*	cimetidine*	unusual
trimethoprim*	clarithromycin*		
chloramphenicol*			
ciprofloxacin*			
itraconazole, fluconazole*			
rifampicin**			

* Enhance action of drug.
** Antagonise action of drug.

Drug interactions with metformin

Cimetidine increases the serum levels of metformin by competing with metformin for transport across the renal tubules.

CONCLUSION

Dietary management is fundamental to the care of all people with type 2 diabetes. However, a substantial number of people will fail to control their diabetes with diet alone and will require oral hypoglycaemic agents. Exercise and other lifestyle changes are also required to improve metabolic status and reduce long-term cardiovascular disease. Type 2 diabetes is a progressive disease requiring increasing doses of hypoglycaemic agents and additional therapies to maintain glycaemic control.

Tight metabolic control is associated with significant reductions in the incidence of microvascular complications. There is also a reduction in macrovascular disease with reducing HbA1c results. Metformin treatment in obese people with diabetes has been shown to significantly reduce these macrovascular events.

Metformin is the drug of first choice for the obese person with diabetes, and indeed metformin should probably also be used first in non-obese people. Thiazolidinediones are currently not recommended as first-line treatment in the UK unless other medications are contraindicated or not tolerated. This situation might change if these drugs are shown to have beneficial effects on cardiovascular outcomes.

As metabolic control deteriorates, combination therapy using different classes of oral hypoglycaemics will be required. Increasingly, insulin therapy is used to prolong glycaemic control. Insulin is often introduced as a single injection while people are maintained on an oral agent, and only when this combination regimen fails are multiple insulin injections introduced.

REFERENCES

Aguilar C, Reza A, Garcia JE, Rull JA 1992 Biguanide related lactic acidosis: incidence and risk factors. Archives of Medical Research 23:19–24

Apfelbaum M, Vague P, Ziegler O et al 1999 Long-term maintenance of weight loss after a very-low-calorie diet: a randomised blinded trial of the efficacy and tolerability of sibutramine. American Journal of Medicine 106:179–184

Baggio LL, Drucker DJ 2004 Incretin hormones and the treatment of type 2 diabetes Online. Available: www.medscape.com/viewarticle/482591

Bailey CJ 1992 Biguanides and NIDDM. Diabetes Care 15:755–772

Blonk MC, Jacobs MAJM, Biesheuvel EHE et al 1994 Influences on Weight Loss in Type 2 Diabetic Patients: Little Long-term Benefit from Group Behaviour and Exercise Training. Diabetic Medicine 11:449–457

Buse J 2000 Combining insulin and oral agents. American Journal of Medicine 108 (6 suppl 1):23–32

Chan JCN, Chan K-WA, Ho LLT et al 1998 An Asian multicenter clinical trial to assess the efficacy and tolerability of acarbose compared with placebo in Type 2 diabetic patients previously treated with diet. Diabetes Care 21:1058–1061

Chaput E, Saladin R, Silvestre M, Edgar AD 2000 Fenofibrate and rosiglitazone lower serum triglycerides with opposing effects on body weight. Biochemistry and Biophysics Research Communications 271:445–450

Dills DG, Schneider J 1996 Clinical evaluation of glimepiride versus glyburide in NIDDM in a double-blind comparative study. Glimepiride/Glyburide Research Group. Hormones and Metabolic Research 28(9):426–429

Donnan PJ, MacDonald TM, Morris AD 2002 Adherence to prescribed oral hypoglycaemic medication in a population of patients with type 2 diabetes: a retrospective cohort study. Diabetic Medicine 19:279–284

Dujovne CA, Zavirak JH, Rowe E et al 2001 Effects of sibutramine on both body weight and serum lipids; a double blind, randomised, placebo-controlled study in 322 overweight and obese patients with dyslipidaemia. American Heart Journal 142:489–497

Faria AN, Ribeiro Filho FF, Lerarlo DD et al 2002 Effects of sibutramine on the treatment of obesity in patients with arterial hypertension. Arquivos Brasileiros de Cardiologia 78:172–180

Ferner RE, Neil HAW 1988 Sulphonylurea and hypoglycaemia [editorial]. British Medical Journal 296:949–950

Fineman MS, Bicsak TA, Shen LZ et al 2003 Effect on glycaemic control of synthetic exendin-4 (AC2993) additive to existing metformin and/or sulfonylurea treatment in patients with type 2 diabetes. Diabetes Care 26:2370–2377

Finer N, Bloom SR, Frost GS et al 2000 Sibutramine is effective for weight loss and diabetic control in obesity with type 2 diabetes: a randomised double-blinded, placebo-controlled study. Diabetes Obesity and Metabolism 2:105–112

Fujioka K, Seaton TB, Rowe E et al 2000 Weight loss with sibutramine improves glycaemic control and other metabolic parameters in obese patients with type 2 diabetes mellitus. Diabetes Obesity & Metabolism 2:175–187

Garber AJ, Theodore D, Goodman A et al 1997 Efficacy of metformin in type II diabetes: results of a double-blind, placebo-controlled, dose response trial. American Journal of Medicine 103:491–497

Gedulin BR, Rink TJ, Young AA 1997 Dose-response for glucagonostatic effect of amylin in rats. Metabolism 46:67–70

Gordon D 1996 In McDowell J, Gordon D (eds) Diabetes. The patient with non-insulin-dependent-diabetes mellitus. Caring for patients in the community. Churchill Livingstone, London

Greenway F 1999 Obesity medications and the treatment of type 2 diabetes. Diabetes Technology and Therapeutics 1:277–287

Guerre-Millo M, Gervois P, Raspe E et al 2000 Peroxisome proliferator-activated receptor a activators improve insulin sensitivity and reduce adiposity. Journal of Biological Chemistry 275:16638–16642

Halpern A, Mancini MC, Suplicy H et al 2003 Latin-American trial of orlistat for weight loss and improvement in glycaemic profile in obese diabetic patients. Diabetes Obesity and Metabolism 5:180–188

Hanefeld M, Sachse G 2002 The effects of orlistat on body weight and glycaemic control in overweight patients with type 2 diabetes: a randomized, placebo-controlled trial. Diabetes Obesity and Metabolism 4:415–423

Harrower A, Wong C 1990 Comparison of secondary failure rate between three second generation sulphonylureas. Diabetes Research 13:19–21

Hazenburg BP 2000 Randomised, double-blind, placebo-controlled, multicenter study of sibutramine in obese hypertensive patients. Cardiology 94:152–158

Helmrich JE, Ragland DR, Leung RW et al 1991 Physical activity and reduced occurrence of non-insulin-dependent diabetes mellitus. New England Journal of Medicine 325:147–152

Holman RR, Cull C, Turner R et al 1999 (UKPDS 44) A randomized double-blind trial of acerbose in Type 2 diabetes shows improved glycaemic control over 3 years. Diabetes Care 22:960–964

Hu FB, Manson JE, Stampfer MJ et al 2001 Diet, lifestyle, and the risk of type 2 diabetes mellitus in women. New England Journal of Medicine 345:790–797

Jackson SM, Parhami F, Xi XP et al 1999 Peroxisome proliferator-activated receptor activators target human endothelial cells to inhibit leukocyte–endothelial cell interaction. Arteriosclerosis Thrombosis and Vascular Biology 19:2094–2104

Jariwala S, Mather R, Walker L et al 2003 Long-term glycaemic control with rosiglitazone in combination with metformin. Diabetic Medicine 20(suppl 2):poster 277

Johnson JL, Wolf SL, Kabali M 1996 Efficacy of insulin and sulphonylurea combination therapy in type II diabetes. A meta-analysis of the randomized placebo-controlled trials. Archives of Internal Medicine 156(3):259–264

Kelley DE, Bray GA, Pi-Sunyer FX et al 2002 Clinical efficacy of orlistat therapy in overweight and obese patients with insulin-treated type 2 diabetes: a 1-year randomized controlled trial. Diabetes Care 25:1033–1041

Kelley DE, Kuller LH, McKolanis TM et al 2004 Effects of moderate weight loss and orlistat on insulin resistance, regional adiposity and fatty acids in type 2 diabetes. Diabetes Care 27:33–40

Koller E, Schneider B, Bennett K et al 2001 Clozapine-associated diabetes. American Journal of Medicine 111:716–723

Lindstrom J, Tuomilehto J, Spenglert M for the Finnish Acarbose Study Group 2000 Acarbose treatment does not change the habitual diet of patients with type 2 diabetes mellitus. Diabetic Medicine 17:20–25

Manson JE, Rimm EB, Stampfer MJ et al 1991 Physical activity and incidence of non-insulin-dependent diabetes mellitus in women. Lancet 338:774–778

Marx N, Sukhova GK, Collins T et al 1999 PPAR alpha activators inhibit cytokine-induced vascular cell adhesion molecule-1 expression in human endothelial cells. Circulation 99:3125–3131

Mathews DR, Bakst A, Weston WM et al 1999 Rosiglitazone decreases insulin resistance and improves beta cell function in patients with type 2 diabetes. Diabetologia 42(suppl 1): A228, abstract 858

Melander A, Bitzen P-O, Faber O, Groop L 1989 Sulphonylurea antidiabetic drugs: an update of their clinical pharmacology and rational therapeutic use. Drugs 37:58–72

McMahon FG, Fujioka K, Singh BN et al 2000 Efficacy and safety of sibutramine in obese white and African American patients with hypertension:a 1-year, double-blind, placebo-controlled, multicenter trial. Archives of Internal Medicine 160:2185–2191

Miles JM, Leiter L, Hollander P et al 2002 Effects of orlistat in overweight and obese patients with type 2 diabetes treated with metformin. Diabetes Care 25:1123–1128

National Institute for Health and Clinical Excellence (NICE) 2004 National clinical guidelines for type 2 diabetes. Online. Available: www.nice.org.uk/pdf/NICE_full_blood_glucose [accessed 18 September 2004]

Newcomer JW, Haupt DW, Fucetola R et al 2002 Abnormalities in glucose regulation during antipsychotic treatment of schizophrenia. Archives of General Psychiatry 59:337–345

Riddle MC, Rosenstock J, Gerlich J 2003 The treat-to-target trial: randomized addition of glargine or human nph insulin to oral therapy of type 2 diabetes patients. Diabetes Care 26(11):3080–3086

Rosenstock J 2000 Improved insulin sensitivity and beta cell responsivity suggested by HOMA analysis of pioglitazone therapy. Diabetologia 443(suppl 1):A192

Scheen AJ, Finer N, Hollander P et al for RIO-Diabetes Study Group. Efficacy and tolerability of rimonabant in overweight or obese patients with type 2 diabetes: a randomised controlled study. Lancet 2006; 368:1660–1672.

Scorpiglione N, Belfiglio M, Carinci F et al 1999 The effectiveness, safety and epidemiology of the use of acarbose in the treatment of patients with type II diabetes mellitus. A model of medicine-based evidence. European Journal of Clinical Pharmacology 55:239–249

Scott R, Lintott CJ, Zimmet P et al 1999 Will acerbose improve the metabolic abnormalities of insulin-resistant type 2 diabetes mellitus. Diabetes Research and Clinical Practice 43:179–185

Seigler DE, Olsson GM, Skyler JS 1992 Morning versus bedtime isophane insulin in type 2 (non-insulin dependent) diabetes mellitus. Diabetic Medicine 9:826–833

Serrano-Rios M, Melchionda N, Moreno-Carretero E 2002 Role of sibutramine in the treatment of obese type 2 diabetic patients receiving sulphonylurea therapy. Diabetic Medicine 19:119–124

Sharma AM 2001 Sibutramine in overweight/obese hypertensive patients. International Journal of Obesity 25(suppl 4) S20–S23

Sonnenberg GE, Carg DC, Weilder DJ et al 1997 Short term comparison of once- versus twice-daily administration of glimepiride in patients with non-insulin-dependent diabetes mellitus. The Annals of Pharmacotherapy 31:671–676

Stevens V, Obarzanek E, Cook N et al 2001 Long-term weight loss and changes in blood pressure: Results of the trial of hypertension prevention, phase II. Annals of Internal Medicine 134:1–11

Thomson RG, Peterson J, Gottlieb A, Mullane J 1997 Effects of pramlintide, an analog of human amylin, on plasma glucose profiles in patients with insulin-dependent diabetes mellitus: results of a multicenter trial. Diabetes 46:632–636

Thomson RG, Pearson LRN, Schoenfeld SL et al 1998 Pramlintide, a synthetic analog of human amylin, improves the metabolic profile of patients with type 2 diabetes using insulin. Diabetes Care 21:987–993

Tong PC, Lee ZS, Sea MM et al 2002 The effect of orlistat-induced weight loss, without concomitant hypocaloric diet, on cardiovascular risk factors and insulin sensitivity in young obese Chinese subjects with or without type 2 diabetes. Archives of Internal Medicine 162:2428–2435

Tontonoz P, Hu E, Graves RA et al 1994 mPPARγ2: tissue-specific regulator of an adipocyte enhancer. Genes and Development 8:1224–1234

Torgeson JS, Hauptman J, Boldrin MN et al 2004 Xenical in the prevention of diabetes in obese subjects (XENDOS Study). A randomized study of orlistat as an adjunct to lifestyle changes for the prevention of type 2 diabetes in obese patients. Diabetes Care 27:155–161

UK Prospective Diabetes Study (UKPDS) Group 1990 Response of fasting plasma glucose to diet therapy in newly presenting type II diabetic patients (UKPDS 7). Metabolism 39:905–912

UK Prospective Diabetes Study (UKPDS) Group 1998a Intensive blood-glucose control with sulphonylureas or insulin compared with conventional treatment and risk of complications in patients with type 2 diabetes (UKPDS 33). Lancet 352:837–853

UK Prospective Diabetes Study (UKPDS) Group 1998b Effect of intensive blood-glucose control with metformin on complications in overweight patients with type 2 diabetes (UKPDS 34). Lancet 352:854–865

Vidal-Puig AJ, Considine PV, Jimenez-Linan M et al 1997 Peroxisome proliferator-activated receptor gene expression in human tissues. Effects of obesity, weight loss, and regulation by insulin and glucocorticoids. Journal of Clinical Investigation 99:2416–2422

Young A, Moore C, Herich J, Beaumont K 2000 In Poyner D, Marshall I, Brain SD (eds) CGRP family: calcitonin gene-related peptide (CGRP), amylin, and adrenomedullin. Landes Bioscience, Georgetown, TX, p 91–102

The person with type 1 diabetes

Derek Gordon and Florence Brown

INTRODUCTION

The history of the discovery of insulin in 1921 is one of intrigue, personality clashes and betrayal, and of a medical student on a summer job placement achieving the Nobel Prize. Without insulin, newly diagnosed children and young adults with diabetes faced a slow, wasting disease that could be treated only by a starvation diet and that led to an inevitable, early death. The discovery of insulin offered a chance of life to those previously living without hope.

EPIDEMIOLOGY

Type 1 diabetes accounts for approximately 10% of all people with diabetes and affects 10–20 million people worldwide. Type 1 diabetes generally affects people under the age of 40 years and 40% develop it before the age of 20 years. One of the most striking characteristics of type 1 diabetes is the large geographic variability in incidence. The Scandinavian countries and the Mediterranean island of Sardinia have the highest incidences in the world, whereas Oriental populations have the lowest incidences. The reasons for such geographical differences are not known.

The incidence of type 1 diabetes has increased by 3–5% over recent decades and the disease is occurring more frequently in younger children in particular. The cause for these changes is also unknown.

THE CLINICAL PRESENTATION OF TYPE 1 DIABETES

Case study 5.1

Tom is an 18-year-old who has presented to his GP with a 3-week history of thirst. He was drinking up to 2 litres of carbonated drinks per day. He had noticed that he was passing much more urine than normal and was getting up through the night on at least three occasions. During this period of time his weight had fallen by about 4 kg. He had become increasingly tired and lethargic and had also noticed that his vision had become blurred. He also admitted to painful cracking of the foreskin. Glycosuria was confirmed as 2% and there was 3+++ of ketonuria using urine testing strips. The diagnosis of type 1 diabetes was confirmed by measurement of plasma glucose of 23.0 mmol/L. Tom was referred immediately by telephone to the local consultant diabetologist, who arranged to see him that day and insulin treatment was started.

People presenting with type 1 diabetes typically give a short and dramatic history of polydipsia, polyuria and weight loss. The lack of insulin causes a rise in blood glucose, which acts as an osmotic diuretic causing polyuria and polydipsia. In an attempt to provide energy, the body mobilises its glucose and fat reserves and, in so doing, switches into ketone production (see Chapter 1). This accounts for the acute weight loss, tiredness and lethargy. Left untreated, the person would develop diabetic ketoacidosis and coma. Nowadays, this is less frequently seen due to heightened awareness of the early diabetic symptoms by healthcare workers and the public in general.

Tom's blurred vision was due to the presence of glucose in the lens of the eye. This causes alteration in the shape of the lens and subsequent blurring of vision due to altered refraction. This corrects itself as, with treatment, blood glucose levels return to normal, but it can take up to 6 weeks before the blurring disappears. People who are newly diagnosed with diabetes should be advised not to get their eyes tested for glasses for up to 3 months from diagnosis or 2 months from the time that their diabetes is stable.

The presence of sugar in the urine encourages the development of penile thrush, as in Tom's case. Reducing glycosuria will eliminate the growth of organisms. In the meantime, however, Tom will also require appropriate antifungal treatment.

At the hospital clinic, Tom would be seen by the diabetes specialist team and have blood samples taken for glucose, urea and electrolytes including bicarbonate, liver function tests, full blood count and glycated haemoglobin (HbA1c). The possibility of diabetic ketoacidosis (DKA) needs to be considered. DKA is a medical emergency and requires hospital admission.

The dietician would assess Tom's current diet and recommend dietary changes in the light of his history, lifestyle and estimated energy consumption. The DNS would start insulin therapy and teach Tom how to perform home blood glucose monitoring (HBGM) and arrange to see him frequently to continue his stabilisation and education. Tom would then enter a full education programme involving all the members of the healthcare team. This might continue over several weeks or months (see Chapter 11).

> Question 'Will my children get diabetes?'

A frequently asked question following a diagnosis of diabetes is whether other family members will be affected. In areas of the world where the risk of diabetes is moderate (e.g. the UK) the risk of developing type 1 diabetes by age 20 years is approximately 1 : 300. The risk is increased to 1 : 50 for children of women with type 1 diabetes and as high as 1 : 15 if a person's father has type 1 diabetes. It is also estimated that by the age of 60 years approximately 10% of first-degree relatives will develop type 1 diabetes. If a child has type 1 diabetes then there is a 1 : 10 chance that another sibling will also be diagnosed with type 1 diabetes.

LESS TYPICAL PRESENTATIONS

Type 1 diabetes can affect people over the age of 40 years and can even occur in the elderly. It is now recognised that it can present with less acute symptoms. It can sometimes be difficult to decide in both young and older people whether they have type 1 or type 2 diabetes at the time of presentation. When the type of diabetes is in doubt, the diagnosis of type 1 diabetes should be considered if:

- ketonuria is detected, or
- weight loss is marked, or
- the person does not have features of the metabolic syndrome (see Chapter 4) or other contributing illness.

THE AIMS OF INSULIN THERAPY

- To preserve life.
- To relieve the symptoms of hyperglycaemia, i.e. polydipsia, polyuria, lethargy and weight loss.
- To restore 'normal metabolism'.
- To prevent diabetic ketoacidosis.

The development of diabetes is associated with many subtle changes in metabolism, for example, lipids, blood clotting and connective tissue biochemistry. Many of these secondary changes in metabolism are responsible for the long-term complications of diabetes. The Diabetes Control and Complications Trial (DCCT) (DCCT Research Group 1993), as well as a number of smaller studies, have clearly demonstrated the beneficial effects of improved diabetic control in preventing the microvascular complications of diabetes (Wang et al 1993).

THE DIABETES CONTROL AND COMPLICATIONS TRIAL

Nearly 1500 people with type 1 diabetes were recruited from 29 diabetic clinics across the USA to take part in the Diabetes Control and Complications Trial (The DCCT Research Group 1993). People were randomly allocated to receive up to 10 years' conventional or intensified treatment. Conventional treatment consisted of one or two daily injections of insulin and education about diet and exercise. People were reviewed every 3 months. Intensified treatment aimed for long-term near-normoglycaemia with at least four home blood glucose assessments a day, three or more insulin injections daily and monthly visits to a clinic with further advice freely available by telephone between clinics.

The trial was halted prematurely after people had been followed-up for periods ranging between 3 and 9 years. Those individuals in the intensively treated group maintained significantly better metabolic control throughout the study period. However, despite the intensive treatment, only 5% of this group attained the goal of near-normoglycaemia throughout the study.

Nevertheless, the study dramatically demonstrated that improving diabetic control was associated with a significant reduction in the risks of developing diabetic complications or their progression. The reduction of 2% in HbA1c in the intensively treated group of individuals was associated with:

- 76% reduction in the risk of newly developing retinopathy and 54% reduction in the progression of retinopathy
- 39% reduction in the incidence of microalbuminuria and 54% reduction in progression to proteinuria
- 60% reduction in development of neuropathy.

This improvement was apparent at all levels of metabolic control. In other words, a reduction in HbA1c from 16% to 14% was associated with the same improvement in outcome as a reduction from 10% to 8%. Nevertheless, it remains the case that those people with poorest control have the greatest risk of complications.

Targets for glycaemic control

The DCCT has implied that there is no threshold figure of HbA1c below which complications do not occur. However, on the basis of epidemiological studies in the DCCT and UK Prospective Diabetes Study (see Chapter 4), the microvascular risk appeared to be low once an average HbA1c was around 7.0–8.0% while macrovascular risk continued to fall with HbA1c levels down to 6.0–7.0% (DCCT standardised). This has led the National Institute for Health and Clinical Excellence (NICE) to make the following recommendations (NICE 2004):

- Adults with type 1 diabetes should be advised that maintaining a DCCT-harmonised HbA1c below 7.5% is likely to minimise their risk of developing diabetic eye, kidney or nerve damage in the longer term.
- Adults with type 1 diabetes who want to achieve an HbA1c down to, or towards 7.5% should be given all appropriate support in their efforts to do so.
- Where there is evidence of increased arterial risk (identified by raised albumin excretion rate, features of the metabolic syndrome, or other arterial risk factors) people with type 1 diabetes should be advised that approaching lower HbA1c level (for example 6.5%) might be of benefit.

Tight (meaning the achievement of normoglycaemia) metabolic control has its downsides. People in the DCCT intensively treated group gained weight and experienced three times as many episodes of severe hypoglycaemia as the conventionally treated group. It should be remembered that many people with type 1 diabetes fear severe hypoglycaemia more than complications in middle or late life.

Tight metabolic control might not be appropriate for the following groups of people:

- people with loss of warning signs of impending hypoglycaemic attack
- young children, particularly under the age of 7 years, when hypoglycaemia can be associated with damage to the developing brain
- frail, elderly people or those with limited life expectancy in whom the rigors associated with close metabolic control, would not be appropriate
- people who have limited abilities to treat hypoglycaemia independently.

Self-monitoring of blood glucose

Self-monitoring of blood glucose was an integral part of the intensive treatment group in the DCCT. However, self-monitoring is only likely to affect blood glucose control when used to inform self-management of diabetes. In clinical practice there is often little relationship between frequency of blood glucose self-monitoring and frequency of insulin dose self-adjustment (Gordon et al 1991).

NICE has therefore made several recommendations, including the following:

- Self-monitoring of blood glucose levels should be used as part of an integrated package that includes appropriate insulin regimens and education to help inform choice and achievement of optimal diabetes outcomes.
- Adults with type 1 diabetes should be advised that the optimal frequency of self-monitoring will depend on:
  - the characteristics of their blood glucose control
  - the insulin regimen
  - personal preference in using the results to achieve the desired lifestyle.

Chapter 7 further expands on the evidence base for blood glucose monitoring.

CURRENTLY AVAILABLE INSULINS

Insulins with different chemical structures, depending on their source and manufacture, are available:

- Bovine (Wockhardt UK)
- Porcine (Wockhardt UK)
- 'Human' (NovoNordisk, Lilly, Sanofi-Aventis)
- Insulin analogues (NovoNordisk, Lilly, Sanofi-Aventis).

ANIMAL INSULINS

The chemical structures of these insulins differ from human insulin by a few amino acids. Bovine insulin differs from human insulin in three of its 51 amino acids, and is thus more likely to cause antibodies to be formed against it. Porcine insulin differs in only one amino acid residue (alanine in place of threonine).

'HUMAN' INSULINS

There are two different methods by which 'human' insulin is produced. Porcine insulin can be chemically altered by replacing the alanine amino acid with threonine (enzymically modified pro-insulin: emp insulin).

Alternatively, 'human' insulin can be produced by introducing the gene for human insulin into bacteria or yeast (prb: proinsulin recombinant bacteria, or pyr: proinsulin recombinant yeast insulins). The organisms are cultured in huge vats and the insulin is harvested and purified.

Following the introduction of 'human' insulins there was much concern about altered warning signs of hypoglycaemia and an increased reported incidence of severe hypoglycaemic episodes with the newer insulins. However, a subsequent literature survey of 39 studies and 12 epidemiological reports concluded that there were no significant differences in the physiological responses to hypoglycaemia or the frequency of hypoglycaemic episodes between human and porcine insulins (Jogensen et al 1994). However, a number of individuals with long-term diabetes remain unhappy about taking human insulin. Healthcare professionals should remain receptive to these views and individuals should be able to continue to use porcine or bovine insulins.

INSULIN ANALOGUES

An analogue is a chemical with a similar, but not identical, molecular structure to another chemical. Insulin analogues have been produced in order to develop insulins which have novel properties. Box 5.1 lists the insulin analogues that are now available in the UK.

Box 5.1
Insulin analogues
currently available in
the UK

Short-acting analogues

- Insulin lispro (Lilly)
- Insulin aspart (Novo Nordisk)
- Insulin glulisine (Sanofi-Aventis)

Long-acting insulin analogues

- Insulin glargine (Sanofi-Aventis)
- Insulin detemir (NovoNordisk)

Characteristics of the short-acting insulin analogues

The currently available short-acting insulin analogues have been created by making amino acid substitutions at one or more sites in the insulin molecule. Insulin molecules normally aggregate together forming hexamers, that is, six molecules of insulin loosely bound together. In this form the hexamer is too large to cross from the subcutaneous site into the circulation. The hexamers must first separate into dimers and then into single insulin molecules before absorption into the bloodstream can occur. This process takes some time and delays the onset of action of the conventional insulins. However, the analogue insulins have been designed to prevent this aggregation and formation of hexamers. This means that when the short-acting insulin analogues are injected into the subcutaneous space they are absorbed much more rapidly.

The short-acting insulin analogues therefore have a more rapid onset of action and a shorter duration of action than the conventional insulins (Mudaliar et al 1999, Nielsen et al 1995; Table 5.1). These insulins therefore have the advantage that they can be injected immediately before, or indeed immediately after, eating. Their peak serum concentration coincides with the postprandial rise in blood glucose and a meta-analysis of several studies has shown that rapid-acting insulin analogues are more effective than short-acting 'human' insulin in improving postprandial glucose control, without an increase in the rate of hypoglycaemic episodes (Davey et al 1997). The shorter duration of action should help to prevent hypoglycaemic episodes occurring before the next meal. People perceive an improvement in their quality of life with rapid-acting analogues due to the increased flexibility of injection times and less frequent hypoglycaemic episodes.

Characteristics of the long-acting insulin analogues

Insulin glargine has also been produced by altering the amino acid sequence of human insulin. The substitution of an asparagine amino acid by glycine and the addition of two arginine amino acids to the end of the insulin β chain results in the insulin becoming more soluble at acid pH. When the insulin is injected into the relatively alkaline, subcutaneous space the insulin glargine (Lantus, Sanofi-Aventis) forms microprecipitates. These tiny crystals are absorbed slowly and at a

Table 5.1
Duration of action
of insulins

Insulin type	Onset of action	Peak action	Duration
Soluble (human)			
Human Actrapid	30 minutes	2–4 hours	5–8 hours
Humulin S			
Insuman Rapid			
Short-acting analogues			
Insulin lispro (Humalog)	5–10 minutes	30–90 minutes	2–4 hours
Insulin aspart (NovoRapid)			
Insulin glulisine (Apidra)			
Isophane (Human)			
Humulin I	2 hours	6–12 hours	18–24 hours
Insulatard			
Insuman Basal			
Insulin Zn suspension			
Hypurin Bovine Lente	2 hours	8–12 hours	30 hours
Long-acting analogues			
Insulin glargine (Lantus)	1–3 hours	Flat with no peak	24 hours
Insulin detemir (Levemir)	1–3 hours	6–7 hours	20–24 hours

Note: with the exception of Hypurin Bovine Lente, bovine and porcine insulins have been excluded from the table.

constant rate into the blood stream. The characteristics of its action profile are shown in Table 5.1. Insulin glargine has a 'peakless' action and is, therefore, ideal insulin to act as basal therapy.

Insulin detemir has a fatty-acid side chain added to the insulin molecule. This allows it to bind to albumin, which again slows its rate of release into the blood and produces a flat and 'peakless' blood concentration curve following injection. Insulin detemir has a shorter duration of action than insulin glargine (see Table 5.1) and may require to be injected twice daily for people with type 1 diabetes.

A further property of the long-acting insulin analogues is the reproducible blood profile from one injection to another. Insulin detemir has a lower coefficient of variation (23–27%) than insulin glargine (36–48%) and both are lower than isophane insulin (46–68%) (Vague et al 2003). (Coefficient of variation is a mathematical measure of variability.) People develop more confidence in their insulins when the effect on blood glucose levels becomes more reproducible from day to day.

INHALED INSULINS

Alternatives modes of delivery of insulin (without requiring painful, skin injections) have been sought for many years but with little success until recently. Insulin in a dry powder form, which allows the insulin particles to be delivered to the lung alveoli, has now been developed. The insulin thus inhaled can be rapidly absorbed across the thin alveolar walls into the circulation. Exubera (Pfizer and Sanofi-Aventis) is the first inhaled insulin to come to market.

When Exubera is inhaled, blood insulin levels rise rapidly and in a similar fashion when tested against the short-acting insulin analogue, insulin lispro. Its duration of action is, however, prolonged and simulates that of the older soluble insulins (Rave et al 2005). Several studies have now demonstrated the efficacy of inhaled insulin in people with both type I and type 2 diabetes (Hollander et al 2004, Quattrin et al 2004, Skyler et al 2005).

Inhaled insulin is contraindicated for people who smoke and should not be introduced until cigarette smoking has ceased for at least 6 months. It is also not suitable for people with poorly controlled asthma or chronic obstructive airways disease. Inhalation is associated with coughing at the time of inhalation but this does not appear to be a major problem. Inhaled insulin is also associated with deterioration in lung function as measured by forced expiratory volume in 1 second (FEV_1) and carbon monoxide diffusing capacity (DL_{CO}). However, these changes are small, of dubious clinical significance, and thought to be of a temporary nature.

Freemantle and colleagues (Freemantle et al 2005) have demonstrated increased acceptability of inhaled insulin over conventional insulin delivery when offered to people with type 2 diabetes. It is likely that inhaled insulin delivery will prove popular with people who have diabetes. However, long-acting, background insulin will still be required to be given as subcutaneous injections.

FORMULATIONS OF INJECTED INSULIN

All conventional insulins are currently available in three broad types of formulation, classed according to their duration of action (see Table 5.1).

First there is unmodified or soluble insulin, which is short-acting and lasts for 5–8 hours when injected subcutaneously. These should be injected approximately half an hour before eating so that the peak action occurs at the same time as the postprandial rise in blood glucose. The peak action of soluble insulin is 1–6 hours.

Second are the intermediate-acting insulins (called isophane insulin in the UK and NPH insulin outside the UK). The action of this insulin is extended by complexing the insulin molecule with protamine (a large protein) and zinc. The mixture of neutral (or soluble) insulin with protamine and zinc was invented by Hagedorn and the point where this complex is chemically formed is termed the 'isophane ratio'; hence the names, isophane or Neutral Protamine Hagedorn (NPH) insulin. The insulin–protamine–zinc complex is absorbed more slowly, extending its duration of action to between 18 and 24 hours. The peak action of isophane insulins is usually 2–12 hours.

Finally, there are the long-acting or lente insulins. If the insulin is mixed with zinc alone, it forms large insulin–zinc crystals, which are slow to dissolve. Thus the action of crystalline zinc insulins can be extended beyond 24 hours and peak action does not begin for at least 4 hours. The lente insulins have fallen out of favour, following the introduction of the long-acting analogues, and the only one remaining in the UK is Hypurin Bovine Lente.

INSULIN REGIMENS

Insulin therapy aims to mimic the insulin response in people without diabetes (Fig. 5.1). It is evident that mealtimes are followed by immediate and sharp increases in insulin secretion as the pancreatic beta cells respond rapidly to rising blood levels of glucose. During the night and between meals there is a constant or basal secretion of insulin.

Conventional insulin therapy has attempted in several ways to simulate this physiological process.

ONCE-DAILY INJECTIONS

A once-daily injection of either isophane insulin or a long-acting insulin analogue taken along with oral hypoglycaemic agents is becoming increasingly popular for people with type 2 diabetes. The insulin acts as a background while the oral agents are used to produce prandial rises in insulin or increased insulin sensitivity (see Chapter 4). Such a regimen would be unsuitable for people with type 1 diabetes. Those people on once-daily insulin injections will, however, represent a significant proportion of the caseload of community nurses who visit the frail and elderly with diabetes in their homes and administer their insulin injections.

TWICE-DAILY INJECTIONS

Twice-daily insulin regimens are appropriate for people who consider the number of daily injections an important issue in the quality of their lives. Similarly, people who find adherence to more complex regimens difficult will probably achieve better glycaemic control on this less rigorous regimen. In the twice-daily routine, the person injects a mixture of short-acting and intermediate-acting insulin before breakfast and also before the evening meal.

The profile of blood glucose levels produced by such a regimen differs significantly from physiological concentrations. Even with the newer insulin analogues, which can produce rapid rises in insulin in the postprandial period, the insulin profile between meals and during the night does not simulate normal physiology.

Fig. 5.1
(A) Insulin concentrations in the blood of normal non-diabetic subjects. Shaded areas represent one standard deviation above and below the mean for observations in six normal subjects. Arrows indicate timing of insulin injections for those with diabetes. (B and C) Insulin therapy: once-daily regimen and twice-daily regimen (arrows indicate insulin injections).

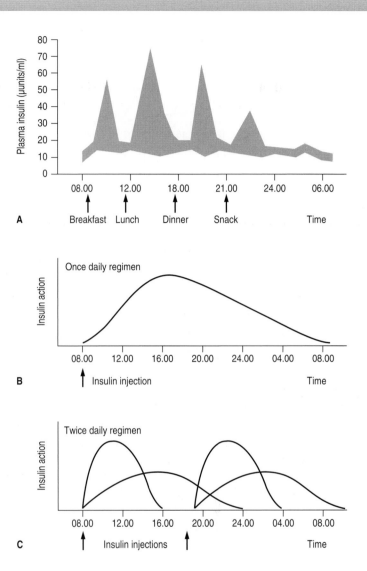

Insulin concentrations are higher than required during the evening but gradually fall throughout the night following the evening dose of insulin. This means that most people on this regimen need an evening snack before going to bed to prevent nocturnal hypoglycaemia.

MULTIPLE INSULIN INJECTIONS

Alternative insulin regimens have been introduced in recent years. In particular, the system of multiple insulin injections has gained favour and is widely prescribed (Fig. 5.2). People inject short-acting insulin or insulin analogues before the three main meals of the day and usually take a further injection of isophane insulin or a

Fig. 5.2
Insulin therapy:
multiple injection
regimen (arrows
indicate insulin
injections).

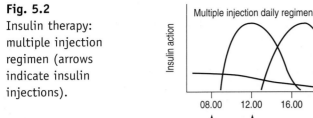
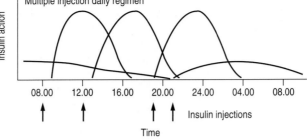

long-acting insulin analogue just before retiring to bed. Those using short-acting analogues might need two isophane injections daily or a long-acting insulin analogue. This is because the duration of action of the short-acting analogue is such that pre-meal blood glucose levels might rise if not covered adequately by background insulin.

Isophane insulins peak during the night and wear off by the following morning. The introduction of long-acting insulin analogues, which provide a peakless profile of blood insulin levels, has resulted in improved glycaemic control overnight. Long-acting insulin analogues can be used when nocturnal hypoglycaemia or fasting hyperglycaemia is a problem.

The major advantage of multiple injection regimens is the flexibility that it provides. Mealtimes do not have to be adhered to rigidly. People can anticipate altered activity (they might want to take part in a sporting activity) and can plan if they are eating more or less than usual or at different times, by making suitable adjustments to their insulin dosage. The use of insulin pen devices has allowed people to carry their insulin with them in an acceptable form and to inject with relative convenience. Many people work complex shift systems and require the flexibility of a multiple injection regimen. An alternative to multiple insulin injection regimens is insulin pump therapy.

CONTINUOUS SUBCUTANEOUS INSULIN INFUSION (CSII OR 'INSULIN PUMP THERAPY')

Case study 5.2

James is a 52-year-old man with type 1 diabetes of 21 years' duration. In the previous year, he had become prone to severe hypoglycaemia with no known cause. James would become disorientated and display bizarre behaviour whereby people thought he was either drunk or under the influence of drugs. James gave up his job and became depressed and withdrawn, especially when the efforts of the diabetes

Case study 5.2
Continued

team to find a suitable insulin regimen were exhausted. Finally, James was offered insulin pump therapy, which had a transforming effect on his blood glucose profiles. He was able to reduce his 24-hour insulin dose by 50% and maintain blood glucose levels within the normal range without hypoglycaemia. His mood improved and he was able to return to work and lead a more normal life.

This case study demonstrates a rather dramatic example of the potential benefits of CSII. Insulin pump therapy was developed during the 1980s. Early pumps were difficult to use, bulky in size and unreliable. Sudden pump failure could precipitate severe diabetic ketoacidosis over a short time. This is due to the fact that there is no reserve of insulin in the subcutaneous space and blood insulin levels would fall rapidly if the pump failed to deliver insulin and hence blood glucose would rise quickly. For these reasons, the CSII fell out of favour in the UK. However, in recent years pump technology has improved and pumps are more sophisticated and easier to use; they are also smaller and more reliable. This has resulted in a resurgence of interest in pump treatment.

Studies that have randomly allocated people with type 1 diabetes to either multiple insulin injection regimens or CSII have demonstrated small improvements in glycaemic control in the CSII groups. HbA1c levels on average were about 0.6% lower using CSII. However, a meta-analysis of eight studies by the NICE Assessment Group showed that this improvement was not maintained at 6 months (NICE 2003).

People on CSII after 4 months of treatment required approximately 12 units/day less insulin than those using a multiple insulin injection regime. However, longer-term studies showed little difference in insulin dosage requirements.

Randomly controlled trials have failed to show any significant differences in the frequency of hypoglycaemic episodes between the two treatment modalities (Weissberg-Benchell et al 2003). However, observational studies that have reported on individuals chosen for CSII on clinical grounds have demonstrated significant reductions in the number of hypoglycaemic events in those people. This is clearly demonstrated in James' case and would suggest that a subset of people who are susceptible to hypoglycaemia or diabetic ketoacidosis with conventional insulin treatments do particularly well with CSII (Rodrigues et al 2005).

CSII therapy demands a high level of commitment both from individuals with diabetes and from the diabetes team. However, individuals using pump therapy become expert in self-management and might require less input from the team over time.

For pump therapy to be successful, individuals will require to blood test at least four times per day, estimate carbohydrate consumption daily, move the cannula site every 2–3 days and learn how to programme the pump. The diabetes team should be trained to assess the person's suitability for CSII and must be able to provide education and ongoing assistance to those people using pumps.

This has led NICE to provide guidelines for CSII treatment, which include:

- CSII should be recommended for people with type 1 diabetes if multiple injection therapy has failed; and
- Those receiving the treatment have the commitment and competence to use the therapy effectively.

Failure of multiple injection therapy is considered to be failure to achieve target HbA1c without disabling hypoglycaemia occurring.

NICE has estimated that approximately 1–2% of people with type 1 diabetes may be suitable for CSII. This number may increase if pump therapy proves to be useful in children and if individual demand increases. Currently, pump use in the UK is restricted by cost factors and most people either buy their own pumps or are dependent on charity funding to sponsor the pumps. However, as a result of the recent NICE recommendations, most health authorities and health boards in the UK have made limited financial provision for CSII for those who need it.

HYPOGLYCAEMIA

Case study 5.3

Natasha is 25 years old and has had type 1 diabetes since she was four. Natasha's diabetes was easily controlled during the first 12 months following diagnosis. This was because she entered a 'honeymoon' phase when there was some return of pancreatic function. However, her control deteriorated during early childhood when she refused to eat and her exercise activity was very variable. She started to menstruate at the age of 12 years and during her teenage years there was a further deterioration in metabolic control. However, over recent years, Natasha has taken much better care of her diabetes. Her HbA1c levels have fallen to 7.1–7.5% over the past 3 years.

At her most recent clinic visit, Natasha reported that she had had four recent severe hypoglycaemic episodes requiring another person to help her. On one occasion she awoke during the night to find the paramedics at her bedside. Her current insulin regimen is Human Mixtard 30, taking 24 units before breakfast and 18 units before her evening meal.

Natasha has begun to experience unexpected and severe hypoglycaemic episodes. This can be due to one of several causes:

- more insulin than is required
- not enough carbohydrate or abnormal absorption of carbohydrate from the gut
- exercise, especially exercise she is not used to
- alcoholism or binge drinking
- endocrine changes: pregnancy, Addison's disease, hypopituitarism
- renal failure
- overused injection sites.

Natasha should be asked about her injection technique and asked to demonstrate this. Her pen device should be checked to ensure that it is working correctly. Injection sites should be examined to ensure there is no lipohypertrophy that might be causing irregular insulin absorption and, if necessary, rotation round her injection sites encouraged. Natasha would be asked to describe her usual mealtimes, with their average content and any missed snacks.

MALABSORPTION

Coeliac disease is slightly more common in people with type 1 diabetes and is often diagnosed late. The malabsorption of this condition can contribute to hypoglycaemia (Buysschaert 2003). Natasha should therefore be asked about symptoms of tiredness (caused by anaemia), abdominal bloating and discomfort and diarrhoea.

DELAYED GASTRIC EMPTYING

Impaired gastric emptying (gastroparesis) is present in 30–50% of people with long-standing type 1 diabetes and, for obvious reasons, might result in hypoglycaemic episodes.

EXERCISE

Exercise can affect glucose levels differently depending on blood insulin levels and the type of exercise. If the person lacks insulin, hepatic glucose production is increased and a progressive rise in blood glucose levels occurs. If the person has adequate levels of insulin in their system, hepatic glucose production is inhibited. Exercise enhances insulin sensitivity and peripheral uptake of glucose is increased resulting in hypoglycaemia if extra food is not taken. Prolonged moderate exercise involving mainly lower limbs, such as jogging, can result in hypoglycaemia during exercise or delayed hypoglycaemia that occurs typically 6–15 hours after exercise had ceased (Gallen 2005). Exercise that involves short bursts of anaerobic exercise can cause hyperglycaemia as can high intensity but short duration exercise (Gallen 2005).

Gallen (2005) suggests that in prolonged exercise long-acting analogues might increase the risk of hypoglycaemia and a switch to isophane insulin may be necessary. He recommends exercise should start with a blood glucose of around 7–10 mmol/L and that glucose be taken in regular small amounts when blood glucose starts to fall. Sports drinks contain around 6 g carbohydrate per 100 ml, as well as containing some sodium and potassium, which are useful for fluid replacement. Another factor contributing to hypoglycaemia might be the more rapid absorption of insulin from the limb involved in exercise. Injection of insulin into a subcutaneous site not involved in the exercise might be a safer option.

Levels of exercise vary. It is therefore important to know each person individually, as any increase in normal activity might be construed as exercise for that person and could result in apparent unexplained hypoglycaemia. As a young woman, Natasha might now have a partner and be engaging in sexual activity, which might be the cause of her nocturnal hypoglycaemia. Hence, education must be tailormade for the individual within the context of his or her lifestyle and significant others.

ALCOHOL

Alcohol inhibits gluconeogenesis and glycogenolysis, so that when alcohol is consumed in large amounts and food intake is inadequate hypoglycaemia can occur (van de Wiel 2004). The situation is especially serious if hepatic stores of glycogen are depleted. Under this circumstance, chronic alcohol abuse can lead to hypoglycaemia, which can sometimes be fatal. A modest intake of alcohol impairs the ability to perceive and interpret the symptoms of hypoglycaemia (Cheyne et al 2004). This is another reason why some people with type 1 diabetes experience hypoglycaemia after drinking alcohol.

ENDOCRINE CHANGES

Hypoglycaemia is common during the early weeks of pregnancy when insulin requirements may drop. The possibility of pregnancy should therefore be considered in any female of child-bearing age who presents with recurrent hypoglycaemic episodes or reducing insulin requirements.

Cortisol, adrenaline and growth hormone are hormones that antagonise the effects of insulin. If the blood levels of these hormones are reduced, insulin action will be unopposed and hypoglycaemia more likely to occur.

Addison's disease, an autoimmune condition, is more commonly found in people with type 1 diabetes than the general population. This condition results in reduced secretion of cortisol from the diseased adrenal glands while people with hypopituitarism will have low circulating concentrations of cortisol and growth hormone. Although these conditions are fairly rare, Natasha should be examined for signs of Addison's disease and hypopituitarism and if indicated she may require endocrine investigation to exclude hormone deficiency.

Hypothyroidism, or an underactive thyroid gland, is not uncommonly co-incidentally found in people with diabetes. Hypoglycaemic unawareness in the person with type 1 diabetes should lead to hypothyroidism being excluded by biochemical testing. If found, it is readily treated with oral Levothyroxine.

LOSS OF WARNING SYMPTOMS OF HYPOGLYCAEMIA

The effect of tight glycaemic control

A fall in blood glucose stimulates the sympathetic nervous system, which in turn causes release of adrenaline from the adrenal glands. The combined effects of sympathetic nerve stimulation and increased blood levels of adrenaline cause the heart to beat faster and more powerfully, resulting in palpitations, increased sweating and tremor of the muscles. These symptoms contribute to hypoglycaemic awareness.

However the brain does not behave normally during hypoglycaemia and these adrenergic symptoms may not be recognised. Indeed healthcare professionals should be alert for this especially when hypoglycaemia is emphatically denied! Failure of the person with diabetes to recognise this is called hypoglycaemic unawareness and in this circumstance blood glucose can fall to levels that cause disabling neuroglycopaenia. Depriving the brain of glucose results in cognitive dysfunction and, as glucose levels continue to fall, reduced conscious level, convulsions and coma.

Hypoglycaemia also stimulates the release of glucagon, cortisol and growth hormone. These counter-regulatory hormones act to antagonise the action of insulin and help to restore normal blood glucose concentrations. A single episode of hypoglycaemia can reduce the neuroendocrine response to a subsequent episode occurring within 24 hours (Heller & Cryer 1991). Therefore, one hypoglycaemic episode makes a second episode within the following 24 hours more likely.

The blood glucose levels that trigger a counter-regulatory response and the onset of hypoglycaemia symptoms are not static. They are influenced by the prevailing standard of glycaemic control. The tighter the control, the lower is the blood glucose threshold that stimulates a neuroendocrine response (Widom & Simonson 1990). It is, therefore, not unusual for people with tight metabolic control to lose the warning symptoms of hypoglycaemia. This can lead to a three-fold increase in the incidence of severe hypoglycaemia (Gold et al 1994). In this situation, people usually regain their warning symptoms if they relax their glycaemic control and eliminate blood glucose levels of less that 4 mmol/L (Amiel 2001).

Autonomic neuropathy

For many years, autonomic neuropathy was considered to be the principal cause of impaired awareness of hypoglycaemia. However, several studies have now discounted this theory. People with autonomic neuropathy experience typical autonomic symptoms during hypoglycaemia (Hepburn et al 1993) and no relationship has been demonstrated between autonomic dysfunction and hypoglycaemic symptoms (Damholt et al 2001).

Renal failure

Deteriorating renal function is associated with decreased insulin requirement. This is because the kidneys are responsible for the excretion of insulin from the body and reduced function results in prolonged insulin action. This in turn can result in unexpected hypoglycaemic events. Other causes of the increased risk of hypoglycaemia in people with renal failure include anorexia and gastroparesis. Anyone with renal failure and diabetes would be referred to secondary care specialists for management.

TREATMENT OF HYPOGLYCAEMIA

For people with impaired awareness of hypoglycaemia, it is important to relax glycaemic control otherwise their lives can be blighted by frequent and severe episodes of hypoglycaemia. Relaxing control should result in a rise in the glucose level at which a counter-regulatory response occurs.

Case study 5.4

Cecilia is a 39-year-old woman who is brought to the accident and emergency department having been found in an unconscious condition in the street. She smelled of alcohol. The paramedic who had been called to the incident noted that she looked pale and was sweating profusely. Her pulse rate was 110 beats per minute. An insulin injection device was found in her jacket pocket identifying her as having diabetes. The paramedic subsequently checked Cecilia's blood glucose and, having found it to be 1.9 mmol/L, gave her a subcutaneous injection of glucagon. Cecilia's conscious level rapidly improved and she was able to drink the glucose drink offered. Cecilia was assessed in the accident and emergency department for any continuing hypoglycaemia over a few hours. She was referred to the diabetes nurse specialist for support in recognising and treating hypoglycaemia.

The management of acute hypoglycaemia depends on the severity of the episode (MacCuish 1993). When early symptoms of hypoglycaemia are recognised, the treatment is to eat carbohydrate in the form of glucose tablets or confectionary (sweets, biscuits or chocolates). Drinks with high glucose content are also suitable. At least 20 g of carbohydrate should be consumed.

When hypoglycaemia is more profound, the person might be unaware of his or her condition and refuse to eat or drink. Under this circumstance, a glucose gel such as HypoGel (Diabetic Bio-diagnostics) can be squeezed into the side of the mouth; jam or honey would be suitable alternatives. In the drowsy or unconscious person who cannot swallow, glucagon (GlucGen HypoKit 1 mg) can be given by subcutaneous or intramuscular injection and can be administered by family members or paramedics. Alternatively, when suitable personnel are available, dextrose (20–50 ml of 50% solution) can be administered intravenously. Cecilia was treated appropriately and was followed-up to ensure that she is aware of what causes hypoglycaemia and how she can prevent this occurring in the future.

Pancreatic and islet cell transplantation

Whole pancreas transplants   Transplantation of whole pancreases has been undertaken since the mid-1970s and this operation, in the right hands, can be associated with high success rates. Data from centres around the world now show that 82% of people remain free of insulin therapy 1 year after transplantation (Gruessner & Sutherland 1997). However, this is a major operation, which is associated with significant mortality. In addition, these people also require long-term immunosuppressive therapy to prevent rejection of the foreign pancreas. The side effects of immunosuppression are not inconsiderable. Pancreas transplantation is, therefore, never going to be a cure for most people with type 1 diabetes. In the UK, pancreas transplantation is undertaken at a few centres and is restricted to people with diabetes who are also undergoing, or have successfully undergone, kidney transplants.

Islet cell transplants Islet cell transplantation has distinct advantages over whole pancreas transplants. It is a fairly simple procedure; the islet cells are injected under local anaesthetic directly into the portal vein. Thereafter the cells travel to the liver where they seed themselves and grow.

The first reported islet cell transplant was in 1977. Early experience with islet cell transplants, however, was not encouraging with only a small number of people cured of their diabetes. In the early 1990s, people invariably needed to go back on insulin within 1 week of transplantation. It was not until the year 2000 that a Canadian doctor reported remarkable success rates in seven people who remained insulin free following islet cell transplantation (Shapiro et al 2000).

The success of Shapiro and colleagues is attributed to a number of factors. Shapiro realised that people were receiving insufficient numbers of islet cells and injected cells from two or three donor pancreases into each individual. Previous immunosuppressive regimes contained high doses of steroids, which are diabetogenic. Shapiro's group uses more modern immunosuppressive drugs, which has allowed them to forego steroids. Finally, Shapiro recognised that chemicals that were previously used to extract the islet cells from the pancreas were, in fact, toxic to the cells and developed 'more gentle' techniques for isolating the islet cells.

It has been estimated that, with the number of donor pancreases available in the UK and the need for multiple donors for each person, only 90 individuals could be treated per year.

INSULIN ADJUSTMENT

People who inject insulin are encouraged to adjust their insulin depending on their day-to-day needs, which take into account diet, activity and information from blood glucose results as well as out-of-the-ordinary events such as illness, stress and exercise. Target blood glucose levels should be agreed between the clinician and the person with diabetes and this will guide the individual on what to aim for in terms of insulin adjustment. An understanding of how insulin works and knowing that insulin can work idiosyncratically in particular people is also helpful. For example a long-acting analogue insulin such as glargine can last 24 hours in some but only 18 hours in others. This will have implications for the timing of insulin injection.

Insulin adjustment is not in itself difficult but there seems to be reluctance by insulin-taking individuals to take on this responsibility. Part of the reason might be clinicians' enthusiasm to adjust insulin, which leads to disempowerment of the individual. However, it is also been acknowledged that it has proved difficult for individuals to apply their knowledge of insulin adjustment and this will require more creative and sustained educational strategies for teaching this skill (Bonnet et al 2001). One of the other reasons for not adjusting insulin includes fear of hypoglycaemia (Reach et al 2005).

A key question the clinician might ask the person with diabetes is:

> *'What would you do?'*

This question will not only enable insulin adjustment skills to be demonstrated but facilitate the confidence required to maintain this skill. Development of confidence or self-efficacy is crucial in encouraging the individual to feel competent at adjusting his or her own insulin.

Before adjusting insulin, whether by the clinician or the individual taking insulin, it is important to consider the reasons why blood glucose levels may be outside the target range. Another question could be:

> *'What do you think may be the reasons for your high/low blood glucose readings?'*
> *or:*
> *'When you think about the way you manage your diabetes, is there anything you could do differently that would get these levels back to where you want them to be?'*

This could lead to the individual considering other options to insulin adjustment, such as a change in dietary intake or activity levels. If no other changes can be made, then what are the considerations when adjusting insulin?

There is sometimes confusion around insulin adjustment when the dose of insulin is adjusted according to the blood glucose level at the time the insulin is due. This method of insulin adjustment leads to erratic results whereby frequent adjustment causes either hyperglycaemia or hypoglycaemia. Adjustment should occur only when a pattern of results is established ideally over 2–3 days and the insulin is thereafter adjusted to prevent the occurrence of either hyperglycaemia or hypoglycaemia and not in response to a single high or low result. The exception to this is if correction doses are recommended as part of an integrated package of self-management (see below).

The following points should be observed when considering insulin dose adjustment:

- When possible, insulin should be adjusted after a pattern of blood glucose results has emerged. For example, if the fasting blood glucose is high for three consecutive mornings then it is rational to increase either the basal insulin in a basal–bolus regimen or the evening insulin if the individual is on a twice daily fixed mixture of insulin.
- Traditionally, insulin has been adjusted by 2–4 units per dose, depending on type of insulin and level of blood glucose. If the individual takes large doses of insulin, e.g. 50 units or more at a time, then the adjustment might need to be 4 or more units to have any impact. Likewise, those on smaller doses, e.g. less

than 20 units per day, will respond to smaller insulin dose changes, e.g. 1 unit at a time.

- Structured diabetes education programmes such as DAFNE (2002) match insulin doses precisely to carbohydrate intake with each individual learning his or her own insulin to carbohydrate ratio (see Chapter 11). Adjustment can take place proactively to accommodate varying meal sizes, exercise, alcohol or illness but patterns of blood glucose results over days are also observed to make sure that the matching has been accurate.
- Structured diabetes education programmes also include correction doses to be taken at normal times of insulin injections rather than being additional. If the blood glucose level is found to be higher than the target range then the individual can take additional insulin to achieve the target blood glucose. Again, this is done in a precise manner and not through guesswork. Correction doses should be a temporary measure because if the blood glucose is consistently above the target then the appropriate insulin taken at the previous mealtime or the basal insulin will be increased to achieve the target level.

NURSE PRESCRIBING

In the UK, following successful completion of the nurse prescribing course, a nurse can become an independent nurse prescriber and/or a supplementary prescriber. Independent prescribing is limited to around 110 medical conditions and there are about 240 prescription-only drugs listed in the Nurse Prescribers' Extended Formulary. Independent prescribing is not appropriate for complex medical conditions or for individuals that have several medical conditions.

Supplementary nurse prescribing is more suited for those with chronic long-term conditions, including diabetes. Supplementary prescribing involves a voluntary partnership between the independent prescriber (medical) and the supplementary prescriber (nurse), who draw up a clinical management plan (CMP) that is agreed by the person with the condition. There are no legal restrictions on what conditions can be treated by a supplementary prescriber but the development of a clinical management plan for each person is a legal requirement. The CMP will include (Kyne-Grzebalski 2005):

- identification of the medicines, including the dosage, frequency and formulation. This can be drawn from existing protocols
- when to refer to the independent prescriber
- documentation of known drug sensitivities and how to report adverse reactions
- documentation of start dates and dates for review.

In the main, nurse prescribing has been shown to be beneficial both for individuals with a chronic condition and for clinicians, although further research is needed in this relatively new development in nursing (Latter & Courtenay 2004).

INSULIN INJECTION TECHNIQUE AND EQUIPMENT

PEN DEVICES

Most people on insulin therapy in the UK are using pen injector devices. These are available on prescription and are usually manufactured by the insulin companies for use with specific insulins, although some independent pharmaceutical companies also manufacture insulin pen devices. Pen devices are available either prefilled, so that the entire device is discarded once used, or as reusable devices, where insulin cartridges are inserted.

Insulin pens will dial up ½-, 1- or 2-unit increments at a time and have a clicking mechanism that enables those with poor vision to dial up their dose by counting the clicks. Needles for insulin pens are also available on prescription and come in a range of sizes between 5 and 12.7 mm. Most popular are 6 mm and 8 mm. Insulin pens are easier to use than drawing up insulin into a syringe. However, many people still prefer to continue to use syringes.

INJECTION TECHNIQUE

Insulin should be injected into subcutaneous tissue at a 90-degree angle for optimal absorption. Skin preparation is unnecessary, other than making sure that the area of injection is visually clean. In those with little fat then the flesh might need to be pinched up, otherwise, whether the flesh is pinched or not is a matter of preference. The needle should be left in place for the count of 10 to allow the insulin to complete its flow through the pen.

DISPOSAL OF NEEDLES

Needles can be destroyed after use by the BD Safe-Clip device, which is available on prescription. Alternatively, used needles can be disposed of in a screw-top jar that is sealed and wrapped, or a ring-pull can that is crushed and disposed of in the normal way.

INJECTION SITES

Injection sites should be rotated between upper arms, abdomen, thighs and buttocks to avoid the development of fatty tissue growth, known as lipohypertrophy.

Lipohypertrophy, if it develops, will cause erratic absorption of insulin leading to unpredictable blood glucose levels, including hypoglycaemia. Overused injection sites should be avoided for at least a year or more. Individuals might not notice that sites have become overused and so part of the annual review should include a physical examination of injection sites.

STORAGE OF INSULIN

Insulin not in use should be stored in a refrigerator but not allowed to freeze. Otherwise insulin is safe at room temperature for about 1 month. Exposure to heat will also reduce the potency of insulin action so care needs to be taken during warm weather and especially if on holiday in hotter climates.

CONCLUSION

The importance of tight metabolic control and the use of intensive insulin therapy and monitoring to prevent the long-term complications of diabetes are now well understood. The development of insulin analogues enabled the production of blood insulin profiles that more accurately simulate the natural secretion of insulin by the human pancreas. However, it is yet to be shown that these newer insulins result in significantly better diabetes control. The development of modern insulin pumps has allowed the introduction of more reliable continuous subcutaneous insulin infusion regimens. Intensive therapy also relies upon education and self-empowerment of individuals with diabetes. The DAFNE project, through education of individuals with diabetes, encourages people to more accurately match their insulin requirements to their diet and exercise schedule and so learn how to control their blood glucose levels. As the targets for HbA 1c levels are set lower and lower, the incidence of hypoglycaemic events increases. There is therefore a need for education of individuals, their families, friends and health professionals of the problems associated with hypoglycaemia. The value of increased nurse prescribing in diabetes is yet to be evaluated but is likely to lessen the burden on physicians and improve the knowledge-base of people with diabetes. The importance of the diabetes team for aiding the person with diabetes to achieve optimal health has never been greater.

REFERENCES

Amiel SA 2001 Hypoglycaemia unawareness: a reversible problem? Diabetic Medicine 18(suppl 1):11–14

Bonnet C, Gagnayre R, d'Ivernois JF 2001 Difficulties of diabetic patients in learning about their illness. Patient Education and Counselling 42:159–164

Buysschaert M 2003 Coeliac disease in patients with type 1 diabetes mellitus and autoimmune thyroid disorders. Acta Gastroenterologica Belgica 66(3):237–240

Cheyne EH, Sherwin RS, Lunt MJ et al 2004 Influence of alcohol on cognitive performance during mild hypoglycaemia; implications for type 1 diabetes. Diabetic Medicine 21(3):230–237

DAFNE Study Group 2002 Training in flexible, intensive insulin management to enable dietary freedom in people with type 1 diabetes: dose adjustment for normal eating (DAFNE) randomised controlled trial. British Medical Journal 325(7367):746

Davey P, Grainger D, MacMillan J et al 1997 Clinical outcomes with insulin lispro compared with human regular insulin: a meta-analysis. Clinical Therapeutics 19:656–674

Damholt MB, Christensen NJ, Hilsted J 2001 Neuroendocrine responses to hypoglycaemia decrease within the first year after diagnosis of type 1 diabetes. Scandinavian Journal of Clinical and Laboratory Investigation 61(7):531–537

Diabetes Control and Complications Trial (DCCT) Research Group 1993 The effect of intensive treatment of diabetes on the development and progression of long-term complications in insulin-dependent diabetes mellitus. New England Journal of Medicine 329(14):977–986

Freemantle N, Blonde L, Duhot D et al 2005 Availability of inhaled insulin promotes greater perceived acceptance of insulin therapy in patients with type 2 diabetes. Diabetes Care 28:427–428

Gallen I 2005 The management of insulin treated diabetes and sport. Practical Diabetes International 22(8):307–312

Gold AE, MacLeod KM, Frier BM 1994 Frequency of severe hypoglycaemia in patients with type 1 diabetes with impaired awareness of hypoglycaemia. Diabetes Care 17:697–703

Gordon D, Semple CG, Paterson KR 1991 Do different frequencies of self-monitoring of blood glucose influence control in type 1 diabetic patients? Diabetic Medicine 8:679–682

Gruessner A, Sutherland DER 1997 Pancreas transplantation in the United States (US) and non-US as reported to the United Network for Organ Sharing (UNOS) and the International Pancreas Transplant Registry (IPTR). In Cecka JM, Terasaki PI (eds) Clinical transplants 1996. UCLA Tissue Typing Laboratory, Los Angeles, p 47–67

Heller SR, Cryer PE 1991 Reduced neuroendocrine and symptomatic responses to subsequent hypoglycaemia after one episode of hypoglycaemia in non-diabetic humans. Diabetes 40:223–226

Hepburn DA, MacLeod KM, Frier BM 1993 Physiological, symptomatic and hormonal responses to acute hypoglycaemia in type 1 diabetic patients with autonomic neuropathy. Diabetic Medicine 10(10):940–949

Hollander PA, Blonde L, Rowe R et al 2004 Efficacy and safety of inhaled insulin (Exubera) compared with subcutaneous insulin therapy in patients with type 2 diabetes: results of a 6-month, randomized, comparative trial. Diabetes Care 27(10):2356–2362

Jogensen LN, Dejgaard A, Pramming SK 1994 Human insulin and hypoglycaemia: a literature survey. Diabetic Medicine 11(10):925–934

Kyne-Grzebalski D 2005 Nurse prescribing: the process, preparation and its impact on diabetes care. Practical Diabetes International 22(8):277–278

Latter S, Courtenay M 2004 Effectiveness of nurse prescribing: a review of the literature. Journal of Clinical Nursing 15(17):56–61

MacCuish AC 1993 Treatment of hypoglycaemia. In: Frier BM, Fisher, BM (eds) Hypoglycaemia and diabetes: clinical and physiological aspects. Edward Arnold, London, p 212–221

Mudaliar SR, Lindeberg FA, Joyce M et al 1999 Insulin-Aspart (B28 Asp-insulin): a fast-acting analogue of human insulin. Diabetes Care 22(9):1501–1506

National Institute for Health and Clinical Excellence (NICE) 2003 Technology appraisal guidance no. 57. Guidance on the use of continuous subcutaneous insulin infusion for diabetes. NICE, London

National Institute for Health and Clinical Excellence (NICE) 2004 Type 1 diabetes: diagnosis and management of type 1 diabetes in adults. Clinical guideline no. 15. NICE, London. Online. Available: www.nice.org.uk/pdf/CG015_fullguideline_adults_main_section.pdf

Nielsen FS, Jorgensen LN, Ipsen M et al 1995 Long-term comparison of human insulin ana-logue B10Asp and soluble human insulin in IDDM patients on a basal/bolus insulin regimen. Diabetologia 38:592–598

Quattrin T, Belanger A, Bohannon NJV, Schwartz SL for the Exubera Phase III Study Group 2004 Efficacy and safety of inhaled insulin (Exubera) compared with subcutaneous insulin therapy in patients with type 1 diabetes. Results of a 6-month, randomised, comparative trial. Diabetes Care 27:2622–2627

Rave K, Bott S, Heinemann L et al 2005 Time action profile of inhaled insulin in compari-son with subcutaneously injected insulin lispro and regular human insulin. Diabetes Care 28(50):1077–1082

Reach G, Zerrouki A, Leclercq D, d'Ivernois JF 2005 Adjusting insulin doses: from knowl-edge to decision. Patient Education and Counselling 56:98–103

Rodrigues IA, Reid HA, Ismail K, Amiel SA 2005 Indications and efficacy of continuous subcutaneous insulin infusion (CSII) therapy in Type 1 diabetes mellitus: a clinical audit in a specialist service. Diabetic Medicine 22(7):842–849

Shapiro AMJ, Lakey JRT, Ryan EA et al 2000 Islet transplantation in seven patients with Type 1 diabetes mellitus using a glucocorticoid free immunosuppressive regimen. New England Journal of Medicine 343:230–280

Scottish Intercollegiate Guidelines Network (SIGN) 2001 SIGN 55: management of diabetes. SIGN, Edinburgh

Skyler JS, Weinstock RS, Raskin P et al 2005 Use of inhaled insulin in a basal/bolus insulin regimen in type 1 diabetic subjects. A 6-month, randomized, comparative trial. Diabetes Care 28:1630–1635

van de Wiel A 2004 Diabetes mellitus and alcohol. Diabetes/Metabolism Research Reviews 20(4):263–267

Vague P, Selam JL, Skeie S et al 2003 Insulin detemir is associated with more predictable gly-caemic control and reduced risk of hypoglycaemia than NPH insulin in patients with type 1 diabetes on a basal-bolus regimen with premeal insulin aspart. Diabetes Care 26(3):590–596

Wang PH, Lau J, Chalmers TC, Zinman B 1993 Intensive blood-glucose control and dia-betes: a meta-analysis. Annals of Internal Medicine 119:71

Weissberg-Benchell J, Antisdel-Lomglio J, Seshadri R 2003 Insulin pump therapy: a meta-analysis. Diabetes Care 26(4):1079–1087

Widom B, Simonson DC 1990 Glycaemic control and neuropsychological function during hypoglycaemia in patients with insulin-dependent diabetes mellitus. Annals of Internal Medicine 112(12):904–912

6 Food for life

June Gordon

DIET AND DIABETES – FROM PAST TO PRESENT

Diabetes is one of the oldest diseases known to man and historically diet has been linked with both its cause and cure. For centuries little was known about the disease and the search for a dietary cure relied on trial and error. When it was discovered that the urine of people with diabetes was sweet, it was thought that the diet should be rich in carbohydrate to make up for these urinary losses. An alternative view was that the body could not cope with carbohydrate foods and that they should therefore be avoided.

Dietary advice fluctuated between the two extremes of high-carbohydrate 'cures' (based on skimmed milk and oatmeal) to low-carbohydrate diets of meat and boiled vegetables. Even after the discovery of insulin in 1921, carbohydrate restriction was advocated.

Today, diet still plays a central role in the management of diabetes, but the composition has changed considerably and recommendations are now in line with those for a healthy diet for the general population. There are, however, some important differences in emphasis for those with diabetes, which warrant intervention and monitoring to ensure that the nutritional objectives are met.

THE IMPORTANCE OF DIET

Diet is an essential component of diabetes management and it is said to be the cornerstone of treatment. For many it is the only form of treatment required. Approximately 80% of people diagnosed will have type 2 diabetes and will be controlled on either diet alone or diet and oral hypoglycaemic agents or diet and insulin therapy. The remaining 20% will have type 1 diabetes and will be controlled on diet and insulin injections. Hence, food choice and eating habits are important aspects of management of diabetes.

THE ROLE OF THE HEALTHCARE PROFESSIONAL IN PROVIDING DIETARY ADVICE

The clinical standards for diabetes (Clinical Standards Board for Scotland (CSBS) 2001) state that it is desirable that people with diabetes have appropriate access to key personnel, including dieticians. Both the UK Prospective Diabetes Study (UKPDS; see Chapter 4) and the Diabetes Control and Complications Trial (DCCT; see Chapter 5) demonstrate the value of dietetic intervention from diagnosis onwards. However, this advice should be part of a comprehensive management plan (Scottish Intercollegiate Guidelines Network (SIGN) 2001). The first 3 months from diagnosis have been shown to be vitally important in determining the response to dietary intervention (UKPDS 1990). Given the projected increase in type 2 diabetes, the ideal that dietary information be given only by a diabetes specialist dietician is unlikely to be met (Dyson 2003) and there might be a delay before newly diagnosed individuals have access to a dietician. In these cases, the healthcare professional will be required to give first-line advice. Suitable advice to give to a person newly diagnosed with diabetes is given in Box 6.1.

The frequency of visits to a dietician will depend on available resources and local policies and protocols. Some hospital and community dietetic departments

Box 6.1

Initial dietary advice suitable for a person newly diagnosed with diabetes before his or her appointment with a dietician

- Quench thirst with water or sugar-free drinks, e.g. diet lemonades or low-calorie diluting drinks
- Have regular meals, avoiding fried or very sugary foods
- Eat plenty of vegetables with cereal, bread, pasta, potato, rice or chapatti as the main part of the meal
- Have meat, fish, chicken, eggs or pulses as a small part of each meal

Diabetes UK produces general diet information leaflets, which can be useful as first-line advice.

produce training packs and run training courses for other healthcare professionals involved in diabetes care. Whatever the situation, it is worth making contact with the local dieticians, as good communication can only benefit the individual as well as ensure consistency of advice. Other healthcare professionals can play a vital role in providing general dietary guidance. They can also reinforce dietetic advice and identify specific situations where more detailed information is required and refer on as appropriate.

THE AIMS AND GOALS OF DIETARY ADVICE

The immediate treatment aim is to control hyperglycaemia; the ultimate aim is to allow the person to lead as normal a life as possible, in good health, and for most people to achieve a weight as close as possible to the 'ideal'. The overall aims and goals of nutritional advice are summarised in Box 6.2.

Box 6.2
Aims and goals of dietary advice (Diabetes UK 2003)

The aim is to provide those who need advice with the information required to make appropriate choices on the type and quantity of food eaten. The advice must:

- Take account of the individual's personal and cultural preferences, beliefs and lifestyle
- Respect the individual's wishes and willingness to change
- Be adapted to the specific needs of the individual, which might change with time and circumstance, e.g. age, pregnancy, nephropathy, intercurrent illness and other illnesses

The beneficial effects of physical activity in the prevention and management of diabetes and the relationship between exercise, energy balance and body weight are an integral part of nutrition counselling. The goals of dietary advice are to:

- To maintain or improve health through the use of appropriate and healthy food choices
- To achieve and maintain optimal metabolic and physiological outcomes, including:
- reduction of risk for microvascular disease by achieving near normal glycaemia without undue risk of hypoglycaemia
- reduction of risk for macrovascular disease, including management of body weight, dyslipidaemia and hypertension
- To optimise outcomes in diabetic nephropathy and any concomitant disorder such as coeliac disease or cystic fibrosis

CURRENT DIETARY RECOMMENDATIONS

BACKGROUND

Before the 1980s, dietary advice centred on carbohydrate restriction as the only means of controlling blood glucose levels. People were advised to limit their intake of carbohydrate foods such as bread, potatoes, rice, pasta and cereals and to fill up on foods such as meat, cheese, eggs, cream and butter. This resulted in a diet low in carbohydrate but high in fat. Research in the 1970s (Brunzell et al 1974, Simpson et al 1979) showed that high-carbohydrate diets could actually improve diabetic control, providing the carbohydrate was in a complex, high-fibre form. Studies were also beginning to show that reducing fat intake in non-diabetic people resulted in reduced morbidity from cardiovascular disease (Miettinen et al 1977). This led researchers to ask whether the high-fat diet could be contributing to the increased risk of heart disease in people with diabetes.

As a result of this research, guidelines were published in both the USA (American Diabetes Association 1979) and the UK (British Diabetic Association Nutrition Subgroup 1982). These overturned decades of teaching by recommending that people with diabetes should consume a diet high in carbohydrate and low in fat. These were considered to be radical documents, but they were followed by the introduction of almost identical policies by diabetes associations in many other countries. These were also very similar to nutritional guidelines published for the general population in the UK (Department of Health and Social Security (DHSS) 1984) and by the World Health Organization (James et al, WHO 1988) for Europe. This had positive implications in that people with diabetes were no longer being advised to follow a 'special diabetic diet'.

These guidelines have now become established practice throughout Europe and North America, although there have been some shifts in emphasis in the light of new knowledge and clinical experience (American Diabetes Association 2003, Diabetes UK Nutrition Subcommittee 2003, European Association for the Study of Diabetes 2000).

CURRENT RECOMMENDATIONS

The current recommendations on the composition of the diet for diabetes are summarised in Tables 6.1 and 6.2.

The main differences in emphasis from previous recommendations (British Diabetic Association Nutrition Subgroup 1992) are:

■ More flexibility in the proportions of energy from carbohydrate and monoun-saturated fat. Monounsaturated fats are promoted as the main source of dietary fat because of their lower atherogenic potential (Kratz et al 2002). Sources of the different types of fatty acids are shown in Table 6.3.

Table 6.1
Composition of the diet for diabetes (Diabetes UK 2003)

Component	Comment
Protein	
	Not > 1 g per kg body weight
Fat	
Total fat	< 35% of energy intake
Saturated + transunsaturated fat	< 10% of energy intake
N-6 polyunsaturated fat	< 10% of energy intake
N-3 polyunsaturated fat	Eat fish, especially oily fish, once or twice weekly
	Fish oil supplements are not recommended
Cis-monounsaturated fat	10–20% = 60–70% of energy intake
Carbohydrate	
Total carbohydrate	45–60%
Sucrose	Up to 10% of daily energy provided it is eaten in the context of a healthy diet. Those who are overweight or who have raised blood triglyceride levels should consider using non-nutritive sweeteners where appropriate
Fibre	
	No quantitative recommendation
Soluble fibre	Found in foods such as pulses, oats and fruit
	Has beneficial effects on glycaemic and lipid metabolism
Insoluble fibre	Found in wholegrain versions of bread, flour and pasta, brown rice and high fibre breakfast cereals
	Has no direct effects on glycaemic and lipid metabolism but its high satiety content may benefit those trying to lose weight and it is advantageous to gastrointestinal health
Vitamins and antioxidants	
	Encourage foods naturally rich in vitamins and antioxidants
	There is no evidence for the use of supplements and evidence that some are harmful
Salt	
	< 6 g sodium chloride per day

Table 6.2
Food choices in the
diet for diabetes

Choice	Comment
Nutritive sweeteners:	
■ Fructose	No proven advantage over sucrose
■ Sugar alcohols (e.g. sorbitol)	Lower cariogenic effect but no other advantages over sucrose May cause diarrhoea
Non-nutritive (artificial/intense)	Useful in beverages sweeteners Potentially useful in the overweight Safe if acceptable daily intake is not exceeded Heavy users should use a variety of different products
'Diabetic' foods	Unnecessary, expensive Can cause diarrhoea Not recommended
Plant stanols and sterols	Approximately 2 g per day can reduce LDL-cholesterol by 10–15% (see section on dyslipidaemia on p. 146)
Fat replacers and substitutes	Can facilitate weight loss Long-term studies needed
Herbal preparations	No convincing evidence of benefit

Table 6.3
Sources of fatty acids

Type of oil	Example
Cis-monounsaturated	Olive oil Some rapeseed oils Fat spreads derived from olive oil
Trans-unsaturated	Hydrogenated vegetable oils Hard margarine Manufactured foods containing hydrogenated vegetable oils (e.g. pies, pastry, biscuits, cakes) Fat spreads derived from these oils
Polyunsaturated	*N*-6 Corn, sunflower Safflower oil, soya bean oil and seeds *N*-3 Oily fish and marine oils

- Less restriction on the use of sucrose. However, overweight people are advised to limit the use of sucrose where practical.
- More active promotion of carbohydrate foods with a low glycaemic index (GI) (see p. 140).
- Greater emphasis on the benefits of regular exercise.

TRANSLATING RECOMMENDATIONS INTO PRACTICAL ADVICE

The scientific evidence for the effect of diet on diabetes management needs to be translated into practical and realistic advice for the individual. Because the nutritional objectives for those with diabetes are very similar to those advocated for the entire population, dietary guidance should be based on a framework of healthy eating principles such as the *Balance of good health* (Health Education Authority (HEA) 1994) shown in Fig. 6.1. More information on this is given in Box 6.3.

This does not mean, however, that dietary advice is simply a matter of healthy eating guidance; many other issues have to be borne in mind and specific aspects relevant to diabetes will need to be superimposed on this. Table 6.4 shows how it can be adapted for diabetes.

Fig. 6.1
The balance of good health (HEA 1994). Reproduced with kind permission of the Food Standards Agency

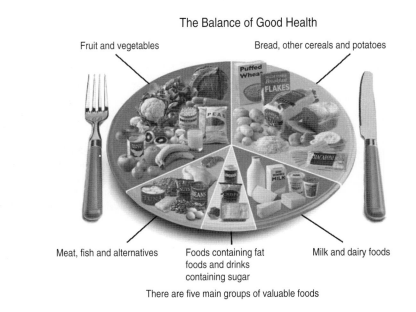

The Balance of Good Health

Fruit and vegetables

Bread, other cereals and potatoes

Meat, fish and alternatives

Foods containing fat foods and drinks containing sugar

Milk and dairy foods

There are five main groups of valuable foods

Box 6.3

The *Balance of good health* plate model

- Primarily a device for encouraging healthy eating practices
- A visual method, with the dinner plate serving as a pie chart. This shows the proportions of the plate that should be covered by the various food groups
- Simple and adaptable; embodies the principles of healthy eating and promotes memory and understanding through visual methods
- Easily implemented in residential and nursing homes

Table 6.4

Adapting the 'balance of good health' model for people with diabetes

Food group	Points to emphasise
Bread, cereal foods and potatoes These should form the largest component of meals and snacks	Quantity and timing: these need to remain fairly constant from day to day Good food choices: pasta, rice, bread, chapattis, potatoes, breakfast cereals (especially oat-based) Reduce the amount of fat added to these foods Wholemeal/wholegrain bread and cereals are high in fibre and have advantages in terms of satiety and helping to prevent constipation
Fruit and vegetables At least 5 servings of a variety of these foods should be eaten every day	These have major health benefits for people with diabetes 1–2 servings of vegetables should be eaten with main meals More use should be made of fresh fruit as a snack or dessert Frozen or canned fruits and vegetables are useful alternatives to fresh varieties Fruit juice should be regarded as a sugar-containing drink and so not consumed on its own – only with meals Encourage consumption of salad or vegetables with manufactured convenience foods or ready meals
Milk and dairy products 2–3 servings daily	Low/reduced-fat varieties of milk, yoghurt, fromage frais, etc., should be chosen Full-fat cheese should be used with care, especially by the overweight; it is best used as part of a meal rather than a snack Cream should only be used as an occasional treat
Meat, fish, pulses and alternatives 2 servings/day	Greater use should be made of pulses (peas, beans and lentils), either as an alternative to meat or as a way of making a smaller quantity of meat go further. Fresh, canned or dried pulses are all suitable Ideally at least 2 portions of fish should be consumed every week, one of which should be oily fish Fat avoidance is important, e.g. meat should be lean: visible meat fat should be trimmed off after cooking. Consumption of meat products (e.g. burgers, pies, sausage rolls) or high-fat meat mixtures (mince) should be kept to a minimum. Poultry is only a low source of fat if the skin is removed and the fat that appears during cooking is discarded

Food group	Points to emphasise
Fat-rich and sugar-rich foods These should be kept to a minimum	*Sugar-rich foods:* The diet does not have to be sugar free, but sugar-rich confectionary and drinks will impair glycaemic control if consumed at inappropriate times or in addition to meals Low-calorie 'diet' soft drinks are good alternatives to their higher-sugar counterparts Either ordinary jam/marmalade or reduced-sugar varieties can be used in small amounts on bread Small amounts of sugar-containing biscuits or cakes can be eaten as scheduled snacks, but higher fibre, lower sugar choices are best, e.g. teabreads, fruit cake, English muffins, plain cakes and biscuits. Those who are overweight should be encouraged to make more use of fruit as snacks Intense artificial sweeteners should be used if sweet-tasting drinks are required *Fat-rich foods:* Sources of fat should be avoided as much as possible Food should be boiled, baked, grilled, dry roasted or microwaved, but not fried Minimum amounts of fat should be spread on bread, added to food or used in cooking. Reduced-fat monounsaturated spread and small amounts of monounsaturated oils (olive or rapeseed or canola) are the best choices High-fat snack foods such as crisps and biscuits should be eaten less often and replaced by healthier alternatives such as fruit, low-fat yoghurt or wholewheat crispbread

Table reproduced from Thomas B (2001).

THE DIETARY MANAGEMENT OF DIABETES

It takes considerable skill to apply the nutritional objectives of diabetes management in a realistic and practical way. Initially, people should be assessed to determine their willingness to change their dietary behaviour (SIGN 2001). A simple, flexible approach is required and counselling skills should be used to motivate the individual to make positive and achievable dietary changes (see Chapter 3). Not everyone will be able (or willing) to achieve all dietary goals and a balance should be found between what is acceptable, achievable and beneficial to that individual person. For most, the actual target will be to make specific dietary changes in the right direction, i.e. towards the ideal. The nature of these changes will vary according to individual nutritional and clinical priorities, habitual diet and lifestyle and the prevalence of risk factors. The focus should always be on modifying an individual's existing eating habits (food choice and the timing of its consumption) in a realistic and achievable way. Pre-printed standardised diet sheets alone are of little benefit in modern day diabetes management. The dietary management of diabetes should take place in the stages outlined in Box 6.4.

Box 6.4
Stages in the dietary
management of diabetes

- Assessment: to decide which aspects of the diet need to be changed and what changes are possible, information will have to be gathered on the person's background and usual eating habits. Nutritional, personal and clinical information will be relevant in determining the advice given
- Education: dietary education is essential to help individuals make the diet and lifestyle changes necessary to optimise diabetic control and long-term health. This cannot be delivered as a single package in a single session. Every one is different in terms of his or her nutritional priorities, dietary targets, pace and degree of change. Education should, therefore, be tailored to the needs of the individual
- Monitoring progress: follow-up and review are essential, but the frequency of this will depend on the type of treatment, the person's ability and confidence, diabetic control and whether or not additional problems such as renal or coeliac disease exist

WEIGHT MANAGEMENT

Approximately 80% of people with type 2 diabetes, and many with type 1 diabetes, are overweight and hence weight loss and stabilisation will be a major priority in their management.

Moderate weight loss of 5–10 kg can help to improve blood glucose and lipid levels, reduce insulin resistance and improve hypertension. It has also been shown that losing weight can improve life expectancy in overweight people with type 2 diabetes by an average of 3–4 months for each 1 kg (2.2 lb) of weight lost (Lean et al 1990). The largest published study to date into weight loss in overweight people with diabetes (Williamson et al 2000) showed that a weight loss of 11% of initial body weight was associated with a reduction in mortality of 25% and in heart disease of 28%. However, losing even small amounts of weight has health benefits. It is therefore worth stressing the benefits of any weight loss and maintenance of this loss for the overweight person with type 2 diabetes.

Assessing body weight and shape

To manage overweight and obesity, it is important to measure and define it in terms of its relative health risk. The body mass index (BMI; Box 6.5) has been adopted widely as the best method of assessing the degree of obesity or overweight.

Ideally, people with diabetes should have a BMI in the 'healthy weight' range, as both diabetes and overweight are risk factors for coronary heart disease. However, BMI does not measure body fat specifically and in recent years there has been a growing interest in the use of waist circumference to determine the risk of obesity (Lean et al 1995). Both diabetes and coronary heart disease are linked with abdominal obesity, where fatty tissue is deposited centrally, giving an apple shape, rather than on the hips and thighs, which gives a pear shape (see Chapter 4). Measuring

Box 6.5

Classification of obesity using the body mass index (WHO 1998)

The body mass index (BMI) is calculated by applying the formula:
$$BMI = Weight\ (in\ kilograms) / Height\ (in\ metres)^2$$
Weight is without shoes and in indoor clothing, and height is without shoes.

- ≤ 18.5   = underweight
- 18.5–24.9   = healthy weight
- 25–29.9   = overweight
- 30–39.9   = moderately obese
- > 40   = severely obese

The ideal range for BMI is, therefore, 18.5–24.9 kg/m².

the waist circumference in addition to BMI can be a useful guide for determining the health risk posed by overweight. Current recommended cut-off points for waist circumference are shown in Table 6.5.

The only way to achieve weight loss is to consume less energy than the body needs and, ideally, to increase physical activity. This will incur an energy deficit, body fat stores will be used as an energy source and weight loss will result.

The person with diabetes who is advised to lose weight should, therefore, be given guidance on a reduced energy intake. This should focus primarily on appropriate food choice, with particular emphasis on avoiding fat-rich, energy-dense foods. Changes in food choices should be incorporated into the general healthy eating framework appropriate for diabetes along with any necessary advice on meal pattern and timing. Modification of existing eating habits will be more successful than handing out standardised pre-printed diet sheets.

Dieticians will tailor individual meal plans for the appropriate degree of energy restriction and many will offer training and provide resources for other healthcare professionals to support them in doing the same. Restricting the energy intake by 500 calories per day should produce a weight loss of 0.5 kg per week. In other words, if a person who usually consumes 2000 kcal per day reduces this by 500 kcal daily to 1500 kcal, that person could expect to lose an average of 0.5 kg per week. Weight loss should be gradual, and any weight-reducing programme should be based on realistic expectations of weight loss: 0.5–1 kg (1–2 lb) per week is ideal. Energy intakes of less than 1000 calories per day are not recommended, as they can

Table 6.5

Waist circumference as a predictor of risk

	Substantially increased risk (Caucasian)	Substantially increased risk (Asian)
Men	≥ 102 (40 inches)	≥ 90 cm (36 inches)
Women	≥ 88 cm (35 inches)	≥ 80 cm (32 inches)

result in loss of lean body tissue. This will affect metabolic rate and can result in less weight being lost in the long term.

It should be remembered that long-term weight control is the primary objective, so any weight loss should be viewed in a positive light.

Case study 6.1

Neil is a 54-year-old married man who has just joined the GP practice. His routine medical examination shows that he has glycosuria and subsequent blood tests confirm that he has type 2 diabetes. He is obese and consumes more than 30 units of alcohol per week. He enjoys a fried breakfast at the weekend, takes three teaspoons of sugar in his tea and drinks sugar-containing fizzy drinks. He admits to smoking 40 cigarettes per day and is unemployed.

In the first instance, Neil will require dietary advice alone for treatment management. There is obviously a lot of scope for improving his diet and there are many aspects to tackle. To summarise the key points, Neil:

- is obese
- probably has a high fat intake
- drinks sugar-containing fizzy drinks
- smokes
- has a high alcohol intake
- is unemployed.

The first priority would be to explain in simple terms what diabetes is and why diet is the main element in Neil's treatment. It is important to emphasise diet and weight loss at this stage and to reinforce this on follow-up. Neil's wife should be included in all educational sessions and they should be encouraged to discuss modifications of diet together.

Dietary management would be in stages (see Box 6.4) starting with assessment of his current diet and his readiness to change (SIGN 2001). Having completed the assessment, the advice should be broken down into stages so that he is not overwhelmed with information and the prospect of too many aspects of dietary change at once. Not all stages should be covered in the first consultation. Small, gradual changes instead of drastic ones tend to be more acceptable and lead to improved adherence.

Healthy eating

It is important to adopt a psychological approach to promote changes in diet (SIGN 2001) and to emphasise that the diet for diabetes is a healthy diet for all the family:

- Advise both Neil and his wife that this healthy way of eating is recommended for the rest of the population and that if they adopt this together they will both receive benefits in terms of reducing the risk of heart disease.

Weight reduction

To emphasise that weight loss will help Neil control his diabetes:

- Explain that weight loss will only be achieved by reducing the energy content of the diet, but that this does not mean strict 'dieting' or starvation.
- Agree a realistic target weight with Neil. Use BMI and measure (or ask him to measure) his waist circumference.
- Break down the weight loss into small goals to make the ultimate goal seem more achievable.
- Offer regular follow-up to give him support and to keep him motivated.

Fat intake

Emphasise the importance of reducing fat intake as follows:

- Recommend that both Neil and his wife use alternative methods of cooking breakfast at the weekend, such as grilling, baking, poaching, steaming or microwaving.
- Suggest that an ideal breakfast should contain mainly complex carbohydrate (e.g. cereal followed by toast), which Neil might be willing to consider eating on weekdays.

Sugar intake

Reduce sugar intake by:

- Suggesting an artificial sweetener as an alternative to sugar and low calorie drinks or water instead of the sucrose-containing ones. Ultimately, Neil might be willing to take tea and coffee without any type of added sweetener.
- Assess the frequency of consumption of confectionary and cakes and suggest alternatives.

Smoking

Bear in mind that Neil is a smoker and that to stop smoking will be a very important aspect of his diabetes management. Neil should be encouraged to stop smoking (SIGN 2001) and if he decides that this is his first priority, support him as follows:

- Emphasise that to prevent further weight gain would be an appropriate goal at this stage. Weight reduction can be tackled at a later stage once he has stopped smoking.
- Point out that Neil might find that he will lose some weight by making changes to his fat and alcohol intake.

Further information on smoking cessation can be found in SIGN 55 (SIGN 2001).

Alcohol intake

To encourage Neil to think about reducing his alcohol intake:

- Ask him if he thinks this amount of alcohol is within recommended limits as he currently exceeds this.
- Explain that his reported intake of 30 units of alcohol per week equates to at least 2400 calories.

- Negotiate a reduction in the amount of alcohol consumed.
- Advise him to avoid the special 'diabetic' beers and lagers that have a high alcohol content and to have ordinary beers and lagers or spirits with low calorie mixers in moderation.
- Advise him that his excessive alcohol intake will actually make him feel unwell and might cause memory loss (SIGN 2001).

Financial implications

As Neil is unemployed, cost could be a major barrier to dietary change. He can be supported in his efforts by:

- Giving practical advice on buying foods that are *not* more expensive, e.g. fresh fruit and vegetables that are in season and on special offer.
- Advising him that he does not need to buy special 'diabetic' foods.
- Suggesting that he makes the complex carbohydrate food the main part of his meal and has a smaller portion of the more expensive protein foods.
- Encouraging him to reduce his alcohol intake and stop smoking.

Neil might be eligible for some of the benefits that are addressed in Chapter 11.

Follow-up

To encourage Neil to make the changes, use a theoretical model with a psychological approach (SIGN 2001):

- Offer regular follow-up so that motivation can be sustained and dietary counselling can continue.
- Reinforce the advice given by the dietician so that the information Neil receives is consistent.
- In consultation with Neil, address each practical step one at a time. Once he has reduced his intake of fried food, replaced the sugar-containing drinks with low-calorie ones and reduced his alcohol intake, consider negotiating an increase in fruit and vegetables, wholemeal bread and wholegrain cereals.
- Encourage his wife to support him in the dietary changes and to adopt these for the family as a whole.
- Always bear in mind that dietary change can be difficult and may be slow.

Neil's case study should help to illustrate the stages in the dietary management for him and to give an example of a realistic means of adapting his diet for weight loss.

CARBOHYDRATE MANAGEMENT

Many factors affect the glycaemic response to foods, e.g. the amount and type of carbohydrate consumed, the effects of cooking or processing on food structure and other meal components such as fat and protein.

To maintain blood sugar levels within the acceptable range there has to be a balance between glucose entering the blood from the gastrointestinal tract and the supply of injected or pancreatically produced insulin available. In the person who does not have diabetes, this happens automatically, but in those with diabetes on hypoglycaemic medication (whether it be sulphonylureas or insulin), the situation is different. Once insulin is injected or an oral hypoglycaemic ingested, its hypoglycaemic action will operate whether or not food has been eaten. Hence, if food is not eaten at the usual time or insufficient food is taken, there is a risk that the person will become hypoglycaemic. Equally, consuming large amounts of carbohydrate at times of low activity of the hypoglycaemic agent will result in higher levels of blood glucose than desired. It is therefore vital that there is a balance between carbohydrate intake and hypoglycaemic medication.

Hypoglycaemia cannot occur in people treated by diet alone (or on metformin). In this situation (as in the person who does not have diabetes), insulin is produced when food is eaten. However, because the ability to produce insulin is limited, it is still important to ensure that carbohydrate intake is evenly spread throughout the day and within the body's ability to handle it.

In practical terms, for people with diabetes, this balance is achieved by regulating the:

- meal pattern
- amount of carbohydrate consumed
- type of carbohydrate consumed.

REGULATING THE MEAL PATTERN

For most people, carbohydrate intake should be fairly evenly distributed throughout the day. Those who have erratic eating habits should be encouraged to adopt a more regular meal pattern to ensure a better and more constant balance between supply and usage of glucose. This can have added benefits in aiding weight loss in those who are overweight. For many, a meal pattern of three evenly sized meals and three snacks is ideal, but this will vary between individuals. Lifestyle might dictate the meal pattern for some and, for people with type 2 diabetes who are overweight, between-meal snacks might need to be discouraged. No matter what, the most important aspect is that the individual's meal pattern stays relatively constant from day to day. Those who are treated with oral hypoglycaemic agents or insulin should also be able to adapt their diet for different circumstances, e.g. exercise or illness.

REGULATING THE AMOUNT OF CARBOHYDRATE CONSUMED

Advice is essential so that an adequate carbohydrate intake can be achieved from day to day, especially for those on sulphonylureas or insulin. Traditionally, the amount of carbohydrate was regulated by various different systems, where foods containing a defined amount of carbohydrate were substituted for one another. This allowed individuals to calculate and usually restrict their intake of carbohydrate. Following the realisation in the 1980s that carbohydrate restriction was both unnecessary and counterproductive, simpler methods of meal planning were introduced:

- The 'carbohydrate exchange' system: this is a system first taught to people more than 30 years ago. People learned the amount of carbohydrate in various foods and how to exchange them for other carbohydrate-containing foods, if desired, to allow variety in the diet while maintaining a fairly consistent carbohydrate intake. For ease of reference, people could eat any type of carbohydrate as long as it was low in sugar and within their set allowance for their meal or snack. Table 6.6 gives some examples of carbohydrate exchanges. The drawbacks of this system are that it does not take into account the glycaemic effect (see p. 139) of a food, nor does it give an indication of protein, fat or energy content, which can draw attention away from these dietary components. The exchange system also tends to result in restriction of carbohydrate, which can result in higher-fat foods being consumed at the expense of carbohydrate.
- Meal planning and household measures: using this system, advice on meal planning would be given, with emphasis on eating regular meals and snacks; eating a variety of foods; controlling energy intake; using appropriate cooking methods; including foods with a low glycaemic index; encouraging high-fibre, low-fat foods and eating more fruit and vegetables (particularly those containing soluble fibre). The person would be given some quantitative guidance on carbohydrate intake (e.g. the amount typically needed at a main meal, late-night snack or to prevent or treat hypoglycaemia), but grams of carbohydrate would not be mentioned.

It is worth remembering that different approaches will be required for different people in different circumstances and from different cultures. People who have had diabetes for many years might have been taught, and still use, the 10-g carbohydrate exchange system. Although it would be reasonable to encourage them to have a better composition of diet, it can be very disturbing for some to be told to abandon a system that they have used with confidence for many years to manage their

Table 6.6

Examples of 10 g carbohydrate exchanges

Food	Amount supplying 10 g carbohydrate
Wholemeal/white bread	1 small slice
Bread roll	Half
Digestive biscuits	1
Apples	1
Tangerines	2
Potatoes	1 egg-sized

diabetes. They should not therefore be forced to change the way in which they do manage the dietary aspects of their diabetes if they do not wish to do so, although many will welcome a more liberal approach.

Some people will feel more comfortable with two fixed daily injections of insulin and a regular meal pattern. Others, by contrast, who are knowledgeable and motivated can, in conjunction with frequent blood glucose monitoring, vary the amount of carbohydrate consumed, or the time at which it is eaten, by adjusting their insulin doses or physical activity or both. In the UK, the results of a trial (DAFNE Study Group 2002) into this liberal approach have been published. This is a 5-day outpatient programme that teaches individuals to adjust their insulin doses to carbohydrate portions by way of carbohydrate to insulin ratio. People are taught to make adjustments on their blood glucose trends associated with food, exercise, alcohol and illness. Although this intensive insulin therapy and carbohydrate counting is time intensive, this style of education helps people understand more about the effects of food on blood glucose levels and be empowered in their self-management (see Chapter 11).

REGULATING THE TYPE OF CARBOHYDRATE: THE GLYCAEMIC INDEX OF FOOD

It used to be thought that if you ate the same amount of carbohydrate – whatever it was – it would have the same effect on your blood glucose levels. It is now known that different carbohydrate-containing foods have different glycaemic responses (Jenkins et al 1984). This means that they have different effects on blood glucose levels, so 10 g of carbohydrate as bread does not have exactly the same effect as 10 g of carbohydrate as fruit or as pasta. Attempts have been made to quantify this effect and to classify foods according to their glycaemic index (GI). This is defined as the glycaemic response to individual foods in relation to that of glucose, i.e. the GI is a measure of how quickly foods containing carbohydrate raise blood glucose levels. Thus choosing slowly absorbed carbohydrates 1can help even-out the blood glucose levels. The glycaemic effect of a carbohydrate food is determined not only by its sugar and fibre content, but also by many physical and chemical characteristics; the way in which an individual food is cooked or processed, or its degree of ripeness, will also affect its GI. The glycaemic response to a single food will also change when it is eaten in combination with other foods, e.g. fat content will delay gastric emptying and therefore delay absorption of carbohydrate; the soluble fibre content of one carbohydrate food will affect the absorption of another. The concept of GI is useful as a pointer to food choice. Foods with consistently low glycaemic effect can be promoted as particularly good choices in preference to those with higher glycaemic potential (Box 6.6). It should be remembered, however, that GI should not be emphasised to such an extent that other important messages concerning meal pattern and overall dietary balance are lost.

Box 6.6
Foods with a low
glycaemic index (GI)

These should be promoted as particularly good food choices:

- Peas, beans and lentils
- Fresh fruit (not over ripe)
- Pasta
- Barley and basmati rice
- Porridge

ADDITIONAL DIETARY CONSIDERATIONS

ORAL HYPOGLYCAEMIC AGENTS

Drugs will be required in the treatment of type 2 diabetes if diet alone fails to control diabetes adequately. Drugs should not, however, be used as an alternative to diet. There are different types of oral hypoglycaemic agents; the modes of action of these are discussed in more detail in Chapter 4.

Sulphonylureas and meglitinides

These act by stimulating insulin production (whereas the glitazones enhance the action of insulin). All increase appetite, which can lead to weight gain and deterioration in glycaemic control. People should be made aware of the possible effects of these drugs and appropriate dietary counselling should be available to prevent or minimise weight gain. Although it is beneficial for everyone to eat regularly, it is especially important for those on sulphonylureas, as hypoglycaemia (see Chapter 11, p. 265) can result if meals are missed. For this reason, individuals should also be advised to avoid drinking alcohol on an empty stomach because of the combined hypoglycaemic effects of alcohol and sulphonylureas.

Meglitinides and glitazones

These work for a relatively shorter time, making the risk of hypoglycaemia less. However, people taking these drugs should still be given advice on the causes, recognition and management of hypoglycaemia.

Metformin

This does not act by stimulating insulin production and hence will not cause hypoglycaemia. It is usually the preferred drug for overweight people with type 2 diabetes, as weight gain is a less common side effect than with other oral hypoglycaemics.

Glucosidase inhibitors

These drugs (e.g. acarbose) act as enzyme inhibitors and delay the digestion and absorption of carbohydrate. This has the effect of reducing the rise in blood glucose levels after a meal. They can be useful for overweight individuals because they do not cause an increase in appetite, but they can cause flatulence, diarrhoea and abdominal distension. Glucosidase inhibitors do not cause hypoglycaemia when used as sole therapy, but if hypoglycaemia does occur when it is being used with another agent, then treatment must be with glucose and not sucrose. This is because this drug would prevent the breakdown and absorption of the sucrose into the bloodstream.

Case study 6.2

> Betty is a 67-year-old woman who is overweight (BMI = 29) and has type 2 diabetes that is controlled by diet. She has had deteriorating glycaemic control over the last few months and it is now thought that she needs the addition of an oral hypoglycaemic agent.

There would be various stages to progress through to determine whether an oral hypoglycaemic agent is in fact required:

- The first step with Betty would be to review her diet to check whether any changes in meal pattern or food consumption could improve her glycaemic control. She might be inadvertently including foods that are making her blood glucose rise (e.g. drinking unsweetened fruit juice between meals, thinking it is a 'healthy' choice). Assessment of her diet and her willingness to make any changes using the information in Table 6.4 would provide useful information as to whether or not there are changes that can be made.
- Betty's recent weight history should be discussed to ascertain whether she has gained weight over the last few months. If this were the case, dietary assessment and subsequent negotiation of dietary targets to facilitate weight loss would be appropriate. Her physical activity should be assessed and any possible increase in this should also be discussed and promoted (SIGN 2001).
- The addition of an oral hypoglycaemic agent might be appropriate if there was no improvement in glycaemic control despite the first two steps. Metformin would be the first drug of choice for Betty because it does not tend to increase appetite. Emphasis should be placed on preventing further weight gain by eating an energy-controlled diet and being as physically active as possible.

INSULIN TREATMENT

Type 2 diabetes controlled with insulin

Insulin therapy will be initiated when oral hypoglycaemic agents are insufficient to achieve good glycaemic control (see Chapter 4). Due to the anabolic effect of insulin, weight gain can be a problem. This potential weight gain should be anticipated and explained to the person so that dietary measures can be discussed and instituted. It might be appropriate for some people with type 2 diabetes to combine insulin with metformin, as the latter improves insulin resistance and has an anorectic effect, thereby reducing the insulin dosage required and minimising the anabolic effect (Relimpio et al 1998, Robinson et al 1998).

Balancing food and insulin in type 1 diabetes

The dietary advice that should be given to a person with type 1 diabetes is basically the same as that for a person with type 2 diabetes as the recommendations apply to diabetes *per se*. Eating regularly is important for people with type 1 diabetes and type 2 diabetes and is particularly relevant for those people using insulin therapy.

The nature of the insulin regimen has to be considered to ensure that food choice and meal timing are compatible with its hypoglycaemic activity. Many insulin preparations are available, each one having a different speed and duration of activity. They can broadly be categorised into short- or intermediate- and long-acting insulins; these are discussed in detail in Chapter 5. It is important that all members of the diabetes team work with the person with diabetes to choose an insulin and dietary regimen best suited to the individual's lifestyle.

Many people are maintained on a combination of insulin preparations to optimise blood glucose control. Most are still managed on a combination of a short-acting and intermediate-acting insulin administered twice a day, but there is an increasing use of multiple injection regimens where one dose of long-acting insulin is injected at bedtime to give a continuous background insulin supply and small amounts of short-acting insulin are given via a pen injector before meals during the day. This gives more flexibility in terms of eating habits and is particularly suitable for adolescents and other people with variable lifestyles. As regimens become more flexible, more knowledge is required about the time–action profiles of different insulins and insulin analogues to give appropriate advice about diet. A dietician with experience in diabetes, whether it be at the hospital diabetes centre or within the primary care setting, would usually be responsible for the dietary education of the person in this respect, but all healthcare professionals involved in diabetes care should be aware of the type of advice that might be given. Insulin is anabolic and progressive weight gain can be a problem when glycaemic control is improved or when insulin replaces oral hypoglycaemics in people with type 2 diabetes.

The advent of easy-to-use blood glucose monitoring devices, together with encouraging individuals to take greater control over their own management, has resulted in greater flexibility in insulin administration with people being taught to alter insulin dosage as circumstances dictate. Similar flexibility also applies to diet. Many people learn to adjust their food intake as part of the overall process of achieving tight glycaemic control (see Chapter 11). However, it is important that the overall diet remains appropriate in terms of energy content and balanced in overall composition.

SPECIFIC CONSIDERATIONS

HYPOGLYCAEMIA

Glucose (10–20 g) is the preferred sugar for the immediate treatment of acute hypoglycaemia because it does not require digestion or metabolism. This could be given in the form of 50–100 mL Lucozade or between three and six glucose tablets. After recovery from hypoglycaemia, a further 10–20 g of slower-acting carbohydrate (e.g. two digestive biscuits) should be given, unless the next meal or snack is due, in which case it should be eaten straight away. See Chapter 11 for further explanation on the treatment of hypoglycaemia.

EXERCISE

Regular exercise has positive benefits in that it can lower blood pressure and blood lipids. It can also reduce insulin requirements and improve overall blood glucose control. For overweight individuals with type 2 diabetes, exercise will have the added benefit of increasing energy expenditure, which, when combined with a healthy diet, should assist weight loss. Regular exercise also helps to maintain lean body mass. This prevents the lowering of metabolic rate, which can be a danger with prolonged dieting.

Exercise and hypoglycaemia

Those whose diabetes is controlled by glucose-lowering medication (whether sulphonylureas, meglitinides or insulin) should be given advice on the prevention of hypoglycaemia during and after exercise (SIGN 2001). Exercise can affect blood glucose levels in two main ways:

1. If a person's blood glucose control is poor and there is insufficient insulin, adrenaline will be released as a result of the exercise and will make the blood glucose rise.
2. If a person's blood glucose is reasonably well controlled this usually implies that there is an adequate supply of insulin. Here the main concern is hypoglycaemia as a result of exercise.

To avoid hypoglycaemia, extra carbohydrate should be taken before the activity. Alternatively, the dosage of insulin or sulphonylurea can be reduced, but care needs to be taken not to reduce this too much. This will be discussed on an individual basis. The amount of extra carbohydrate required will depend on the individual and the type of exercise undertaken. It can be taken as part of the last meal before exercise (e.g. an extra 20 g of complex carbohydrate as digestive biscuits, fruit, yoghurt or nuts and raisins) or as a quick snack immediately before (e.g. 20 g of quicker-acting carbohydrate in the form of a small bar of chocolate). Top-ups of carbohydrate might be required for endurance exercises to prevent hypoglycaemia during the exercise. Extra carbohydrate might also be required after exercising has stopped due to the fact that the hypoglycaemic effect of exercise can last for several hours. It is also worth remembering that everyday activities such as running for the bus or vigorous housework can also cause hypoglycaemia.

ALCOHOL

There is no need for the person with diabetes to avoid alcohol completely, but it can create additional hazards. Alcohol consumption should be restricted to 3–4 units per day in men and 2–3 units per day in women, as in the general population (SIGN 2001). Alcohol can act as a very potent hypoglycaemic agent because it inhibits the formation of glucose by the liver. Glucose-lowering agents (e.g. sulphonylureas or insulin) together with alcohol can have a very serious effect if inadequate carbohydrate is eaten. Delayed hypoglycaemia can occur up to 16 hours after alcohol consumption – a fact that must be emphasised. People should avoid drinking alcohol on an empty stomach and ensure that they have extra carbohydrate to make up for the added hypoglycaemic effect of the alcohol. It is especially important to have a bedtime snack, as alcohol can continue to lower the blood glucose for several hours after alcohol consumption has stopped. Signs of hypoglycaemia can resemble signs of drunkenness; so that alcohol can mask the symptoms, which can therefore go unnoticed. Hence it is also vital that individuals carry identification that they have diabetes.

ILLNESS

Any illness can affect diabetic control. Individuals taking insulin or tablets must continue with these when ill (see Chapter 11). If people are vomiting they should contact their GP, but insulin must never be stopped. The body's natural response to illness is to utilise more glucose. Insulin requirements rise and there is an increased risk of diabetic ketoacidosis. This means that increased doses of insulin or oral hypoglycaemics might be required. Carbohydrate must also be taken in some form and meals can be replaced with liquid, semi-solid or solid foods containing carbohydrate depending on the person's appetite. As a guide, 10 g of carbohydrate should be taken every hour until the person feels better. Regular blood testing is essential in times of illness. Table 6.7 suggests some sources of carbohydrate during illness.

FASTING FOR RELIGIOUS FESTIVALS

During the month of Ramadan, practising Muslims abstain from food and liquids between dawn and sunset, commonly eating one large evening meal after sunset and a light meal before dawn. Fasting is obligatory for all healthy adult Muslims, although people with diabetes are exempt from fasting. Despite this, many choose

Table 6.7
Suggested carbohydrate sources during illness

Food	Amount supplying 10 g carbohydrate
Lucozade	50 mL/2 fl oz
Fruit juice	1 small glass (100 mL/4 fl oz)
Milk	1 cup (200 mL)
Thick soup	1 cup (200 mL)
Ice cream	1 briquette (1 scoop)
Yoghurt	Half tub low fat/1 tub 'diet'

to observe this religious obligation. Fasting can last up to 18 hours a day during the summer months and large quantities of sugary fluids, such as canned juices and fizzy drinks, together with fried foods and carbohydrate-rich meals are taken during the non-fasting hours. Sweet foods may also be specially prepared for Ramadan. Longer gaps between meals and greater amounts of foods (in particular foods high in sugar and starch) mean that people with diabetes can experience large swings in blood glucose levels during Ramadan.

Case study 6.3

Amina is a 56-year-old Muslim woman with type 1 diabetes that is controlled on a twice-daily mix of soluble and intermediate-acting insulin. She asks for advice with regard to her diet and insulin during the period of Ramadan. Although she is aware that she is exempt from fasting, she is choosing to observe this religious obligation.

With the appropriate advice, Amina should be able to undertake the fast safely. Ideally, discussions should take place well in advance of Ramadan as clinic attendance often drops at this time because people avoid exercise to conserve energy. Amina should be encouraged to attend the clinic to discuss monitoring her diabetes with the healthcare team and to be given advice about any changes to her insulin regime. Appointments should not be scheduled for days that she wishes to visit the mosque. Amina should be encouraged to take her blood glucose regularly because she will be at risk of hypoglycaemia. Some Muslims consider blood glucose testing as breaking a fast; however, an educational class designed specifically for self-management during Ramadan explains that this is a myth (Chowdhury et al 2003). Meal times should be discussed to ascertain the exact changes from Amina's current meal pattern and some general dietary guidelines given:

- limit the amount of sweet foods taken after sunset, e.g. only have small amounts of ladoo, jelaibi or burfi
- fill up on starchy foods such as basmati rice, chapati or naan
- include fruits, vegetables, dhal and yoghurt in the meals after sunset and in the early morning

- try to have the early morning meal just before sunrise instead of at midnight. This will spread the energy intake more evenly and result in more balanced blood glucose levels when fasting
- choose water and sugar-free drinks to quench thirst. Avoid adding sugar to drinks and use a sweetener where needed
- limit fried foods such as paratha, puri, samosas, chevera, pakoras, katlamas, fried kebabs and Bombay mix. Measure the amount of oil used in cooking (between one and two tablespoons for a four-person dish).

Amina will also require advice about insulin. The most important message is for her not to stop taking insulin during Ramadan. She would need guidance on how to make appropriate adjustments to her insulin dosage and to negotiate for how long she can safely fast. There are some general guidelines regarding insulin:

- Her insulin could be changed to isophane alone before her morning meal and soluble mixed with a small dose of isophane in the evening. It is strongly recommended that premixed insulins are avoided during fasting, but if the person insists on staying on this, the dose should be changed so that less insulin is given at Sehri (the early morning meal).
- It might be useful to change her onto an insulin analogue as this would allow her to eat immediately after injecting. It is also short acting, which would reduce the risk of hypoglycaemia when fasting.
- She should be advised where possible to rest during the day to avoid low blood glucose levels.
  It would be useful to ask:
- Have you fasted before with diabetes? What happened then? Valuable information can be obtained from past experience.
- Will you have the pre-fast meal in the morning or do you plan to omit this meal?
- Are you prepared to break the fast if you become hypoglycaemic and need sugar? It is recommended that people break their fast if they become hypoglycaemic.

With the appropriate support and guidance, the period of Ramadan should not pose a risk to the person with diabetes (www.diabetes/org.uk/healthcare).

DYSLIPIDAEMIA (RAISED BLOOD LIPID LEVELS)

Altered lipid metabolism occurs in people with both type 1 and type 2 diabetes but the pattern of dyslipidaemia is different. It is often present in people newly diagnosed with diabetes or those with poor glycaemic control. People's lipid profiles should be reassessed after there has been control of hyperglycaemia. In people with type 1 diabetes with adequate control, lipid profiles tend to be similar to those of the non-diabetic population [elevated total and low-density lipoprotein (LDL) cholesterol; see Chapter 8]. As the risk of cardiovascular disease is higher in the population of people with diabetes, it is more important that these elevated levels are detected and corrected, ideally by means of dietary adjustment.

Most people with type 2 diabetes, and some overweight people with type 1 diabetes, have a dyslipidaemia associated with insulin resistance. This is characterised by an increase in triglyceride and harmful LDL cholesterol and a reduction in protective high-density lipoprotein (HDL) cholesterol. This often persists after glycaemic control has been achieved. Lifestyle interventions include weight loss, particularly by reduction of saturated fat (which reduces concentrations of triglyceride, LDL cholesterol and may increase HDL cholesterol). If weight loss is not required, energy from saturated fat can be replaced by carbohydrate or *cis*-monounsaturated fat. Regular physical exercise will help to reduce triglyceride concentrations and to improve insulin sensitivity. Sterols and stanols of plant origin have been shown to lower LDL cholesterol. These are now being incorporated into spreads and other fat-derived products such as yoghurts, semi-skimmed milk, etc., and are marketed as adjuncts to other dietary methods of reducing LDL cholesterol. However, they are very expensive (two to four times more than conventional) and their long-term effects on morbidity and mortality due to coronary heart disease are unknown. Hypertriglyceridaemia is sometimes associated with alcohol consumption and this possibility should always be considered. Fish oil supplements should not be recommended because of potential deleterious effects on LDL cholesterol and glycaemic control (Franz et al 2002).

COELIAC DISEASE

People with type 1 diabetes have a greater risk of developing coeliac disease than the general population, possibly as a result of the presence of HLA-related autoimmune factors common to both conditions (Cronin & Shanahan 1997). Because of this, coeliac disease should be suspected in anyone with diabetes with gastrointestinal symptoms or unexplained anaemia. Coeliac disease is characterised by intolerance to gluten, a protein found in wheat and rye and to similar proteins found in barley and possibly oats. The reaction to gluten damages the mucosal lining of the small intestine, flattening the villi and reducing the ability to absorb nutrients. As a result, symptoms of malabsorption commonly occur, although these can vary in nature and severity. The intolerance is permanent and requires complete and life-long exclusion of gluten from the diet. This not only corrects the histological and clinical consequences but also reduces the risk of long-term detrimental effects on health.

Case study 6.4

Belinda is a 35-year-old woman with type 1 diabetes who presents to her GP with a history of fatigue and unexplained iron-deficiency anaemia. She undergoes blood tests and an intestinal biopsy and is subsequently found to have coeliac disease.

Belinda will need to be referred to a dietician for detailed advice about commencing on a strict gluten-free diet. This is a major undertaking in itself, as it will place a double dietary burden on someone who already has diabetes and it is vital that she receives good dietetic support. There will be additional constraints on food choices many of which are key dietary sources of carbohydrate, such as bread, pasta, breakfast cereals, biscuits and many other manufactured foods. When coeliac disease is untreated, there is an increased risk of hypoglycaemia, and the introduction of a gluten-free diet results in an increase in insulin requirement (Iafusco et al 1998). There should be good liaison within the diabetes team to ensure that the appropriate support and advice is given. Dietetic guidance will be essential to ensure that Belinda's carbohydrate intake is not compromised and that she has appropriate information on avoiding gluten, how to make alternative food choices (such as rice and potatoes) or how to make substitutes in foods (such as specially manufactured gluten-free breads, flours and pasta). It will also be necessary to ensure that Belinda has a balanced diet to maintain health and protect against disease, particularly osteoporosis. She should have regular dietetic follow-up to encourage adherence with the gluten-free diet. The difficulties in following a gluten-free diet, both in terms of family meals and eating away from home, should not be underestimated.

CONCLUSION

Diet is the cornerstone of treatment for diabetes. Nutritional recommendations have changed over the years in the light of new scientific evidence available and are now similar to those for healthy eating for the rest of the population. This still represents a significant deviation from the typical UK diet and many people with diabetes consider diet to be the most difficult and traumatic part of management. All members of the healthcare team should be aware of the current nutritional guidelines for diabetes to ensure that consistent information is given to individuals and the positive aspects of dietary change emphasised. Regular follow-up and support will be vital to encourage the individuals and their families to make the necessary changes. If the whole family is supportive and prepared to make changes towards better eating habits, it can help the individual person follow the appropriate dietary advice. Diabetes should be seen as the catalyst for change, which can ultimately improve the future health of the whole family.

REFERENCES

American Diabetes Association (ADA) 1979 Principles of nutrition and dietary recommendations for individuals with diabetes mellitus. Diabetes 28:1027–1030

American Diabetes Association (ADA) 2003 Evidence-based nutrition principles and recommendations for the treatment and prevention of diabetes and related complications. Position statement. Diabetes Care 26:S51–S61

British Diabetic Association (BDA) Nutrition Subcommittee 1982 Dietary recommendations for diabetics for the 1980s. Human Nutrition: Applied Nutrition 36A:378–394

British Diabetic Association (BDA) Nutrition Subcommittee 1992 Dietary recommendations for people with diabetes: an update for the 1990s. Diabetic Medicine 9(2):189–202

Brunzell JD, Lerner RL, Porte D et al 1974 Effect of a fat-free high carbohydrate diet on diabetic subjects with fasting hyperglycaemia. Diabetes 23:138–142

Chowdhury TA, Hussain HA, Hayes M 2003 An educational class on diabetes self-management during Ramadan. Practical Diabetes International 20(8):306–306a

Clinical Standards Board for Scotland (CSBS) 2001 Clinical standards diabetes. CSBS, Edinburgh

Cronin C, Shanahan F 1997 Insulin-dependent diabetes mellitus and coeliac disease. Lancet 349:1096–1097

DAFNE Study Group 2002 Training in flexible, intensive insulin management to enable dietary freedom in people with type 1 diabetes: dose adjustment for normal eating (DAFNE) randomized controlled trial. British Medical Journal 325:746–749

Department of Health and Social Security (DHSS) Committee on Medical Aspects of Food Policy (COMA) 1984 Diet and cardiovascular disease. Report on health and social subjects 28. HMSO, London

Diabetes UK Nutrition Subcommittee 2003 The implementation of dietary advice for people with diabetes. Diabetic Medicine 20:786–807

Dyson P 2003 The role of nutrition in diabetes. Nursing Standard 17(51):47–53

European Association for the Study of Diabetes, Diabetes and Nutrition Study Group 2000 Recommendations for the nutritional management of patients with diabetes mellitus. European Journal of Clinical Nutrition 54:353–355

Franz MJ, Bantle JP, Beebe CA et al 2002 Evidence based nutrition principles and recommendations for the treatment and prevention of diabetes and related complications. Diabetes Care 25:148–198

Health Education Authority (HEA) 1994 The balance of good health. Introducing the National Food Guide. HEA, London

Iafusco D, Rea F, Prisco F 1998 Hypo and reduction of the insulin requirement as a sign of coeliac disease in children with insulin dependent diabetes mellitus. Diabetes Care 21(8):1379–1380

James WPT, Ferro-Luzzi A, Izaksson B et al 1988 Healthy nutrition. WHO Regional Publications No 24. World Health Organization, Copenhagen

Jenkins DJA, Wolever TM S, Jenkins AL et al 1984 The glycaemic response to carbohydrate foods. Lancet 2:388–391

Kratz M, Cullen P, Kannenberg F et al 2002 Effects of dietary fatty acids on the composition and oxidizability of low density lipoprotein. European Journal of Clinical Nutrition 56:72–81

Lean MEJ, Powrie JK, Anderson AS et al 1990 Obesity, weight loss and prognosis in type 2 diabetes. Diabetic Medicine 7:228–233

Lean MJ, Han TS, Morrison CE 1995 Waist circumference as a measure for indicating need for weight management. British Medical Journal 311:158–161

Miettinen M, Turpeinen O, Karvonen MN et al 1977 Cholesterol-lowering diet and mortality from coronary heart disease. Lancet 2:1418–1419

Relimpio F, Pumar A, Losada Mangas MA et al 1998 Adding metformin versus insulin dose increase in insulin-treated but poorly controlled type 2 diabetes: an open-label randomized trial. Diabetic Medicine 15:997–1002

Robinson AC, Burke J, Robinson S et al 1998 The effects of metformin on glycaemic control and serum lipids in insulin treated NIDDM patients with suboptimal metabolic control. Diabetes Care 21:701–705

Scottish Intercollegiate Guidelines Network (SIGN) 2001 SIGN 55: management of diabetes. SIGN, Edinburgh

Simpson RW, Mann JI, Eaton J et al 1979 High-carbohydrate diets and insulin dependent diabetes. British Medical Journal 2:523–525

Thomas B (ed) 2001 Manual of Dietetic Practice 3rd edn, Blackwell Science, UK.

United Kingdom Prospective Diabetes (UKPDS) Study Group 1990 Response of fasting plasma glucose to diet therapy in newly presenting type 2 diabetic patients (UKPDS 7). Metabolism 39:905–912

Williamson DE, Thompson TJ, Thun M et al 2000 Intentional weight loss and mortality among overweight individuals with diabetes. Diabetes Care 23:1499–1504

WEBSITE ADDRESSES

British Dietetic Association: www.bda.uk.com

Clinical Standards: can be accessed via: www.show.scot.nhs.uk/organisations/orgindex.htm

Coeliac Society: www.coeliac.co.uk

Diabetes UK: www.diabetes.org.uk

Scottish Intercollegiate Guidelines Network (SIGN) guidelines: www.sign.ac.uk

Monitoring diabetes

Joan McDowell and Florence Brown

INTRODUCTION

Research has clearly demonstrated the link between elevated blood glucose levels and diabetic microvascular complications in people with type 1 diabetes (The Diabetes Control and Complications Trial (DCCT) 1993) and type 2 diabetes (UK Prospective Diabetes Study (UKPDS) 1998). There is evidence that elevated blood glucose levels are also linked to macrovascular complications (UKPDS 1998) (see Chapter 8). Self-monitoring, by measuring glucose levels in either blood or urine, can help people with diabetes make sense of and contribute to the decisions about self-management. Self-monitoring improves the individual's understanding of his or her diabetes and assists the person to maintain day-to-day control of his or her blood glucose. This can enable the individual to explore the impact of exercise, diet and treatment on blood glucose levels. The value of self-monitoring of blood glucose in people with type 1 diabetes is well established, however, self-monitoring – especially blood glucose monitoring by people with type 2 diabetes – remains fiercely debated (Gallichan 1997, Reynolds & Strachan 2004, Reynolds & Webb 2006). One of the challenges for both the person with diabetes and the healthcare professional is to make this serious and complicated disease become 'real' so that it can be controlled successfully enough to avoid diabetic complications. It would seem reasonable, therefore, that self-monitoring, which allows the person with diabetes to recognise and correct abnormal results, could be a cornerstone to self-management of diabetes.

The two methods for self-monitoring of glucose in diabetes are through blood glucose monitoring or urine testing for glucose. An alternative to self-monitoring would be to provide a blood test at the surgery or hospital for measurement of glycated haemoglobin (HbA1c) (Owens et al 2005).

This chapter addresses monitoring in type 1 diabetes and discusses some of the controversies of monitoring in type 2 diabetes.

HISTORY OF BLOOD GLUCOSE MONITORING

Self-monitoring of blood glucose (SMBG) became available to people with type 1 diabetes only in the late 1970s, initially with the availability of reagent strips that required a lengthy complex procedure including visual reading of colour change for an accurate result. In the UK, provision of strips came from the hospital pharmacy budget and there was no provision for them in primary care.

In recent years, blood glucose meters have been developed and refined and are available at relatively low cost to individuals or obtainable at no cost from many hospital clinics and GP surgeries. Strips and lancets to prick a finger to obtain a blood sample require to be prescribed by the GP. Alternatively, they can be bought at significant cost from the pharmacist (£15–£25 per box of 50 strips). Results are precise providing technique is accurate although are less exact at whole blood glucose levels less than 3.5 mmols/L. Blood glucose meters have improved significantly over recent years with more sophisticated technology and are easier and quicker to use. The procedure involves obtaining a fingertip drop of blood placing it onto a strip that has been sited or about to be sited, in a meter. The result is available anywhere within 5–30 seconds. More recently, some pharmaceutical companies have modified their meters to accept blood from alternative, less painful sites to the fingertips. The amount of blood required for an accurate result has reduced significantly and is as little as 0.3 microlitres.

URINE TESTING

Before blood glucose monitoring (BGM) becoming available, people with diabetes were asked to perform tests to measure glucose in the urine. As with measuring blood glucose, urine testing has also become a less complex procedure, which involves dipping a reagent strip into urine for 2 seconds then waiting up to 30 seconds for the strip to change colour if glucose is present. No glycosuria indicates that the blood glucose level several hours before was probably under 10 mol/L and likely to be in the acceptable range for preventing long-term complications. People with diabetes do not like urine testing, saying that repeated 'negative' results can lead them to believe that diabetes has gone away (Lawton et al 2004). Urine testing does not give any indication of hypoglycaemia, which can be an immediate complication of too much insulin or oral hypoglycaemic therapy. Caution should be exercised in interpreting urine testing results in the older population. The renal threshold is higher in this group and hence an individual might have a high blood glucose but no glycosuria. In this situation, regular blood glucose monitoring would detect any progressing hyperglycaemia.

HBA1C MEASUREMENT

Alternatives to self-monitoring are to do no monitoring at all and instead have a test performed by the healthcare professional known as a 'long-term' test: glycated haemoglobin or HbA1c. Red blood cells containing haemoglobin are made in the bone marrow, circulate for 120 days and are then removed by the spleen and liver. These millions of red cells have a mean life of around 49 days when prevailing blood glucose binds irreversibly with haemoglobin to form glycated haemoglobin or HbA1c. Measuring glycated haemoglobin is done in most laboratories and the result offers a very good test of how average the blood glucose level has been in the previous seven weeks. The DCCT (1993) demonstrated that to minimise complications in type 1 diabetes, the HbA1c should be below 7.5%. The UKPDS (1998) demonstrated that to minimise complications in type 2 diabetes the HbA1c should be below 7.1%. Nearly all research looking at glycaemic control outcomes uses HbA1c as the outcome measure. The disadvantage of the HbA1c is that it does not indicate swings in blood glucose or hypoglycaemia, nor give immediate feedback to enable the individual to make decisions regarding self-treatment or lifestyle adjustments. It remains debatable as to whether swings in blood glucose levels are damaging (Buse 2003, Davidson 2003).

The Clinical Standards Board for Scotland (2001) recommends an absolute minimum of an annual HbA1c measurement and more often as indicated. The exception to this is in pregnant women with diabetes, in whom it is important to know the trend in glycaemic control on a month-to-month basis. For someone with changing diabetes management the HbA1c would be checked not more than 2-monthly and 3- to 6-monthly in others.

FRUCTOSAMINE

This is another form of assay used to measure glucose binding to proteins in the blood. It reflects the average blood glucose level over the preceding 2–3 weeks. It is really only of value in people who suffer from a haemoglobinopathy in whom an HbA1c measurement is not accurate (Owens et al 2005).

MONITORING IN TYPE 2 DIABETES

In the early years, BGM was taught to people with type 1 diabetes to enable the regulation of glycaemic control through adjustment of insulin by the person with diabetes. In recent years, as the seriousness of type 2 diabetes has become increasingly recognised, so has the move to encourage people with type 2 diabetes to self-monitor (European NIDDM Policy Group 1994).

A major factor contributing to the increase in BGM in type 2 diabetes has been the recognition that type 2 diabetes is a progressive disease that, over time, requires increasing and changing treatment. Although someone with type 2 diabetes might start treatment with a modified diet, the UKPDS (1998) demonstrated progression to one or more types of oral hypoglycaemic agent and then to insulin therapy.

Pharmacists are keen to support people with diabetes and this includes educating individuals on how to use a meter.

CONSENSUS STATEMENTS

The American Diabetes Association declared that SMBG has revolutionised management of diabetes (ADA 2003):

> *Using SMBG, patients with diabetes can work to achieve and maintain specific glycemic goal targets.*

Although the above quote is questionable in terms of the evidence available, the ADA also states that SMBG can monitor the efficacy of diet, medications and exercise. The Association recommends that all people on insulin or oral hypoglycaemic agents should perform SMBG on a daily basis. The number of tests a day should be agreed between the healthcare professional and the individual. The ADA affirms that the role of SMBG in people who control their diabetes with diet alone is not known.

The European consensus guidelines states that urine testing can be useful for people who cannot manage blood testing where this is indicated in people whose glucose control is deteriorating or who take insulin (European Diabetes Policy Group 1999). This suggests that BGM is the first choice of monitoring but it also suggests that self-monitoring in people whose diabetes is stable might be unnecessary.

Within the UK there has been the continued development of a consensus statement around the debate of SMBG and recommendations are presented in Table 7.1 (Owens et al 2005). These recommendations have been developed around current research and expert opinion (Reynolds & Webb 2006).

THE EVIDENCE

A health technology assessment (HTA) systematic review examining blood glucose monitoring in diabetes was published in 2000 (Coster et al 2000). Part of the review related to BGM in type 2 diabetes. Only eight randomised controlled trials (RCTs) in relation to BGM in type 2 diabetes were identified as being robust enough to be included in the review. The eight RCTs included comparisons of blood testing, urine testing and no testing. Interventions were not standardised and training of individuals and adherence were not addressed systematically. No trial required subjects to modify their drug therapy in accordance with self-monitoring results. Six studies were included in a meta-analysis. The review concluded:

> *...that the results do not provide evidence for clinical effectiveness of an item of care with appreciable costs. Further work is needed to evaluate self-monitoring so that resources for diabetes care can be used more efficiently. (Coster et al 2000)*

Table 7.1
Recommendations regarding self-monitoring of blood glucose (SMBG)

Diabetes type	Treatment group	Monitoring regimen
Type 1 diabetes	All people with type 1 diabetes	SMBG should be regarded as an integral part of treating all people with type 1 diabetes People with type 1 diabetes should be educated to SMBG and adjust treatment appropriately The majority of patients with type 1 diabetes should consider SMBG four or more times per day to prevent hypoglycaemia and control hyperglycaemia Avoiding metabolic emergencies such as diabetic ketoacidosis might require frequent SMBG
Diabetic pregnancy	Diabetic pregnancy	Pregnant women with type 1 diabetes, plus those with type 2 diabetes requiring insulin and patients with gestational diabetes requiring insulin should SMBG at least four times per day to include both fasting and post-meal blood glucose measurements In diet-treated patients it may be necessary to SMBG with the same frequency as insulin-treated patients to ensure strict glycaemic control In insulin-treated patients increased frequency of testing may be necessary in the first trimester when the risk of hypoglycaemia is greatest
Type 2 diabetes	Intensive insulin therapy	People who adopt intensive insulin therapies require regular feedback regarding SMBG levels People with type 2 diabetes who use a multiple daily insulin regimen should SMBG in the same way as those with type 1 diabetes Fasting blood glucose should be tested daily during basal insulin dose titration
Type 2 diabetes	Conventional insulin therapy	People with type 2 diabetes who are using a conventional insulin regimen and who have stable control should SMBG two or three times a week People with type 2 diabetes who are using a conventional insulin regimen and who have less stable control should SMBG at least once daily, varying the time of testing between fasting, pre-meal and post-meal Fasting blood glucose should be tested daily during basal insulin dose titration

Table 7.1 (Cont'd)
Recommendations
regarding self-monitoring
of blood glucose (SMBG)

Diabetes type	Treatment group	Monitoring regimen
Type 2 diabetes	Combined insulin and oral antidiabetic therapy	Fasting blood glucose should be tested daily during basal insulin dose titration People with type 2 diabetes who use insulin or oral hypoglycaemic agents should SMBG at least once daily, varying the time of testing between fasting, pre-meal and post-meal
Type 2 diabetes	Diet and exercise	People with type 2 diabetes who have good control on diet and exercise, metformin or glitazone treatment do not need SMBG monitoring, unless they are destabilized by other factors Glycaemic control managed through diet and exercise in people with type 2 diabetes is best monitored through HbA1c testing Patients with type 2 diabetes managed only by diet and exercise do not normally require routine SMBG Informed patients might choose SMBG as a means of monitoring lifestyle changes
Type 2 diabetes	Metformin (± glitazone)	As for diet and exercise
Type 2 diabetes	Glitazone (± metformin)	As for diet and exercise
Type 2 diabetes	Sulphonylurea alone (or in combination with oral antidiabetic agents)	Hypoglycaemia can be more common than assumed in people with type 2 diabetes on sulphonylureas and SMBG will reveal this situation

From Owens et al 2005. Reproduced with permission from SB Communications.

A more recent meta-analysis of SMBG in people with type 2 diabetes not using insulin looked at six RCTs and concluded cautiously that SMBG has a small beneficial effect on glycaemic control but, again, stated that there were methodological issues with the studies (Welschen et al 2005). From these studies it would appear that some people benefit more from SMBG than others; however, the cost of SMBG is very likely to be offset against the longer-term costs of care for the same people (*Bandolier* 2005). Given that BGM in type 2 diabetes remains so controversial, it is prudent at this point to consider why clinicians appear to be ignoring the evidence, or, rather, ignoring the lack of evidence (Barraclough 2003). There are several ways of interpreting 'lack of evidence':

- The research has not measured what it should have measured.
- The intervention might have had positive effects for some, but not all subjects and an RCT would not necessarily identify these differences.
- The research might not have been done.
- There is no supporting evidence, even when trials with adequate power have been properly conducted.
- Some people believe that the only evidence worth considering is that obtained from RCTs.
- Some studies might not have been able to separate other factors that could influence glycaemic control; they might not have had control groups (Gallichan 1997).

Clues about 'other factors' are hinted at in the three qualitative studies described below.

A qualitative study of people with type 1 diabetes found that, although there is no doubt that blood glucose monitoring is acceptable and useful for some, it is clearly difficult and painful, both physically and psychologically, for others (Fox et al 1994). Some people are unable to make the connection between testing and using test results to influence glycaemic control (Fox et al 1994).

A more recent grounded theory study of 40 people with type 2 diabetes diagnosed within the previous 6 months and interviewed twice during a 9-month period found that those who had optimal glycaemic control viewed monitoring in a positive light. However, the reverse was true for those who observed results outside the recommended range (Peel et al 2004). Positive aspects of monitoring were stated as modifying lifestyle and adjusting regimens based on results. Negative aspects identified were: evidence of the existence of their diabetes; additional distress if results were inexplicable; they did not know what to do with the results; monitoring for the benefit of the doctor, which was especially annoying if health professionals did not enquire about results. Not enquiring about results might reflect the reliance of healthcare professionals on HbA1c.

The same research group also recently completed a grounded theory study on urine testing (Lawton et al 2004). Forty people with newly diagnosed type 2 diabetes were interviewed three times over 1 year. They expressed 'profoundly negative views' on urine testing. Urine testing was perceived as less accurate, less hygienic and less convenient than BGM. Negative urine results were seen as an indicator that they did not have diabetes. It is interesting to compare these results with those of a study where a more positive view of urine testing was taken (Miles et al 1997). It suggests differences in diabetes education programmes and might reflect the personal views of the diabetes educators.

The fact that SMBG, from the point of view of the person with diabetes, has many costs and benefits is reflected in a survey of people with type 1 and type 2 diabetes who take insulin in the Tayside Region of Scotland (Evans et al 1999). This study showed that uptake of BGM strips from pharmacists was far below that prescribed, suggesting that people are not testing as often as requested by health professionals.

Another study showed that for those with type 2 diabetes taking insulin, SMBG was a useful aid and improved glycaemic control when insulin adjustment had been taught (Franciosi et al 2001). However, the same study showed that, in those not treated with insulin, SMBG was associated with higher HbA1c levels and higher psychological burden. The authors stated that SMBG should be part of wider educational programme but at the same time recommended that SMBG should be limited to those on insulin therapy.

Conversely, a prospective, multicentre randomised controlled study showed that glycaemic control improved significantly in the intervention group (Schwedes et al 2002). The intervention group received a structured diabetes education programme that included feedback. Participants maintained a diary of eating habits and SMBG results. Self-monitoring resulted in marked improvement in general well-being with significant improvement in the subitems depression and lack of well-being (Schwedes et al 2002). The researchers concluded that meal-related SMBG within a structured counselling programme improved glycaemic control in the majority of the intervention group of this study. The weakness of the study was that the final outcome measures were assessed at 6 months after the completion of the intervention and it is well recognised that an intervention effect can wear off after 6 months. However, the point is that it is still possible for SMBG to be effective if it is presented in the correct context of an effective education programme. In a later study, the same group demonstrated that SMBG was beneficial in the context of a short, structured education programme that included considering options for action (self-reflection) and believing in self-efficacy (self-regulation) (Siebolds et al 2006).

FINANCIAL IMPLICATIONS TO THE HEALTH SERVICES

Blood glucose monitoring is a costly procedure. The publication of the National Institute for Health and Clinical Excellence (NICE) guideline on blood glucose control in type 2 diabetes (NICE 2002) resulted in restrictions by GPs on the prescribing of blood glucose strips. The NICE guideline stated that self-monitoring:

- should not be considered as a stand-alone intervention
- should be taught if the needs and purpose are clear and agreed with the individual
- can be used in conjunction with appropriate therapy as part of integrated care.

Some primary care organisations have interpreted these guidelines to mean that as SMBG in type 2 diabetes has no evidence base, substantial cost savings can be gained from restrictions on prescribing SMBG strips. This has been refuted by Diabetes UK (2004). It is acknowledged that there are resource implications in utilising SMBG. Such resources include the actual equipment for BGM as well as the support required from health professionals to teach the skill and assist individuals to place SMBG within their own lifestyle context.

The NHS National Prescribing Centre (2002) produced a bulletin summarising the evidence for SMBG in type 2 diabetes. The first point was that the NHS spends 40% more on BGM materials than it does on oral hypoglycaemic agents (£90 million versus £64 million in 2001). The bulletin goes on to repeat the recommendations of the NICE report as above but also points out that there is no evidence that BGM is more effective than urine testing. It concludes that measurement of HbA1c is likely to provide more helpful information than day-to-day monitoring. This ignores the fact that SMBG and HbA1c are different measures measuring different aspects of glycaemic control. It is possible for people with diabetes to have HbA1c levels at target but be experiencing both frequent hypoglycaemia and/or hyperglycaemia. The above statement also raises the issue of patient empowerment.

EMPOWERMENT

Empowerment of individuals has been acknowledged at a government level and constitutes a significant role in the Diabetes National Service Framework documents for each country in the United Kingdom (Department of Health (DH) 2003, Northern Ireland Task Force 2003, Scottish Executive Health Department (SEHD) 2002, Welsh Department of Health 2003). However, there is a sense in these documents that a person with diabetes is empowered only if he or she follows the rules of diabetes management. There is a simplicity in the assumption that diabetes education results in optimal glycaemic control. There are all sorts of reasons why people with diabetes do not adhere to the 'rules' of self-management, not least the fear of hypoglycaemia.

A recent study has highlighted that the incidence of severe hypoglycaemia (requiring assistance from another) in people with either type 1 or type 2 diabetes is much higher than previously reported (Leese et al 2003). Severe hypoglycaemia is an accepted reason for not striving for glycaemia in the 'normal' range. Hypoglycaemia has long been recognised as an inevitable side-effect of the sulphonylurea oral agents and insulin therapy. The DCCT (1993) demonstrated that the achievement of near-normal glycaemia was at the expense of a two- to threefold increase in the incidence of severe hypoglycaemia. SMBG has therefore become even more critical for the person aiming for tight glycaemic control, although this is not the target for everyone (see Chapters 4 and 5). SMBG is necessary for the fine-tuning of insulin doses (or sulphonylurea) and allows the person with diabetes to maintain near-normal blood glucose levels with as few episodes of hypoglycaemia as possible.

To ensure appropriate use of the findings, individuals should be reviewed by professionals to discuss the meaning of results and their management options. Without support, people can become distressed by inexplicable results (Peel et al 2004). Whichever form of monitoring a person chooses, he or she should be supported in the choice and encouraged to take an active role in self-management. Self-monitoring should be continually reinforced, and support given to enable the chosen lifestyle changes to occur.

Self-monitoring does not improve a person's diabetes control by itself (NICE 2002). A recent survey undertaken by Diabetes UK (2004) showed that only 28% of the sample of 361 people received any written information about testing. It was also found that key barriers to testing were associated pain, forgetfulness, inconvenience and anger when healthcare professionals appeared to show little interest in their results. The targets agreed should be specific to the individual person and be realistically achievable taking into account a variety of factors, including the risk of hypoglycaemia and diabetes-related complications, as well as the ability to undertake the skill (Home et al 2002). Agreed targets should be documented and an interest shown by the healthcare team in the individual's self-monitoring results (Diabetes UK 2004).

Case study 7.1

Richard is a 56-year-old man who has just been diagnosed as having type 2 diabetes. He has a strong family history of type 2 diabetes and is therefore not totally surprised at the diagnosis. He is aware of the long-term implications of the disease. Richard's initial management is by diet alone. In discussion, he remembers his mother testing her urine for glucose. His brother, who also has type 2 diabetes, has just started testing his own blood glucose levels because his diabetes is going out of control. Richard asks how he ought to be monitoring his diabetes.

Richard appears eager and willing to monitor his diabetes. Through personal experience he is aware of two forms of monitoring. The healthcare professional will discuss with him the advantages and disadvantages of both methods and will facilitate his choice. The challenge is to be sure he is fully informed and to teach him his chosen method, the meaning of his results, how the results relate to his lifestyle and what action to take in relation to his results.

MONITORING OPTIONS

The decision on type of self-monitoring should take place following discussion with the individual. Although the healthcare professional might be constrained by guidelines, the ideal scenario would be that the method chosen is as a result of the individual's understanding of the costs and benefits of each method, including how self-monitoring fits into his or her responsibilities in relation to self-management options. The person with diabetes is entitled to consider no self-monitoring as an option and might choose a periodic HbA1c at the surgery or diabetic clinic.

Whether the person is physically able to undertake the test should be considered. Physical constraints, for example visual deficits or a lack of manual dexterity, can prevent or inhibit testing. A survey undertaken by Diabetes UK demonstrated that a significant number of people had a disability that affected their use of blood glucose meters (Diabetes UK 2004). Equally, an inability to read either the time or results, or a lack of understanding of either spoken or written English, will make monitoring more difficult to teach and to comprehend.

If monitoring is envisaged as being of value only to the healthcare team (either by the healthcare team and/or the individual with diabetes) clinic visits might become more frequent and self-monitoring becomes the focus of the consultation rather than the person with diabetes engaging in problem solving and decision making. Self-monitoring is a first step in facilitating self-empowerment.

URINE TESTING

Urine testing has the advantages of being cheap, easy to use and painless to carry out. Some people with diabetes do, however, find the concept of urine testing 'dirty' or unpleasant. In comparison with blood glucose monitoring, people find urine testing to be less convenient, less hygienic and less accurate (Lawton et al 2004). In the UK, urine testing has been predominantly replaced by BGM (Owens et al 2005); however, it may be the only form of monitoring in some other countries and is therefore included here for clarification.

Testing for glycosuria reflects only what has been happening to the blood glucose since the bladder was last emptied, hence it gives a relatively crude assessment of glycaemic control. It gives no indication of the current blood glucose level, nor does it demonstrate fluctuations in levels. The amount of glycosuria is also influenced by the renal threshold for glucose, which is affected by many factors (Box 7.1). The renal threshold can be visualised as a dam for glucose. It is only when the blood glucose level exceeds the level of the dam that there will be any glycosuria. The double-voided sample is considered more accurate than the first 'stored' sample, especially first thing in the morning. The bladder should be emptied and, after drinking a glass of water, the person encouraged to pass urine that should be the sample used for testing.

Any glycosuria present usually reflects an elevated blood glucose level in the hours before the bladder was last emptied. In an adult this frequently means that the blood glucose has been above 10 mmol/L. A negative result for glycosuria cannot be related to a particular level of blood glucose. A negative result implies only that the blood glucose has probably been below the renal threshold since the last time the patient passed urine; it gives no indication of hypoglycaemia. It is possible that individuals could have glycaemic control that is considered 'too tight', resulting in the increased risk of hypoglycaemia. By contrast, those people who like to have 'a touch of sugar in the urine' might in fact have blood glucose levels well in excess of 10 mmol/L.

Self-monitoring should be supported by a periodic HbA1c to fully inform major therapy changes such as oral hypoglycaemic agents to insulin therapy.

Box 7.1

Factors affecting the renal threshold

- Lower in children and increases with age
- Lower during pregnancy
- Increases with duration of diabetes
- Time of day: it varies throughout the normal day
- Population groups: it varies among different populations
- Medications: ascorbic acid and salicylates give a false-positive result
- Fluid intake and urine concentration

Urine testing procedure

Before proceeding to teach urine testing to Richard (in Case study 7.1), an estimation of his renal threshold should be obtained. This can be done by testing a double-voided urine sample for glucose, and at approximately the same time obtaining a blood glucose result. If the two results are compatible with a renal threshold of 10 mmol/l then, should he so choose, he would be taught this method of monitoring.

The testing of urine with dipsticks is familiar to most healthcare professionals and is given in Boxes 7.2 and 7.3.

Frequency of urine testing and its meaning

There is no consensus on the optimal frequency of urine testing for Richard (case study 7.1); however, it is generally recommended that four tests are performed each week. A pre-breakfast test reflects glycaemic control in the early hours of the morning and is a reflection of adequacy of insulin secretion in the individual. A test 2 hours after the main meal of the day (which may be lunch or evening meal) reflects how well the pancreas copes with a carbohydrate load. Testing at these times twice a week gives an overall guide of glycaemic control. The person should be taught how to record these results and advised to bring this record book to each clinic attendance. The significance of the results should be discussed.

Box 7.2
Equipment for urine testing

- Disposable gloves for the healthcare professional
- A clean container for the sample (optional)
- Urine testing dipsticks
- A watch or clock with a second hand
- Diary to record results

Box 7.3
Procedure for urine testing

- The healthcare professional wears gloves
- The expiry date of the urine testing strips is checked
- The urine to be tested should be the second sample passed at the required time and collected in a clean container
- One urine testing strip should be removed from the container and the lid replaced securely
- The strip should be dipped briefly into the urine sample and the time noted. When removing the strip it should be wiped along the rim of the container to remove any excess urine. Alternatively, the strip can be passed through the stream of urine at time of voiding and the time noted
- After the appropriate time, the colour reaction is compared with the side of the container according to the manufacturer's instructions. Individuals with colour blindness might not be able to assess colour change
- Results should be recorded and reviewed at every consultation
- Store the urine test strips container in a safe, dry place away from children

Deteriorating control evident in the postprandial test reflects a lack of ability to respond to a carbohydrate load but this might be modified by diet and/or exercise. Any persistent glycosuria in the fasting samples indicates that the blood glucose level has been elevated overnight and this may or may not be modifiable by lifestyle factors but in particular may require medication.

SELF-MONITORING OF BLOOD GLUCOSE

When presenting monitoring management options to Richard, it would be pointed out that recent recommendations state that SMBG is not necessary (see Table 7.1). Whereas SMBG has the advantage of being accurate when the procedure is done properly, it does reflect the blood glucose concentration at a precise time. SMBG would also allow Richard to evaluate the effects of diet, exercise and lifestyle interventions on his blood glucose levels. Recent improvements in technology have made the procedure less complex: smaller amounts of blood are required and finger-pricking is less painful. If Richard asked to undertake SMBG, he should be facilitated in this choice. The equipment and procedure for undertaking SMBG are detailed in Boxes 7.4 and 7.5.

Box 7.4
Equipment for SMBG

- Disposable gloves for the healthcare professional
- A finger-pricking device
- Cotton wool or paper tissues
- A watch or clock with a second hand (if not using a timed meter)
- Blood glucose testing strips
- Disposal container for lancet
- Meter
- Diary to record results

Box 7.5
Procedure for SMBG

- The healthcare professional wears gloves
- The expiry date of the blood testing strips must be checked
- The person with diabetes washes his or her hands in warm water and dried. This not only cleanses the skin but also promotes blood flow to the fingertips
- To reduce the pain, the finger can be pricked on the side, using an appropriate device. Testing can be rotated around all the fingers but avoiding thumb and forefinger
- The drop of blood is applied to the blood glucose testing strip according to the manufacturer's instructions
- The process is timed accurately
- Results should be recorded and referred to at every consultation
- The testing sticks container should be stored in a safe, dry place away from children

SMBG procedure

Visual reading of strips is no longer an option in the UK; however, strips for visual reading only are still available in other countries. Principles for SMBG, whether by meter or visually read remain the same. The procedure has to be carried out precisely as outlined in Box 7.5 to obtain an accurate result.

Testing can be rotated around all the fingers but the thumbs and forefingers can become tender as these are used most in day-to-day activities. It is recommended that people do not squeeze their fingers to acquire a drop of blood as this can produce a mixture of serous fluid and blood and this may alter the result (*Balance* 2000). The blood drop is applied to the blood glucose test strip according to the manufacturer's instructions and this will stimulate the timing mechanism on the blood glucose meter. Too little blood can result in a falsely low result and if a meter is not being used, a watch with a seconds hand should be used to ensure accurate timings before reading results.

Learning new skills requires practice. To help eliminate error in this procedure, the person should be taught how to perform SMBG, observed doing so, encouraged to practice (initially using glucose solution, which is included with the meter) and demonstrate the skill to the healthcare professional. Thereafter, an annual reassessment can be carried out, which would include technique and also a quality check of the meter itself.

Bringing blood monitoring equipment to all consultations will allow facilitation of any problem solving that people might require in relation to SMBG. This could include checking SMBG technique and cleaning and checking of the meter. Many people find the recording of results in a diary tedious and yet checking back in the memory bank of the meter can be frustrating because it can be difficult to see patterns of blood glucose results. Many pharmaceutical companies provide software that can be used by the individual with diabetes or the diabetic clinic to download results from the memory of the meter.

Finger-pricking lancets should be disposed of safely inside a firm plastic container, which should be secured before being deposited in the dustbin. In some areas, sharps containers are issued and local policies have been established whereby people deposit used lancets and needles at the local health centre. Finger-pricking devices are usually included with the purchase of a meter or can be purchased separately from manufacturers. To prevent cross-infection, finger-pricking devices should be used only by its owner and in accordance with the instructions of the manufacturer.

Frequency of SBMBG and its meaning

A recent consensus guideline on SMBG for all people with diabetes has been published (Owens et al 2005; see Table 7.1). In deciding on the frequency and timing of tests for those with type 1 diabetes and those with type 2 diabetes the authors took into account the differences between patterns in glycaemia in both conditions.

Type 1 diabetes is characterised by blood glucose levels that can range from hypoglycaemia to hyperglycaemia, often with little pattern from day to day. This has particularly been observed by continuous glucose monitoring systems (Sachedina & Pickup 2003). This means that a single blood glucose measure cannot relate to HbA1c results and the more erratic the blood glucose profile then the more frequent SMBG needs to be performed. This is necessary to understand treatment requirements and also for the individual to avoid extremes of blood glucose that might impair performance during day-to-day tasks such as driving. It is recommended that people with type 1 diabetes should consider SMBG at least four times per day.

People with type 2 diabetes are recommended to self-monitor their blood glucose according to their treatment regimen (see Table 7.1). The table gives recommendations and obviously individuals have to choose whether to follow them. In people with type 2 diabetes who are treated only with diet, both fasting and postprandial blood glucose levels are elevated but are also predictable from day to day (Pickup 2003). A more recent study has found that the correlation depends on the level of glycaemic control. The higher the fasting blood glucose, the more likely it is to relate to HbA1c. Owens et al (2005) conclude that a fasting blood glucose is a better measure of overall glycaemic control where control is suboptimal and that a postprandial blood glucose measure is better in those who have optimal glycaemic control.

Case study 7.2

Duncan has found it hard to accept his diagnosis of type 2 diabetes. He questioned his GP about the possibility that his diagnosis was a mistake. He had no symptoms and indeed felt very well. His GP suggested that performing blood glucose monitoring might enable Duncan to gain a sense of what happened to his blood glucose under varying lifestyle conditions. Duncan agreed to give this a try and after being taught how to SMBG by the community nurse he returned for a review, full of enthusiasm about what he had discovered. He had observed that his blood glucose levels rose above the target range 2 hours after a meal. He had also observed that his blood glucose level dropped in the late afternoon following a brisk walk. He had noted that during a period of illness his blood glucose levels rose despite his appetite being diminished. He found these results motivating in terms of the choices he could make about lifestyle and also precipitated questions such as glycaemic control in relation to illness, etc.

Although urine testing is easier to perform than SMBG, SMBG gives a more accurate picture of blood glucose levels at any particular point in time. Duncan might have seen some of the above changes if he had performed urine testing but not in the precise more quantifiable way that allowed him to see the impact of all lifestyle behaviours. Additionally, SMBG helped Duncan to accept that his diabetes was a reality.

Is SMBG for everyone?

SMBG is recommended as an integral part of treatment for everyone with type 1 diabetes. For those who are reluctant to SMBG, it is further recommended that they undertake SMBG for 2 weeks before any clinic appointment to facilitate the decision making at that meeting (Owens et al 2005).

SMBG is also recommended for those people who are heading towards the maximum dose of oral agents and/or whose control is suboptimal. There might be times when people with type 2 diabetes seem to be failing on oral hypoglycemic agents but in fact might be able to improve things with lifestyle adjustments. SMBG can be motivating in maintaining behaviour change but can also help the individual to accept that having done his or her best with lifestyle changes then insulin therapy might be the inevitable therapeutic option.

SMBG should also be considered in the younger person with type 2 diabetes who, by virtue of the age of onset of the disease, are more likely to live with the disease for longer and require insulin therapy at some point.

In those for whom there would not appear to be any real benefits from close monitoring of diabetes control, for example, someone with a reluctance to self monitor, no risk of hypoglycaemia, stable glycaemic control with an HbA1c level that is agreed to be optimal, then HbA1c alone might be an acceptable option (Owens et al 2005).

INTERPRETING FASTING/RANDOM GLUCOSE RESULTS IN THE CLINIC

To acquire some objective assessment of glycaemic control in the clinic, a fasting blood glucose or a random blood glucose can be checked.

In type 1 diabetes, blood glucose profiles can show considerable variation throughout the day. This is because the primary causation of type 1 diabetes is lack of endogenous insulin and blood glucose is reliant on the balancing act between food, exercise, stress levels and insulin injections.

Most people with type 2 diabetes retain some secretion of insulin from their beta cells and are in fact insulin resistant as opposed to insulin deficient, hence a 24-hour glucose profile of the person with type 2 diabetes is very similar to the normal person's profile, although the levels are significantly higher. A fasting blood glucose or random blood glucose will give a fairly accurate reflection of glucose levels throughout the day (Pickup 2003). As the fasting blood glucose is less likely to be influenced by what has recently been eaten, this result is probably the most important.

METERS FOR THE VISUALLY IMPAIRED

In the UK, meters for the visually impaired has been an area of neglect. After many years, when no speaking meters were available, there is now the new SensoCard Plus Meter from Cobolt Systems Ltd. The SensoCard speaks instructions for the user and also speaks the result. The meter has recently come down in price and strips are available on prescription. Control solution to check the meter is working properly and software to download results to a computer are also available from the company (www.cobolt.co.uk)

Roche-Diagnostics also have a meter called Compact Plus which has an Acoustic Mode that can be activated for people who are visually impaired. The Acoustic Mode delivers a sequence of beeps which represent the results and the various error messages. Roche-Diagnostics are also expecting to launch the Voice Mate in the near future. This device obviously has a speaking mechanism to enable use by the visually impaired (www.roche-diagnostics.co.uk).

People with visual impairment can find it difficult to use finger-pricking devices and accurately apply a drop of blood to a test strip. However, in reality, they often find their own way to overcome these obstacles.

CONTINUOUS GLUCOSE MONITORING

Continuous monitoring of glucose levels over a 2–3 day period is a relatively new technique that is now available in some secondary care centres. Two systems are currently available, the Menarini Glucoday and the Roche MiniMed Glucose Monitoring System. Both involve passing a very fine catheter subcutaneously into the abdomen and measuring the interstitial fluid glucose levels. This can be a useful procedure for people with diabetes who have inexplicable patterns. It is particularly useful for detecting patterns of asymptomatic hypoglycaemia.

TESTING FOR KETONES

Whereas testing for glycosuria has been largely superseded by SMBG, there is still an important place for blood or urine testing for ketones.

All people taking sulphonylurea agents or insulin therapy should be advised to increase the frequency of their blood or urine monitoring during an illness. Those on insulin should also test their blood or urine for ketones 4-hourly, as they are at risk of developing diabetic ketoacidosis. They should seek help if any ketones appear in their blood or urine or if they do not feel better within 24 hours.

Growing children and teenagers are most prone to developing diabetic ketoacidosis because of high levels of growth hormone, which antagonises the action of insulin. As in all people with type 1 diabetes, a prompt and substantial increase in insulin dose might avert hospital admission.

As ketone testing strips are probably used infrequently, people need to be reminded to acquire new sticks before their old ones have gone beyond the expiry date. Some modern blood glucose meters are also able to measure blood ketones as well as blood glucose. This can be an advantage, as the people at most risk of diabetic ketoacidosis are most likely to have access to blood glucose monitoring already and so this eliminates the need to test for urine ketones.

OTHER FACTORS THAT CAN INFLUENCE MONITORING OF DIABETES

Some people are meticulous in their monitoring and insulin dose adjustment yet never achieve optimal diabetic control. Polonsky (2002), in addressing the issue of burnout in people with diabetes, describes this as a situation where the person feels overwhelmed and defeated. People experience frustration and feelings of failure. Glycaemic control is worse and self-care deteriorates.

It is easy to understand that monitoring can contribute to these feelings, especially if the individual has not had the problem-solving education required to know how to act on suboptimal blood glucose levels. Some people need to take a break from diabetes by stopping monitoring for a while. Polonsky (2002) suggests that healthcare professionals need to be aware of burnout and suggests strategies to support people with diabetes if they have reached this stage. This includes establishing a strong collaborative relationship, negotiating person-centred goals and engaging the individual in active problem solving (see Chapter 3). A systematic review and meta-analysis of RCTs of psychological interventions in people with type 2 diabetes showed that these not only improved glycaemic control but also reduced psychological distress (Ismail et al 2004).

QUALITY ASSURANCE

Quality assurance is important because mistakes can lead to inappropriate treatment and management. It is the responsibility of the healthcare team to ensure that clinical measurements are as reliable and accurate as possible, as clinical decisions are made on this basis. Quality assurance relates not only to professionals but also to the individuals with diabetes who are self-monitoring (Seley & Quigley 2000).

Quality control of blood glucose monitoring in community practice is therefore of the utmost importance. It should assess two components of testing:

1 the testing skills of the personnel
2 the accuracy and performance of the testing equipment.

Most biochemistry departments have now implemented a quality assurance system for blood glucose meters and training of personnel within their areas. Training in technique and regular assessment of performance is essential. One way of assessing skill is by peer assessment. Asking a colleague to assess another colleague's technique according to the agreed standard will identify any areas of possible improvement.

Alternatively, solutions of known glucose concentration could be 'tested' to evaluate performance of either a meter or the individual performing the test. Each manufacturer gives different instructions for the use of their product. The healthcare team must be aware of the differences between the products and be competent in their practice.

The frequency of quality control can be determined by local practices but a weekly calibration and checking of meters used in practice is not uncommon. A record should be kept of the quality control results to assist with audit of this practice.

CONCLUSION

People with diabetes are encouraged to self-monitor either their blood or urine for glucose. Blood glucose testing gives a more precise result. The frequency of monitoring is variable but the timing depends on whether the person has type 1 diabetes or type 2 diabetes treated without insulin.

Despite self-monitoring, people with diabetes do not appear to be adjusting their therapy in the light of their results. Structured education programmes are widely recommended in guidelines and research. In these, self-monitoring is put into a context that enables people with diabetes to understand its value on a personal level. People require ongoing support and encouragement from all members of the healthcare team to build their confidence in therapy and lifestyle adjustments. Self-monitoring remains difficult for some individuals and the role of the healthcare professional is to assist with strategies that will help the individual overcome some of the barriers.

Some people will be dependent on others to monitor their diabetes for them. This will include those who are community nurse dependent and those with visual, literacy or language problems.

The healthcare team and the person with diabetes have various tests available to them to assess glycaemic control. These measure different parameters and should be used to acquire an overall picture of an individual's glycaemic control.

REFERENCES

American Diabetes Association (ADA) 2003 Position statement. Tests of glycemia in diabetes. Diabetes Care 26:S106–S108

Balance 2000 Accurate glucose tests. March–April: 66–69

Bandolier 2005 Glucose monitoring in type 2 diabetes. Online. Available: www.jr2.ox.ac.uk/bandolier/band134/b134-2.html

Barraclough K 2003 There is no evidence that... British Medical Journal 326(7398):1095

Buse JB 2003 Should postprandial glucose be routinely measured and treated to a particular target? No! Diabetes Care 26:1615–1618

Clinical Standards Board for Scotland (CSBS) 2001 Clinical standards for diabetes. CSBS, Edinburgh

Coster S, Gulliford MC, Seed PT et al 2000 Self-monitoring in type 2 diabetes mellitus: a meta analysis. Diabetic Medicine 17:755–761

Davidson J 2003 Should postprandial glucose be routinely measured and treated as a particular target? Yes! Diabetes Care 26:1919–1921

Department of Health (DH) 2003 National service framework for diabetes DH, London. Online. Available: www.publications.doh.gov.uk/nsf/diabetes/

Diabetes Control and Complications Trial (DCCT) Research Group 1993 The effect of intensive treatment of diabetes on the development and progression of long-term complications in insulin-dependent diabetes mellitus. New England Journal of Medicine 329:977–986

Diabetes UK 2004 What's the point? Survey of attitudes among non-testers. Online. Available: www.diabetes.org.uk/infocentre/htm

European Diabetes Policy Group 1999 A desktop guide to type 2 diabetes mellitus. Diabetic Medicine 16 September 1999 16(9):716–730

European NIDDM Policy Group 1994 A desktop guide of non-insulin dependent diabetes mellitus: an update. Diabetic Medicine 11:899–909

Evans JMM, Newton RW, Ruta DA et al 1999 Frequency of blood glucose monitoring in relation to glycaemic control: observational study with diabetes database. British Medical Journal 319:83–86

Fox C, Wade G, Fox A 1994 What makes people with diabetes measure their blood glucose? Practical Diabetes International 11(6):74–76

Franciosi M, Pellegrini F, De Beradis G et al 2001 The impact of blood glucose self monitoring on metabolic control and quality of life in type 2 diabetic patients. Diabetes Care 24:1870–1977

Gallichan M 1997 Self-monitoring of glucose by people with diabetes: evidence based practice. British Medical Journal 314:964–967

Home P, Chacra A, Chan J et al 2002 Considerations on blood glucose management in type 2 diabetes mellitus. Diabetes Metabolism Research and Reviews 18(4):273–285

Ismail K, Winkley K, Rabe-Hesketh S 2004 Systematic review and meta-analysis of randomized controlled trials of psychological interventions to improve glycaemic control in patients with type 2 diabetes. Lancet 363:1589–1597

Lawton J, Peel E, Douglas M, Parry O 2004 'Urine testing is a waste of time': newly diagnosed type 2 diabetes patients' perceptions of self-monitoring. Diabetic Medicine 21(9):1045–1048

Leese GP, Wag J, Broomhall J et al 2003 Frequency of severe hypoglycaemia requiring emergency treatment in type 1 and type 2 diabetes. Diabetes Care 26:1176–1180

Miles P, Everett J, Murphy J, Kerr D 1997 Comparison of blood or urine testing by patients with newly diagnosed non-insulin dependent diabetes: patient survey after randomised crossover trial. British Medical Journal 315(7104):348–352

National Institute for Health and Clinical Excellence (NICE) 2002 Management of type 2 diabetes – managing blood glucose levels. Guideline G. NICE, London. Online. Available: www.nice.org.uk/page.aspx?o=213902

Northern Ireland Task Force 2003 The Report of the Joint Clinical Resource Efficiency Support Team (CREST) Diabetes UK Taskforce on diabetes: a blueprint for diabetes care in Northern Ireland in the 21st century. Online. Available: www.diabetes.org. uk/frameworks/frameworks.htm

Owens D, Pickup J, Barnett AH et al 2005 The continuing debate on self-monitoring of blood glucose in diabetes. Diabetes and Primary Care 7:9–21

Peel E, Parry O, Douglas M, Lawton J 2004 Blood glucose self-monitoring in non-insulin treated type 2 diabetes: qualitative study of patient's perspectives. British Journal of General Practice 54:183–188

Pickup JC 2003 Diabetic control and its measurement. In Pickup JC and Williams G (eds) Textbook of diabetes, 3rd edn. Blackwell Publishing, Oxford p 34.1–34.17

Polonsky WH 2002 Understanding and treating patients with diabetes burnout. In Anderson BJ, Rubin RR (eds) Practical psychology for diabetes clinicians. American Diabetes Association, Alexandria, TX

Reynolds RM, Strachan MWJ 2004 Home blood glucose monitoring in type 2 diabetes. British Medical Journal 329:754–755

Reynolds RM, Webb DJ 2006 Recommendations and conclusions from a mini-symposium on self-blood glucose monitoring. Journal of the Royal College of Physicians Edinburgh 36:155–158

Sachedina N, Pickup JC 2003 Performance assessment of the Meditronic-MiniMed Continuous Glucose Monitoring System and its use for measurement of glycaemic control in type 1 diabetic subjects. Diabetic Medicine 20:1012–1015

Schwedes U, Siebolds M, Mertes G 2002 Meal related structured self-monitoring of blood glucose: effect on diabetes control in non-insulin treated type 2 diabetic patients. Diabetes Care 25:1928–1932

Scottish Executive Health Department (SEHD) NHS Scotland 2002 Scottish diabetes framework. SEHD, Edinburgh

Seley JJ, Quigley L 2000 Blood glucose testing. American Journal of Nursing 100(8): 24A–24E

Siebolds M, Gaedeke O, Schwedes U and on behalf of the SMBG Study Group 2006 Self-monitoring of blood glucose-psychological aspects relevant to changes in HbA1c in type 2 diabetic patients treated with diet or diet plus oral antidiabetic medication. Patient Education and Counseling 62(1):104–110

The NHS National Prescribing Centre 2002 When and how should patients with diabetes mellitus test blood glucose. MeReC Bulletin 13(1). Online. Available: www.npc.co.uk

United Kingdom Prospective Diabetes (UKPDS) Study Group 1998 Intensive blood glucose control with sulphonylureas or insulin compared with conventional treatment and risk of complications in patients with type 2 diabetes (UKPDS 33). Lancet 352(9131):837–853

Welschen LMC, Bloemendal E, Nijpels G et al 2005 Self-monitoring of blood glucose in patients with type 2 diabetes who are not using insulin: a systematic review. Diabetes Care 28(6):1510–1517

Welsh Department of Health 2003 National service framework for diabetes standards in Wales. Online. Available: www.wales.nhs.uk/sites3/documents/334/diabetes-standards-wales.pdf

Cardiovascular risk reduction

Claire McDougall and Miles Fisher

INTRODUCTION

Diabetes is now one of the most common non-communicable diseases and poses one of the most challenging health problems worldwide. Modernisation and Westernisation of lifestyles are the underlying cultural processes driving the escalating diabetes epidemic. In 2000 the estimated worldwide prevalence of type 2 diabetes was 151 million adults, compared to 135 million in 1995 and 30 million in 1985 (Harris et al 1998). It is estimated that this prevalence will increase to 300 million people worldwide in 2025, with the steepest increases in rates of diabetes being in developing countries due to their rapidly changing economies and lifestyles (King et al 1998).

The burden of macrovascular disease in people with diabetes has been recognised for many years. It is well established that people with type 1 and type 2 diabetes have an increased risk of atherosclerotic cardiovascular disease (CVD). People with diabetes have a higher incidence of morbidity and mortality from coronary heart disease (CHD), and there is also evidence suggesting an increased risk of stroke and peripheral vascular disease in these people.

Epidemiological studies from around the world have confirmed the excessive cardiovascular morbidity and mortality in people with diabetes compared to non-diabetic subjects in the same geographical area over the same time period. Data from the Framingham cohort, in the USA (Kannel & McGee 1979), which first examined this issue, demonstrated an increase in CVD in people with diabetes compared to people who did not have diabetes in the study population.

There were higher rates of CHD, congestive cardiac failure, stroke, peripheral vascular disease and cardiovascular death within the subgroup of people with diabetes. Although this group was small, and there might have been discrepancies in the diagnostic criteria for diabetes, several other larger studies have mirrored these findings.

Another study from the USA (Wingard et al 1993) demonstrated the increased prevalence of coronary heart disease in different age groups. The rate of CHD was increased 14-fold in the 18–44-years age group, threefold in the 45–64-years age group and doubled in those people over the age of 65 years. Two further studies have also shown that whereas the *absolute* rates of CVD are higher in men with diabetes, the *relative* risk of CVD is higher in women with diabetes (Jousilahti et al 1999, Manson et al 1990), so it is sometimes stated that 'women with diabetes lose the protection of their gender'.

The age-adjusted mortality has also been shown to be greater in diabetic populations. A meta-analysis of ten observational studies (Lee et al 2000) revealed a relative risk of death of 1.9 for men and 2.6 for women, when compared with their non-diabetic counterparts.

The South Tees Mortality Study (Roper et al 2002) looked at death rates in a cohort of 4842 people with type 2 diabetes and found that one-quarter was dead within 6 years, the majority from cardiovascular causes. Cardiovascular mortality was significantly increased in both sexes and all age groups, but it was particularly evident in middle-aged women with diabetes. Relative death rates for age band 40 to 59 years were 5.47 and 5.60 for men and women, respectively.

Despite the accumulation of this evidence over the past three decades, reducing the risk of cardiovascular disease in the person with diabetes remains a major challenge. This chapter examines a multifactorial approach to reducing cardiovascular morbidity and mortality in the person with diabetes and includes detailed examination of several recent studies that have helped provide evidence for this approach.

GLYCAEMIC CONTROL

Controversy remains regarding the extent to which hyperglycaemia contributes to the high prevalence of CVD in people with type 1 and type 2 diabetes and there is relatively little convincing evidence to suggest that aggressively managing hyperglycaemia reduces cardiovascular risk in people with diabetes mellitus. One study in 1971 even suggested that, far from being protective, lowering plasma glucose using the sulphonylurea, tolbutamide, had toxic effects on the myocardium (University Group Diabetes Program 1970). Although this study has subsequently been criticised for poor study design and the results of other studies have contradicted this evidence, other controversial issues arose in this field in the 1980s. The association between elevated plasma insulin levels and coronary heart disease in insulin-resistant people, for example, led some investigators to suggest that insulin itself might be atherogenic, given that insulin stimulates both smooth muscle proliferation and lipid synthesis. Over the past decade, however, more evidence has been published that has further increased our understanding about the relationship between CVD and glycaemic control.

UNITED KINGDOM PROSPECTIVE DIABETES STUDY

The long-awaited results from the United Kingdom Prospective Diabetes Study (UKPDS) were published in 1998 (UKPDS Study Group 1998a, 1998b, 1998c, 1998d). This randomised, controlled trial of people newly diagnosed with type 2 diabetes refuted the suggestion that treatment with either sulphonylureas or insulin therapy was associated with increased cardiovascular risk (UKPDS Study Group 1998a). Subjects in the main study were randomised either to conventional treatment with diet or to intensive treatment with either sulphonylurea or insulin therapy. There was a significant reduction in HbA1c in the intensive treatment group and a 25% risk reduction in microvascular endpoints (neuropathy, nephropathy and retinopathy and need for laser treatment). However, despite small reductions in macrovascular endpoints, such as myocardial infarction (MI), these results did not reach statistical significance. These people have been followed for a few years since the end of the UKPDS and the reduction in MI with intensive treatment based on sulphonylureas or insulin therapy is now statistically significant.

Interestingly, a substudy from the UKPDS group in overweight individuals indicated that treatment with metformin led to a reduction in cardiovascular events, including MIs and diabetes-related deaths (UKPDS Study Group 1998b). Because MI was such a common cause of death in these individuals, the reduction in MIs was also mirrored by a reduction in total mortality. This unexpected finding was not fully anticipated by the UKPDS investigators and the results remain difficult to explain. The number of people receiving metformin was small ($n = 342$) and this might have exaggerated the degree of benefit. The reductions in events could not be explained on the basis of reductions in HbA1c, suggesting that metformin might have extended benefits that were not directly related to glucose-lowering effects of the drug. Metformin has a relatively minor effect in reducing insulin resistance at the level of the liver, and this is one possible explanation.

DIABETES CONTROL AND COMPLICATIONS TRIAL

The results of the Diabetes Control and Complications Trial (DCCT), a multicentre trial, which randomised 1141 people with type 1 diabetes to usual care or intensive insulin therapy, mirrored to some extent the findings from the UKPDS Study. There was a significant reduction in microvascular endpoints in the intensive treatment group compared to the conventionally treated group (DCCT Research Group 1995). Although there was a trend towards a reduction in cardiovascular disease in the intensive treated group, again this did not reach statistical significance. This might be due to the small number of events that actually occurred throughout the period of follow-up (40 in the control group; 23 in the treatment group), which is attributable to the young age of the population studied (13–39 years). A subsequent meta-analysis, including data from DCCT and several smaller studies, demonstrated a significant reduction in the number of macrovascular events, but no significant effect on the number of people developing macrovascular disease, or on macrovascular mortality (Lawson et al 1999).

Therefore, although the results from the UKPDS and DCCT trials were beneficial in so much as they proved that treatment with insulin or sulphonylureas reduced microvascular events and did not lead to an *increase* in cardiovascular disease, to date, no study has demonstrated that intensive management of hyperglycaemia reduces the risk of CHD. However, in addition to the evidence that metformin might reduce the incidence of macrovascular complications, the thiazolidinediones, a new group of oral agents, have also been shown to have extended benefits beyond glucose lowering, including favourable affects on blood pressure, lipids and microalbuminuria, as well as reductions in novel cardiovascular risk markers such as C-reactive protein (CRP) (Haffner et al 2002). Whether this translates into clinical benefit in terms of a reduction in cardiovascular events is currently being tested in large studies with rosiglitazone and pioglitazone, respectively.

Case study 8.1

Alan attends his GP's surgery for routine review. He is 52 years old, works as a taxi driver and takes no regular exercise. He is known to have hypertension and coronary heart disease, having suffered a myocardial infarct 2 years earlier. He is overweight, with a body mass index of 28, and he has hyperlipidaemia with elevation of triglycerides and total cholesterol, discovered when screened following his heart attack. His lipid profile results 18 months previously were: triglycerides 3.7 mmol/L, total cholesterol 7.9 mmol/L and HDL cholesterol 0.6 mmol/L. He has symptoms of peripheral vascular disease, with claudication after walking about 500 yards. Despite advice from his GP, Alan continues to eat a diet high in fat and he smokes 30 cigarettes per day. He drinks less than 10 units of alcohol per week.

Alan's present medications are: glyceryl trinitrate spray, isosorbide mononitrate, and atenolol for his angina along with bendroflumethiazide for hypertension control, aspirin 75 mg and simvastatin 20 mg.

At this GP attendance, Alan reports that he has noticed increasing tiredness over the past few months and more recently he has been more thirsty. His GP checks a urine sample, which confirms the presence of glycosuria, and a random blood glucose is measured at 18.2 mmol/L. Alan's blood pressure is measured at 166/94 mmHg. His HbA1c comes back at 8.8%, and his lipid profile shows a total cholesterol of 5.9 mmol/L and HDL cholesterol 0.8 mmol/L.

PRACTICAL ASPECTS OF GLUCOSE LOWERING THERAPY IN PEOPLE WITH DIABETES

Based on the results of the UKPDS, Alan should initially be treated with lifestyle measures. If, as is likely, he is unable to reach the target HbA1c with lifestyle measures alone, then metformin would be the drug of first choice. It would be helpful, however, to have an echocardiogram to be certain that he does not have cardiac failure, as this would be a contraindication to the use of metformin. An echocardiogram would also establish the best secondary preventive therapies. If significant left ventricular dysfunction is present, a thiazolidinedione is also contraindicated because of the side effect of fluid retention, so a sulphonylurea would be indicated.

DYSLIPIDAEMIA

Hyperlipidaemia is also a risk factor for atherosclerotic cardiovascular disease. In the general population, the Multiple Risk Factor Intervention Trial (MRFIT) demonstrated that the incidence of ischaemic events increases proportionally with elevations in serum low-density lipoprotein (LDL) cholesterol, and conversely with reductions in serum high-density lipoprotein (HDL) cholesterol concentrations (Stamler et al 1993). This study also showed that the absolute increase in risk of a cardiovascular event per unit rise in serum cholesterol was steeper in people with diabetes than in those without.

Well-controlled type 1 diabetes is associated with serum lipids similar to that of the general population. Poor glycaemic control, increasing age, obesity and the presence of nephropathy all lead to an increase in serum triglyceride and very low-density lipoprotein (VLDL) concentrations in type 1 diabetes. Type 2 diabetes is also associated with an unfavourable lipid profile; although the level of total and LDL cholesterol might be within normal limits, the HDL concentration tends to be low with elevated triglycerides. In addition, the distribution of LDL subfractions is altered so that small, dense LDL particles predominate and these are thought to be more atherogenic. This pattern of dyslipidaemia is also seen in those people without frank diabetes who have the 'metabolic syndrome' and who also have an increased risk of cardiovascular disease (see Chapter 4).

It is interesting to remember that as recently as 10 years ago lipid-lowering agents were thought to have few beneficial effects on cardiovascular mortality in the general population and the data from one meta-analysis even suggested that there was an increased risk of suicide and accidental death in people who were receiving lipid-lowering agents (Davey Smith & Pekkanen 1992). The advent of the HMG CoA reductase inhibitors (statins) revolutionised lipid-lowering therapy and the evidence that has emerged over the past decade for reducing serum total and LDL cholesterol is compelling and has dramatically changed clinical practice. This has included subgroup analysis of large studies containing many people with diabetes and, more recently, studies performed exclusively in people with diabetes.

SECONDARY PREVENTION STUDIES

Three major studies published in the 1990s, in which more than 15 000 people participated, looked at the issue of secondary prevention of atherosclerotic CVD using statin therapy: the Scandinavian Simvastatin Survival Study (4S) (Scandinavian Simvastatin Survival Study Group 1994), the Cholesterol and Recurrent Events (CARE) Trial (Sacks et al 1996) and the Long-term Intervention with Pravastatin in Ischaemic Disease (LIPID) Study (LIPID Study Group 1998).

Data from the 4S and CARE, which were conducted in the US and Canada, and from the LIPID Study, which was carried out in Australia and New Zealand, were consistent. Reducing LDL and total cholesterol is associated with reductions in all-cause mortality, CHD-related deaths and major coronary events (first MI, unstable angina). As a result, statin therapy in people with a history of coronary heart disease is normal practice.

PRIMARY PREVENTION STUDIES

Also in the 1990s, two large studies also examined the issue of the role of statins in the primary prevention of coronary heart disease. Data from the West of Scotland Coronary Prevention Study (WOSCOPS) and the Airforce/Texas Coronary Atherosclerosis Prevention Study (AFCAPS/TexCAPS) suggested that statin therapy was also of benefit in people with no history of CVD (Shepherd et al 1995, Downs et al 1998). People with a wide range of cardiovascular risk were included in these studies and all people appeared to benefit. Few people with diabetes were included in these studies so no meaningful analysis could be made of the data from these small subgroups.

However, despite the large numbers of people in these five studies, relatively few individuals with diabetes were included. A total of 2000 people with diabetes were included in these five cohorts and, until recently, clinical practice was based on data from these small diabetic subgroups. Over the last few years, however, further studies have been published that have greatly enhanced our knowledge of the effects of lipid-lowering in the population of people with diabetes.

The Heart Protection Study

The Heart Protection Study (HPS) was a large randomised study designed to address the question of whether lowering LDL cholesterol below previously accepted thresholds in people at high risk of cardiovascular disease would confer added benefit (Heart Protection Society Collaborative Group 2002). In particular, its aim was to study the effects of lipid lowering within subgroups for which there was limited existing evidence including people with diabetes, women, the elderly and those with non-coronary occlusive arterial disease.

There were 5963 people with diabetes within the study group and 90% of these were classified as having type 2 diabetes. There were highly significant reductions in serum total LDL cholesterol concentrations and a corresponding 22% reduction in first major vascular event in the simvastatin-treated group when compared to the placebo group. These figures are similar to the reductions seen with simvastatin in the non-diabetic, high-risk people studied.

An even greater reduction was seen in the group with diabetes but without previous coronary or occlusive vascular disease. A total of 2912 diabetic people had no cardiovascular disease and simvastatin reduced the primary endpoint of first major vascular event from 13.5% to 9.3%, and of first major coronary event from 6.5% to 3.7%. This effect was still seen regardless of age, sex, blood pressure, body mass index (BMI), HBA1c and, most importantly, initial LDL cholesterol, with similar levels of relative risk reduction in those with high serum cholesterol levels compared to those individuals with 'normal' cholesterol levels (Collins et al 2003).

ALLHAT-LLA and ASCOT-LLA

The Antihypertensive and Lipid-Lowering treatment to prevent Heart Attack Trial–Lipid Lowering Arm (ALLHAT-LLA) was a non-blinded, randomised study with one arm examining the benefits of cholesterol lowering with 40 mg of pravastatin in modestly hypertensive people with one or more coronary heart disease risk factors. The other arm of the study compared the effects of two different antihypertensive regimes (The ALLHAT Officers and Coordinators for the ALLHAT Collaborative Research Group 2002a).

In this trial, the primary endpoint of all-cause mortality was not altered significantly by treatment with pravastatin, unlike other primary prevention trials. There was a non-statistically significant reduction in rates of CHD and stroke. These rather disappointing results were thought to be due to a lower than average compliance rate in the treatment group (70–75%) and high use of open-label statins in the placebo group, leading to a smaller reduction in both total and LDL cholesterol than observed in the other large intervention trials. In total, 3638 people with type 2 diabetes took part in the study (35% of the cohort) and there were no differences in the rates of the primary or secondary endpoints in this subgroup.

Published shortly after ALLHAT in 2003, the Anglo-Scandinavian Cardiac Outcomes Trial – Lipid Lowering Arm (ASCOT-LLA) was a similarly designed study, again with one arm, looking at cholesterol lowering, this time with 10 mg of atorvastatin in people with hypertension and who were at high risk, but had no previous history of CHD (Sever et al 2003). The results of this study revealed a 36% reduction in non-fatal MI and fatal CHD in the active treatment group. However, treatment with atorvastatin in the subgroup with diabetes (25% of the total cohort) did not lead to a statistically significant reduction in primary endpoint. This might have been due to the higher use of open-label statins within the placebo group with diabetes than among the group who did not have diabetes.

Collaborative Atorvastatin Diabetes Study (CARDS)

Until very recently, no study had shown the benefits of cholesterol lowering in a cohort containing only individuals with diabetes. This evidence has now been provided by the Collaborative Atorvastatin Diabetes Study (CARDS), a multicentre, double-blind trial that examined the effects of cholesterol lowering in 2838 people with type 2 diabetes and low LDL-cholesterol (median 3.1 mmol/L) randomised to atorvastatin 10 mg/day or placebo (Colhoun et al 2004).

The study was stopped early in June 2003 when the second interim analysis showed a significant benefit in people taking atorvastatin. After a median follow-up of about 4 years, daily treatment with atorvastatin 10 mg reduced the risk of acute coronary events by 36% (absolute risk reduction 1.9%; $P = 0.013$) and stroke – the single biggest cause of disability among adults – was reduced by 48% (absolute risk reduction 1.3%; $P = 0.016$). Importantly, the benefit to people was observed irrespective of their LDL-cholesterol or triglyceride levels at the start of the study.

CARDS also reinforces the long-term safety profile of statins. The study showed no significant differences in treatment-related events or liver enzyme abnormalities and no cases of muscle symptoms or rhabdomyolysis. Discontinuation rates associated with treatment-related events were low in both groups.

SHOULD EVERYONE WITH DIABETES RECEIVE A STATIN?

These more recent studies add weight to the argument for treating people with diabetes with statins to reduce cardiovascular risk. Before the availability of these data, it was necessary to extrapolate data from the older studies to the population of people with diabetes in order that they could enjoy the benefits of lipid-lowering therapy. However, the issue of whether or not all people with diabetes should receive statin therapy remains controversial.

Some believe that everyone with type 2 diabetes should be treated as if they had pre-existing CHD, and one large study based on data from Finland suggested that a person with diabetes was at greater risk of suffering from a coronary event than a person without diabetes who has previously had a similar event (Haffner et al 1998). A similar study carried out in Tayside, however, has suggested that, while certainly at higher risk of CHD than the general population, people with diabetes without known cardiovascular disease are not more likely to suffer an event than a person who has pre-existing cardiovascular disease (Evans et al 2002). Several recent guidelines suggest that all people with diabetes are treated as a CHD equivalent, and so should be given a statin. Although all people with diabetes would gain from the widespread use of statins, the issues of cost and compliance need to be considered carefully before adopting such a 'blanket' prescribing policy.

A further issue that remains unresolved is the use of statins in people with type 1 diabetes. This group has a much higher incidence of CHD than their counterparts who do not have diabetes. Despite this, however, diabetes is usually diagnosed at a young age when the absolute incidence of CHD is negligible. The benefit of statin therapy in type 1 diabetes has not been proven given the very small numbers of these people included in statin trials. The timing of initiation of therapy also remains unresolved in people with type 1 diabetes, and there is still a need for further information regarding the benefits of statins in people with diabetes but who do not have CHD, particularly people with type 1 diabetes and younger people with type 2 diabetes.

A further cloudy issue in the management of dyslipidaemia is how far cholesterol should be lowered. Although the Heart Protection Study provided some indication as to target levels of cholesterol it was not specifically designed to identify this. A recent novel analysis of the reduction of CHD events with all forms of lipid-lowering therapy (Brady & Betteridge 2003) has shown that the lower the cholesterol the greater the reduction in CHD events, and the same is true for an analysis of the reduction of CHD events in people with diabetes. The Pravastatin or Atorvastatin Evaluation and Infection Therapy (PROVE-IT) Study (Cannon et al 2004) has demonstrated that high-dose atorvastatin is better than a less efficacious dose of pravastatin in reducing major cardiovascular events or death in patients with acute coronary syndromes; 18% of the cohort had diabetes but the reduction in diabetic subjects did not reach statistical significance.

OTHER DRUGS

Fibrates are also available as lipid-lowering therapy. They cause a reduction in serum triglycerides and elevations in HDL cholesterol with little impact on LDL cholesterol. Given that the major lipid abnormalities seen in people with diabetes are a reduction in HDL cholesterol and elevated serum triglycerides, it would seem likely that fibrates would be a more reasonable choice of lipid-lowering therapy in the person with diabetes. A randomised double-blind placebo-controlled trial has studied the effect of fibrates on progression of coronary artery disease in people with type 2 diabetes (Diabetes Atherosclerosis Intervention Study Investigators 2001) and demonstrated a 28% reduction in triglycerides and 6% increase in HDL cholesterol, with no significant change in LDL cholesterol. There was a significant reduction in coronary artery plaque progression in the fenofibrate-treated group compared to the placebo group. There was also a reduction in clinical endpoints in the treated group, although the study did not have statistical power to analyse these data. This is currently being examined in a larger randomised, prospective study of fenofibrate in people with diabetes examining harder cardiovascular end points.

The Veterans Affairs High-density lipoprotein cholesterol Intervention Trial (VA-HIT) Study Group carried out a randomised double-blind placebo controlled trial looking at the effect of treatment with gemfibrozil in 2500 men with established CHD and reduced HDL cholesterol and normal levels of LDL cholesterol (Rubins et al 1999). This cohort had a large diabetes subgroup. The study demonstrated that HDL cholesterol increased and triglycerides were significantly reduced in the gemfibrozil treated group. There was also a 22% relative risk reduction in primary endpoints in the treatment group and a 41% relative risk reduction in CHD related death in the subgroup of people with diabetes.

Although these studies look promising, larger studies looking at the effects of fibrates on clinical endpoints are necessary. No large study has looked at the combined effect of a fibrate and a statin and, although this might seem like the ideal combination in the person with diabetes, given the typical lipid profile, there are concerns regarding the safety of these agents in combination in terms of rhabdomyolysis.

Ezetimibe is a novel lipid-lowering agent that acts by selectively inhibiting cholesterol absorption without disrupting the absorption of fat soluble vitamins.

It reduces LDL cholesterol by 15–20% and is mainly used in people who are intolerant of statins (especially at higher doses), or as combination therapy in people who are failing to reach target serum cholesterol levels despite high dose statins.

PRACTICAL ASPECTS OF LIPID-LOWERING THERAPY IN PEOPLE WITH DIABETES

Based on the evidence described above, all people with diabetes with existing cardiovascular disease (coronary heart disease, cerebrovascular or peripheral vascular disease) should be treated with either simvastatin 40 mg or pravastatin 40 mg as a starting dose. People with diabetes without known cardiovascular disease should be treated with either simvastatin 40 mg or atorvastatin 10 mg if they are at high risk, and this will include nearly everyone over 40 years of age. Cholesterol targets should be at least less than 5.0 mmol/L in both situations, and can be lowered with time. The dose can be increased if the target cholesterol is not reached or the person's medication can be switched to rosuvastatin, which is a newer, more potent statin, a fibrate or ezetimibe can be added. Fibrates can also be added if raised triglycerides or a low HDL cholesterol is part of the problem, but the use of these drugs combined with a statin will usually be following advice from secondary care.

In our earlier case study, Alan has a history of MI and is already on simvastatin. His total cholesterol is not to target and the dose of simvastatin that was used in the most recent studies was higher. The first step would be to increase the simvastatin to 40 mg. If a repeat cholesterol is still not less than 5.0 mmol/L there are three treatment options: increase the simvastatin to 80 mg with possible side effects, switch to a more potent statin such as atorvastatin or rosuvastatin, or add ezetimibe.

Case study 8.2

Mumazza, an Asian woman aged 58, has presented to her GP with symptoms of thirst, polyuria and polydipsia. Her body mass index is 28 and blood pressure is 144/92 mmHg. She has no past medical history of note and takes no medications. Her mother had died at the age of 74, diabetes had been diagnosed in the months before her death. Mumazza is a non-smoker and takes no alcohol. Investigations confirmed the clinical suspicion of type 2 diabetes with a random blood glucose of 14.4 mmol/L and an HbA1c of 8.2%. Total cholesterol was 6.1 mmol/L with an HDL cholesterol of 0.9 mmol/L and triglycerides of 4.3 mmol/L. Mumazza was given dietary advice by a dietician, instruction in urine testing and reviewed 8 weeks later. At this review, she had lost weight and home urine testing was all negative. Her HbA1c was down to 6.8% and her blood pressure was 142/92 mmHg. Lipid estimation showed a total cholesterol of 5.2 mmol/L, HDL cholesterol of 1.0 mmol/L and triglycerides were 2.8 mmol/L. Mumazza has no known heart disease and her total cholesterol is only modestly increased. Nonetheless, her cardiovascular risk would be substantially reduced with either atorvastatin 10 mg or simvastatin 40 mg.

HYPERTENSION

Hypertension is commonly associated with both types 1 and 2 diabetes. It is estimated that 10–30% of people with type 1 diabetes and over 50% of people with type 2 diabetes are hypertensive, which is double the prevalence than in the general population. It is estimated that 40% of people with type 2 diabetes are hypertensive by the age of 45, this figure rising to 60% at 75 years (Hypertension in Diabetes Study (HDS) 1993a).

The pathophysiology of hypertension in diabetes is multifactorial, with issues such as alterations in vascular reactivity to pressor agents and changes in the renin–angiotensin system being thought to be responsible in type 1 diabetes. Although all these factors can also operate in type 2 diabetes, additional factors are at play, such as central obesity, renovascular disease and insulin resistance.

It is well known that there is an additive effect of coexistent hypertension on CHD outcomes in people with diabetes. Data from the Framingham Study suggested that people with type 2 diabetes and hypertension had a higher incidence of CHD than those with diabetes alone (Garcia et al 1974). This has been confirmed by two larger studies.

In the UKPDS cohort, 35% of men and 46% of women were hypertensive at the start of the study (although this is likely to be an underestimation given that hypertension was defined as a mean blood pressure of > 160/90 mmHg). It was noted that people with hypertension were three times more likely to have had a previous cardiovascular event (Hypertension in Diabetes Study (HDS) 1993a) and had a much greater prevalence of ECG features of coronary heart disease at entry to the study. Also, over 4.6 years of follow-up, the presence of hypertension predicted an increase in the incidence of cardiovascular events (Hypertension in Diabetes Study (HDS) 1993b).

The MRFIT Study (Stamler et al 1993) also demonstrated the synergistic effect of hypertension and diabetes on cardiovascular risk. Over 5000 men with diabetes participated in the study and were noted to have a mortality rate three times higher than their counterparts without diabetes. The presence of hypertension predicted CHD and stroke mortality, especially in those people who had hypercholesterolaemia or were smokers.

REDUCING BLOOD PRESSURE: THE EFFECT ON CARDIOVASCULAR DISEASE

A large number of studies dating back to the 1970s have looked at the issue of treating blood pressure in the context of reducing cardiovascular risk. Most of these studies were published in the late 1980s and confirmed that blood pressure reduction in the general population did indeed reduce the risk of coronary heart disease and stroke. Men and women of all ages were shown to benefit from blood-pressure reduction. The majority of these early studies used thiazide diuretics and beta-blockers.

Over the past few years, however, further studies have examined other issues in the treatment of hypertension. Two major trials looked at the effect of blood-pressure lowering on intensive targets. The Hypertension Optimal Treatment (HOT) Trial was designed to address the question of how far blood pressure should be lowered to achieve the most benefit in terms of cardiovascular disease, i.e. are there additional benefits or risks in lowering blood pressure to fully normotensive levels or is there little benefit in lowering diastolic blood pressure to below 90 mmHg (Hansson et al 1998)? Interestingly, although the study showed that reducing blood pressure to within normotensive limits did not confer any additional benefit in terms of cardiovascular morbidity in people without diabetes, this was not true for the subgroup of people who had diabetes, in whom additional benefit was seen (Hansson et al 1998). Indeed, it was observed in the subgroup of people with diabetes that active lowering to within normal limits conferred additional benefits. These results have formed the basis for most guidelines in treatment of hypertension in diabetes.

A further randomised controlled trial from the UKPDS Study, also published in 1998, randomised 1148 people with type 2 diabetes and hypertension to either tight or less tight blood pressure control. Data from this study (the Hypertension in Diabetes Study) confirmed the beneficial effects of tight blood pressure control on cardiovascular disease in people with type 2 diabetes (UKPDS Study Group 1998a).

The Losartan Intervention For Endpoint reduction in hypertension (LIFE) Trial (Dahlof et al 2002) compared losartan- and atenolol-based therapy in 9193 people with hypertension and left ventricular hypertrophy. The primary composite endpoint was cardiovascular death, MI and stroke. Losartan reduced the primary endpoint significantly, with significant reductions in stroke but not in MI or cardiovascular death. In all, 1195 people with pre-existing diabetes were included in the study, and the results were published separately (Lindholm et al 2002). In people with diabetes, losartan caused significant reductions in the composite endpoint and in cardiovascular and total mortality compared to atenolol, but the reduction in strokes and MI was not significant.

The Antihypertensive and Lipid-Lowering treatment to prevent Heart Attack Trial (ALLHAT) also set out to establish the relative benefit of various drugs in certain high-risk groups such as the elderly, black people and people with diabetes. A total of 33 357 participants (12 062 with type 2 diabetes) from North America, all of whom had at least one other risk factor for CVD, were randomly assigned to chlorthalidone, lisinopril, amlodipine or doxazosin (The ALLHAT Officers and Coordinators for the ALLHAT Collaborative Research Group 2002b). The doxazosin arm of the trial was discontinued early because there was a clear benefit of chlorthalidone over doxazosin. The main study revealed no significant differences between the groups in terms of the primary outcome measures of death due to CHD or non-fatal MI, with chlorthalidone being superior to lisinopril and amlodipine in terms of reduction in stroke, combined CHD and CVD.

CURRENT GUIDELINES AND LIMITATIONS

A large number of studies have therefore proved the efficacy and safety of all antihypertensive classes in people with diabetes (Table 8.1). A number of guidelines have been published in response to these data (Krans et al 1995, Ramsay

Table 8.1
Treatment of
hypertension in people
with diabetes

	Drug	Study
Of proven macrovascular benefit		
ACE inhibitors	captopril	CAPP
	enalapril	Syst-EUR
	fosinopril	FACET
	lisinopril	GISSI-3
Angiotensin receptor blockers	losartan	LIFE
Beta-blockers	atenolol	HDS
Calcium channel blockers	amlodipine	FACET
	felodipine	HOT
	nitrendipine	Syst-EURO
Diuretics	chlorthalidone	ALLHAT
	hydrochlorothiazide	MIDAS
Of uncertain macrovascular benefit		
Alpha-blockers	doxazosin	ALLHAT
Calcium channel blockers	isradipine	MIDAS
	nisoldipine	ABCD

et al 1999, The Joint National Committee on Prevention, Detection, Evaluation and Treatment of High Blood Pressure 1997). The majority of these suggest that clinicians aim for a target blood pressure of < 140/80 mmHg (some even lower) in people with diabetes. Although the evidence overwhelmingly suggests that this is the correct course of action, these targets are often very difficult to achieve. This was well demonstrated in the UKPDS/HDS studies in which, despite regular visits and intensive treatment with at least three agents in 29% of situations, only 56% of hypertensive individuals reached a target blood pressure of < 150/85 mmHg.

The UKPDS also examined the efficacy of different antihypertensive agents in reducing macrovascular and microvascular complications in type 2 diabetes (UKPDS Study Group 1998b). In this study, both captopril and atenolol were equally effective in reducing blood pressure and rates of macrovascular endpoints. It was previously perceived that beta-blockers might reduce hypoglycaemic awareness, although in practice this has not proved problematic. In both groups, however, approximately one-third of people required three or more antihypertensive agents. This highlights the fact that first choice of antihypertensive agent in this group is often academic, given that many agents have to be prescribed in a stepwise fashion, often leading to issues with adherence and polypharmacy. However, following the results of the ALLHAT Study, many clinicians would advocate using a thiazide diuretic as a first-line agent in treating hypertension in people with diabetes. Angiotensin-converting enzyme (ACE) inhibitors are also useful in people with diabetes because of their reno- and cardioprotective effects (see below). Calcium channel antagonists were thought to be unsafe in people with diabetes but the results of the HOT Trial, the Systolic Hypertension in Europe (SYST-EUR) Trial and from A Coronary disease Trial Investigating Outcome with Nifedipine gastrointestinal therapeutic system (ACTION) do not support this hypothesis (Poole-Wilson et al 2004).

PRACTICAL ASPECTS OF BLOOD PRESSURE LOWERING THERAPY IN PEOPLE WITH DIABETES

Based on the evidence described above, everyone with diabetes should have their blood pressure estimated at least once a year. People with a raised systolic blood pressure over 140 mmHg or a raised diastolic blood pressure over 90 mmHg should initially be offered lifestyle measures, but this is unlikely to be adequate by itself and often multiple hypotensive agents will be required. The early use of diuretics and either ACE inhibitors or angiotensin receptor antagonists is suggested; and calcium channel blockers, beta-blockers or alpha-blockers can be added at a later stage if targets are not reached or if patients cannot tolerate other agents.

Alan, presented earlier in case study 8.1 (p. 176), has treated hypertension that is not to target on a combination of a diuretic and a beta-blocker. The beta-blocker should be continued because Alan has established coronary heart disease. An ACE inhibitor should be added both to reduce blood pressure and for maximum cardioprotection (see below). Mumazza (case study 8.2, p. 182) has two blood pressure readings that are raised. If hypertension is confirmed on subsequent readings, an ACE inhibitor would be the drug of first choice, with the addition of a diuretic if targets were not reached.

NON-PHARMACOLOGICAL MEANS OF REDUCING BLOOD PRESSURE

It seems likely that, although there is no direct evidence that reducing blood pressure through lifestyle measures reduces the risk of CVD, these should be the first line of management in hypertension both in the general population and in people who have diabetes.

Excess body fat is the most important factor causing a predisposition to hypertension (Stamler 1991). Weight loss has been proven in a population with diabetes to reduce both insulin resistance and blood pressure (Su et al 1995) and should be encouraged in people with type 2 diabetes.

There is also a clear linear relationship between alcohol consumption, blood pressure levels and the prevalence of hypertension in populations, and people with diabetes and hypertension should be advised to limit their alcohol intake. In addition, lowering dietary salt intake has been shown to reduce the need for antihypertensive therapy (Whelton et al 1998), and such dietary advice should be offered.

PHARMACOLOGICAL TREATMENT OF CARDIOVASCULAR DISEASE

ACE INHIBITORS AND ANGIOTENSIN RECEPTOR BLOCKERS

ACE inhibitors were initially introduced for the treatment of hypertension, including people with diabetes. Subsequent studies demonstrated that ACE inhibitors had additional benefit in reducing the deterioration in renal function in people with type 1 diabetes with diabetic nephropathy. In the field of cardiology, they are now well established as treatment for congestive cardiac failure, improving both morbidity and mortality. An unexpected finding in several of the heart failure studies was that the use of ACE inhibitors was associated in a reduction in acute vascular events, including MIs. This subgroup analysis formed the rationale for the HOPE (Heart Outcomes Protection Evaluation) Study, in which people with existing cardiovascular disease, or people with diabetes with a high cardiovascular risk, were treated with ramipril or placebo (Heart Outcomes Prevention Evaluation (HOPE) Study Investigators 2000). At the end of 5 years, there were significant reductions in stroke, MI and cardiovascular death in the active treatment group.

However, the HOPE study has been severely criticised. Significant differences were seen when blood pressures in the ramipril and control groups were compared, leading some commentators to suggest that the benefit was due to aggressive blood-pressure lowering, similar to levels attained in HOT and UKPDS, in a high-risk group of individuals. Similar results were seen in the EURopean trial On reduction of cardiac events with Perindopril in stable coronary Artery disease (EUROPA) study (EUROPA Investigators 2003). The blood-pressure differences between perindopril and placebo in the EUROPA Study were if anything greater than those seen in HOPE Study. The EUROPA study thus confirms a cardioprotective and vasculoprotective effect of ACE inhibitors in high-risk individuals, including people with diabetes, but does not exclude blood-pressure lowering as a possible mechanism.

Similar benefits in terms of reductions in cardiovascular outcomes have not been shown using angiotensin receptor antagonists (ARAs). Two studies have examined these drugs in people with type 2 diabetes and established diabetic nephropathy (Brenner et al 2001, Lewis et al 2001). Neither of these studies showed an effect on cardiovascular deaths, although both showed that irbesartan and losartan slowed the rate of renal impairment in type 2 diabetes. Should we therefore treat people with type 2 diabetes with ACE inhibitors for cardioprotection and probable renal protection, or should we treat them with ARAs for renal protection and possible cardioprotection? Until well-designed studies have compared ACE inhibitors with ARAs for cardiovascular outcomes, this cannot be answered. From a practical point of view, however, all people with diabetes with existing cardiovascular disease should be treated with an ACE inhibitor, and ACE inhibitors or ARAs provide a firm base for the treatment of hypertension in people with diabetes without existing cardiovascular disease, as described above.

ANTIPLATELET AGENTS

The role of aspirin in the secondary prevention of cardiovascular disease is well established, as in Alan's case presented above. There is much evidence to suggest that treatment with low-dose aspirin in people with or without diabetes with angina reduces the risk of vascular events.

The most convincing evidence of the benefits of aspirin in secondary prevention is the large meta-analysis performed by the Antiplatelet Trialists' Collaboration. This included 29 trials in high-risk people with separate information on diabetes status (Antiplatelet Trialists' Collaboration 1994). The rate of cardiovascular events, including MI, was reduced from 22% to 18% in people with diabetes, and from 16% to 13% in those without diabetes. Similarly, 20% of the people in the Clopidogrel versus Aspirin in Patients at Risk of Ischaemic Events (CAPRIE) Study of clopidogrel had prior diabetes, and the benefit if anything was greater in those individuals with diabetes (CAPRIE Steering Committee 1996).

The evidence for the use of aspirin in the primary prevention of cardiovascular disease is not as clear as in Mumazza's situation (case study 8.2). Two trials published in the 1980s had conflicting results, one suggesting that aspirin was very effective in reducing the risk of first MI, the other demonstrating no benefit (Peto et al 1988, Steering Committee of the Physicians' Health Study Research Group 1989). In the HOT Trial, people were also treated with 75 mg of aspirin or a placebo in addition to their hypotensive therapy. People who received aspirin had a significant reduction in cardiovascular events. It was reported that the relative benefit was similar in people with diabetes, although the specific data for those with diabetes were not provided.

Again from a practical point of view, all people with diabetes and existing cardiovascular disease should be treated with aspirin or clopidogrel; in a small number of individuals both will be used together following an acute coronary syndrome. Most current guidelines suggest the use of aspirin for primary prevention based on risk-table estimations. However, it is unclear how accurate these charts are at calculating the coronary risk in people with diabetes, given that the tables were based on the Framingham data, in which people with diabetes were under-represented. New tables are being devised also taking into account novel risk factors, such as presence of microalbuminuria, which were not previously accounted for.

OBESITY

It is clear that abdominal obesity is closely related with diabetes mellitus. The risk of developing type 2 diabetes increases exponentially with increasing BMI. Individuals with a BMI of 21 are at least risk of developing the condition, whereas the relative risk of those with a BMI > 35 is approximately 100 (Bjorntorp 1991).

Obesity has always been associated with coronary heart disease. Until recently, the role of obesity as an independent risk factor remained controversial because of its co-existence with other traditional risk factors such as diabetes, hypertension and dyslipidaemia. However, several long-term studies have demonstrated that obesity should be considered as an independent risk factor for CVD, and these findings have led to the American Heart Association reclassifying obesity as a modifiable risk factor for coronary heart disease (Jousilahti et al 1999, Manson et al 1990).

As well as reducing the risk of developing diabetes, there is now observational evidence that significant weight loss (approximately 10 kg) in an obese individual is associated with dramatic risk reductions in morbidity and mortality and weight loss in people with diabetes has been shown to increase life expectancy. This approach is now being formally tested in a large, prospective study in the US that is projected to last for at least 10 years.

CONCLUSION

Atherosclerotic cardiovascular disease is a major cause of premature morbidity and mortality in people with diabetes. Appropriate treatment with hypoglycaemic agents, antihypertensive therapy including ACE inhibitors, lipid-lowering therapy, and antiplatelet therapy can reduce or delay the onset of macrovascular disease in people with diabetes.

REFERENCES

ALLHAT Officers and Coordinators for the ALLHAT Collaborative Research Group 2002a Major outcomes in moderately hypercholesterolaemic, hypertensive patients randomized to pravastatin vs usual care. The Antihypertensive and Lipid-Lowering Treatment to Prevent Heart Attack Trial (ALLHAT-LLT). Journal of the American Medical Association 288:2998–3007

ALLHAT Officers and Coordinators for the ALLHAT Collaborative Research Group 2002b Major outcomes in high-risk hypertensive patients randomized to angiotensin-converting enzyme inhibitor or calcium channel blocker vs diuretic. The Antihypertensive and Lipid-Lowering Treatment to Prevent Heart Attack Trial (ALLHAT). Journal of the American Medical Association 283:2981–2997

Antiplatelet Trialists' Collaboration 1994 Collaborative overview of randomised trials of antiplatelet therapy-I: Prevention of death, myocardial infarction, and stroke by prolonged antiplatelet therapy in various categories of patients. British Medical Journal 308:81–106

Bjorntorp P 1991 Metabolic implications of body fat distribution. Diabetes Care 14:1132–1143

Brady AJB, Betteridge DJ 2003 Prevalence and risks of undertreatment with statins. British Journal of Cardiology 10:218–219

Brenner BM, Cooper ME, de Zeeuw D et al for the RENAAL Study Investigators 2001 Effects of losartan on renal and cardiovascular outcomes in patients with type 2 diabetes and nephropathy. New England Journal of Medicine 345:861–869

Cannon CP, Braunwald E, McCabe CH et al for the Pravastatin or Atorvastatin Evaluation and Infection Therapy – Thrombolysis in Myocardial Infaction (22 investigators) 2004 Intensive versus moderate lipid lowering with statins after acute coronary syndromes. New England Journal of Medicine 350:1495–1504

CAPRIE Steering Committee 1996 A randomised, blinded trial of clopidogrel versus aspirin in patients at risk of ischaemic events (CAPRIE). Lancet 348:1329–1339

Colhoun HM, Betteridge DJ, Durrington PN et al on behalf of the CARDS investigators 2004 Primary prevention of cardiovascular disease with atrovastatin in type 2 diabetes in the Collaborative Atorvastatin Diabetes Study (CARDS): multicentre randomised placebo-controlled trial. Lancet 364:685–696

Collins R, Armitage J, Parish S et al for the Heart Protection Study Collaborative Group 2003 MRC/BHF Heart Protection Study of cholesterol-lowering with simvastatin in 5963 people with diabetes: a randomised placebo-controlled trial. Lancet 361:2005–2016

Dahlof B, Devereux RB, Kjeldsen Se et al for the LIFE Study Group 2002 Cardiovascular morbidity and mortality in the losartan intervention for endpoint reduction in hypertension study (LIFE): a randomised trial against atenolol. Lancet 359:995–1003

Davey Smith G, Pekkanen J 1992 Should there be a moratorium on the use of cholesterol lowering drugs? British Medical Journal 304(6842):431–434

Diabetes Atherosclerosis Intervention Study Investigators 2001 Effect of fenofibrate on progression of coronary-artery disease in type 2 diabetes: the Diabetes Athersclerosis Intervention Study, a randomised study. Lancet 357: 905–910

Diabetes Control and Complications Trial (DCCT) Research Group 1995 Effect of intensive diabetes management on macrovascular events and risk factors in the Diabetes Control and Complications Trial. American Journal of Cardiology 75: 894–903

Downs JR, Clearfield M, Weiss S et al 1998 Primary prevention of acute coronary events with lovastatin in men and women with average cholesterol levels: results of the AFCAPS/TexCAPS Air Force/Texas Coronary Atherosclerosis Prevention Study. Journal of the American Medical Association 279: 1615–1622

European Trial on Reduction of Cardiac Events with Perindopril in Stable Coronary Artery Disease (EUROPA) Investigators 2003 Efficacy of perindopril in reduction of cardiovascular events among patients with stable coronary artery disease. Lancet 362:782–788

Evans JM, Wang J, Morris AD 2002 Comparison of cardiovascular risk between patients with type 2 diabetes and those who had had a myocardial infarction: cross sectional and cohort studies. British Medical Journal 324: 939–942

Garcia MJ, McNamara PM, Gordon T, Kannel WB 1974 Morbidity and mortality in diabetics in the Framingham population. Sixteen year follow-up study. Diabetes 23(2):105–111

Haffner SM, Greenberg AS, Weston WM et al 2002 Effect of rosiglitazone treatment on non-traditional markers of cardiovascular disease in patients with type 2 diabetes mellitus. Circulation 106: 679–684

Haffner SM, Lehto S, Ronnemaa T et al 1998 Mortality from coronary heart disease in subjects with type 2 diabetes and in nondiabetic subjects with and without prior myocardial infarction. New England Journal of Medicine 339: 229–234

Hansson L, Zanchetti A, Carruthers SG et al for the HOT Study Group 1998 Effects of intensive blood-pressure lowering and low-dose aspirin in patients with hypertension: principal results of the Hypertension Optimal Treatment (HOT) randomised trial. Lancet 351:1755–1762

Harris, MI, Flegal KM, Cowie CC et al 1998 Prevalence of diabetes, impaired fasting glucose, and impaired glucose tolerance in U.S. adults: the Third National Health and Nutrition Survey, 1988–1994. Diabetes Care 21:518–524

Heart Outcomes Prevention Evaluation (HOPE) study investigators 2000 Effects of ramipril on cardiovascular and microvascular outcomes in people with diabetes mellitus: results of the HOPE study and MICRO-HOPE substudy. Lancet 355:253–259

Heart Protection Study Collaborative Group 2002 MRC/BHF Heart Protection Study of cholesterol lowering with simvastatin in 20,536 high-risk individuals: a randomised placebo-controlled trial. The Lancet 360:7–22

Hypertension in Diabetes Study (HDS) 1993a Hypertension in diabetes study (HDS) I. Prevalence of hypertension in newly presenting type 2 diabetic patients and the association with risk factors for cardiovascular and diabetic complications. Journal of Hypertension 11(3):309–317

Hypertension in Diabetes Study (HDS) 1993b Hypertension in diabetes study (HDS) II. Increased risk of cardiovascular complications in hypertensive type 2 diabetic patients. Journal of Hypertension 11(3):319–325

Joint National Committee on Prevention, Detection, Evaluation and Treatment of High Blood Pressure 1997 The sixth report of the Joint National Committee on prevention, detection, evaluation and treatment of high blood pressure. Archives of Internal Medicine 157:2413–2446

Jousilahti P, Vartiainen E, Tuomilehto S, Puska P 1999 Sex, age, cardiovascular risk factors, and coronary heart disease: a prospective follow-up study of 14 786 middle-aged men and women in Finland. Circulation 99(9):1165–1172

Kannel WB, McGee DL 1979 Diabetes and cardiovascular disease. The Framingham study. Journal of the American Medical Association 241:2035–2038

King H, Aubert RE, Herman WH 1998 Global burden of diabetes, 1995–2025: prevalence, numerical estimates, and projections. Diabetes Care 21:1414–1431

Krans HMJ, Porta M, Keen H, Staehr Johansen K (eds) 1995 Diabetes care and research in Europe: the St Vincent declaration action programme. Implementation document, 2nd edn. Guidelines on cardiovascular disease and stroke. World Health Organisation, Copenhagen

Lawson ML, Gerstein HC, Tsui E, Zinman B 1999 Effect of intensive therapy on early macrovascular disease in young individuals with type 1 diabetes. A systematic review and meta-analysis. Diabetes Care 22(suppl 2):B35–B39

Lee WL, Cheung AM, Cape D, Zinman B 2000 Impact of diabetes on coronary artery disease in women and men: a meta-analysis of prospective studies. Diabetes Care 23:962–968

Lewis EJ, Hunsicker LG, Clarke WR et al for the Collaborative Study Group 2001 Renoprotective effect of the angiotensin-receptor antagonist irbesartan in patients with nephropathy due to type 2 diabetes. New England Journal of Medicine 345:851–860

Lindholm LH, Ibsen H, Dahlof B et al for the LIFE study group 2002 Cardiovascular morbidity and mortality in patients with diabetes in the Losartan Intervention For Endpoint reduction in hypertension study (LIFE): a randomised trial against atenolol. Lancet 359:1004–1010

Long-Term Intervention with Pravastatin in Ischaemic Disease (LIPID) Study Group 1998 Prevention of cardiovascular events and death with pravastatin in patients with coronary heart disease and a broad range of initial cholesterol levels. New England Journal of Medicine 339:1349–1357

Manson JE, Colditz GA, Stampfer MJ et al 1990 A prospective study of obesity and risk of coronary heart disease in women. New England Journal of Medicine 322:882–889

Peto R, Gray R, Collins R et al 1988 Randomised trial of prophylactic daily aspirin in British male doctors. British Medical Journal 296:313–316

Poole-Wilson PA, Lubsen J, Kirwan BA et al on behalf of the ACTION (A Coronary disease Trial Investigating Outcome with Nifedipine gastrointestinal therapeutic system) investigators 2004 Effect of long-acting nifedipine on mortality and cardiovascular morbidity in patients with stable angina requiring treatment (ACTION trial): randomised controlled trial. Lancet 364:849–857

Ramsay LE, Williams B, Johnson GD et al 1999 Guidelines for management of hypertension: report of the third working party of the British Hypertension Society. Journal of Human Hypertension 13:569–592

Roper NA, Bilous RW, Kelly WF et al 2002 Cause-specific mortality in a population with diabetes. South Tees Diabetes Mortality Study. Diabetes Care 25:43–48

Rubins HB, Robins SJ, Collins D et al for the Veterans Affairs High-Density Lipoprotein Cholesterol Intervention Trial Study Group 1999 Gemfibrozil for the secondary prevention of coronary heart disease in men with low levels of high-density lipoprotein cholesterol. New England Journal of Medicine 341:410–418

Sacks FM, Pfeffer MA, Moye LA et al for the Cholesterol and Recurrent Events Trial investigators 1996 The effect of pravastatin on coronary events after myocardial infarction in patients with average cholesterol levels. New England Journal of Medicine 335:1001–1009

Scandinavian Simvastatin Survival Study Group 1994 Randomised trial of cholesterol lowering in 4444 patients with coronary heart disease: the Scandinavian Simvastatin Survival Study (4S). Lancet 344:1383–1389

Sever PS, Dahlöf B, Poulter NR et al for the ASCOT investigators 2003 Prevention of coronary and stroke events with atorvastatin in hypertensive patients who have average or lower-than-average cholesterol concentrations, in the Anglo-Scandinavian Cardiac Outcomes Trial-Lipid Lowering Arm (ASCOT-LLA): a multicentre randomised controlled trial ASCOT-LLA. Lancet 361:1149–1158

Shepherd J, Cobbe SM, Ford I et al for the West of Scotland Coronary Prevention Study Group (WOSCOPS) 1995 Prevention of coronary heart disease with pravastatin in men with hypercholesterolemia. New England Journal of Medicine 333:1301–1307

Stamler J 1991 Epidemiologic findings on body mass and blood pressure in adults. Annals of Epidemiology 1(4):347–632

Stamler J, Vaccaro O, Neaton JD, Wentworth D 1993 Diabetes, other risk factors and 12-year cardiovascular mortality for men in the Multiple Risk Factors Intervention Trial (MRFIT). Diabetes Care 16:434–444

Steering Committee of The Physicians' Health Study Research Group 1989 Final report on the aspirin component of the ongoing Physicians' Health Study. New England Journal of Medicine 321:129–135

Su HY, Sheu WH, Chin HM et al 1995 Effect of weight loss on blood pressure and insulin resistance in normotensive and hypertensive obese individuals. American Journal of Hypertension 8(11):1067–1071

UK Prospective Diabetes Study (UKPDS) Study Group 1998a Tight blood pressure control and risk of macrovascular and microvascular complications in type 2 diabetes (UKPDS 38). British Medical Journal 317:703–713

UK Prospective Diabetes Study (UKPDS) Study Group 1998b. Efficacy of atenolol and captopril in reducing risk of macrovascular and microvascular complications in type 2 diabetes (UKPDS 39). British Medical Journal 317:713–720

UK Prospective Diabetes Study (UKPDS) Study Group 1998c Intensive blood-glucose control with sulphonylureas or insulin compared with conventional treatment and risk of complications in patients with type 2 diabetes (UKPDS 33). Lancet 352:837–853

UK Prospective Diabetes Study (UKPDS) Study Group 1998d Effect of intensive blood-glucose control with metformin on complications in overweight patients with type 2 diabetes (UKPDS 34). Lancet 352:854–865

University Group Diabetes Program 1970 A study of the effects of hypoglycemic agents on vascular complications in patients with adult-onset diabetes mellitus II. Mortality results. Diabetes 19(suppl 2):789–830

Whelton PK, Appel LJ, Espeland MA et al 1998 Sodium reduction and weight loss in the treatment of hypertension in older persons: a randomized controlled trial of nonpharmacologic interventions in the elderly (TONE). TONE Collaborative Research Group. Journal of the American Medical Association 279(11):839–846

Wingard DL, Barret-Connor EL et al 1993 Prevalence of cardiovascular and renal complications in older adults with normal or impaired glucose tolerance or NIDDM. A population-based study. Diabetes Care 16(7):1022–1025

Microvascular disease

Eugene Hughes

Case study 9.1

Diana is a 42-year-old married woman with type 1 diabetes. She has recently moved into the area and applies to join a new GP practice. She makes an appointment to see the GP as she has developed tingling and numbness in both her feet. She complains of a burning discomfort in her legs that is worse during the night and prevents her from sleeping.

Diana has had diabetes for almost 20 years and is on a twice-daily regime of a fixed mixture of insulin (soluble and isophane). She says that her diabetes is satisfactorily controlled and she never has any problems with hypoglycaemia. In conversation, it is clear that she rarely monitors her blood glucose and has not attended a diabetic clinic for more than 8 years. Her previous GP did not run a diabetic clinic and she has not received any screening for diabetic complications during this period of time. Diana's GP finds that her blood glucose is measured at 14.6 mmol/L and her long-term control has been suboptimal indicated by an HbA1c of 10.2%. Diana states that she has never smoked and drinks only three units of alcohol per week.

On examination, Diana has reduced sensation to both light touch and pin-prick testing to mid-calf level in both legs. Her blood pressure is noted to be elevated at 165/95 mmHg; both her urea and creatinine are also elevated at 15.8 mmol/L and 270 micromol/L, respectively. Diana is referred to the local eye-screening clinic and advanced background retinopathy is confirmed.

Diana, after living with diabetes for nearly 20 years, has now developed some of the complications of diabetes namely hypertension, retinopathy, nephropathy and neuropathy. Diana's hypertension would be managed according to the recommendations in Chapter 8.

INTRODUCTION

Microvascular disease occurs in people with both type 1 diabetes and type 2 diabetes. The hallmark of diabetic microvascular disease is microangiopathy (small vessel disease). This is the underlying abnormality that leads to retinopathy, nephropathy and neuropathy.

In microangiopathy, thickening of the capillary basement membrane leads to increased capillary permeability at an early stage. The development of microangiopathy is intricately linked with hyperglycaemia, and the duration of hyperglycaemia is an important determinant of microvascular disease. Individuals with type 1 diabetes can survive for many years without showing any signs of microvascular disease, particularly if they have optimal glycaemic control. Those with type 2 diabetes tend to be older at presentation and, even though they commonly have features of microvascular disease, it is ultimately macrovascular disease that leads to their untimely death. The exact biochemical mechanism of microvascular disease is not within the remit of this chapter; however, the central mechanism appears to relate to the sorbitol pathway. Hyperglycaemia leads to increased accumulation of sorbitol which does not easily cross cell membranes. The biochemical consequences of this directly affect the proteins in the vessel walls (Williams & Pickup 2004).

Diabetic microvascular disease is associated with the development of complications in people with both type 1 and type 2 diabetes. This section discusses the following microvascular complications:

- diabetic retinopathy
- diabetic nephropathy
- diabetic neuropathy
- autonomic neuropathy
- erectile dysfunction (impotence).

For each of these complications, the prevalence, pathological features, screening, protocols for early referral and – where relevant – the implications of the national service framework for diabetes and the general medical services contract for primary care will be considered (Kenny 2004).

DIABETIC RETINOPATHY

THE FACTS

- Diabetes is the most common cause of blindness in people aged 30–69 years and the most common cause of blindness in the working population of developed countries (Cormack et al 2001, Icks et al 1997).

- At the time of diagnosis of type 2 diabetes, 25% of people have a background retinopathy.
- 2% of the UK diabetes population are registered blind.
- The condition is treatable by laser photocoagulation.

FACTORS INFLUENCING THE DEVELOPMENT OF RETINOPATHY

- The duration of diabetes.
- The presence of hypertension.
- The development of chronic renal failure.
- The level of glycaemic control.
- Lifestyle factors including smoking and alcohol.
- Race as it is more common in certain ethnic groups.

It is clear from Diana's case study that she meets three of these: diabetes for almost 20 years; hypertension and poor glycaemic control.

CLASSIFICATION

Diabetic retinopathy is graded into four main categories, depending on the extent of the disease seen on fundal examination.

BACKGROUND RETINOPATHY

As capillaries close, the retina becomes underperfused with blood. Surrounding capillaries dilate in response to this and microaneurysms form. These tiny pin-head red dots are the first lesions to be seen in developing retinopathy. Dilated capillaries are usually leaky and proteinaceous material escapes forming creamy yellow exudates (hard exudates) on the retinal surface. Large blot haemorrhages tend to form at the interface of the well-perfused and ischaemic areas of the retina (Fig. 9.1).

ADVANCED BACKGROUND RETINOPATHY

If extensive leakage from capillaries occurs around the macula, macular oedema develops. As the macula is involved with central vision, oedema of this area can markedly impair vision. The person will usually complain of blurring of vision, particularly central vision, which is used when reading. As more and more capillaries become occluded, large areas of the retina become ischaemic and cotton wool spots (or soft exudates) develop at sites of retinal microinfarction. The veins of the retina also begin to dilate. The veins form loops or show beading and reduplication. The presence of cotton wool spots and venous changes suggest that new vessel formation is imminent. Approximately one-third of people will develop new blood vessel

Fig. 9.1
Fluorescein angiogram
of the retina

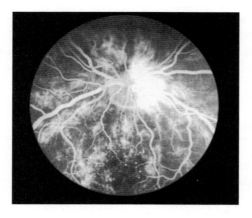

formation within the next 2 years and progress to proliferative retinopathy. People with advanced background retinopathy should therefore be referred to an ophthalmology clinic. Diana was found to have this when she underwent screening.

PROLIFERATIVE RETINOPATHY

Ischaemic areas of the retina subsequently give rise to new blood vessel formation. These new vessels usually arise from veins in the retinal periphery or on the optic disc. At first they lie on the surface of the retina but eventually they grow forwards, attaching themselves to the posterior surface of the vitreous, which lies immediately in front of the retinal surface. As the vitreous detaches, it pulls on the new vessels, causing them to rupture and haemorrhage. Haemorrhaging into the vitreous causes sudden loss of vision as the blood prevents light reaching the retina behind. Vitreous haemorrhages usually clear gradually over a period of days or weeks with vision slowly recovering. Urgent referral to an ophthalmologist is recommended.

ADVANCED RETINOPATHY

Repeated vitreous haemorrhages stimulate fibrous tissue proliferation. Fibrous strands arising in relation to new vessels begin to contract and as this process gradually progresses, the retina become detached with resulting loss of vision.

COMPONENTS OF RETINOPATHY

- Small, round microaneurysms: dots.
- Medium-sized haemorrhages: blots.
- Hard exudates: irregular yellow lipid deposits.
- Cotton wool spots: white indistinct ischaemic areas.
- New vessels: fine tangled loops of vessels.

SUMMARY OF CLASSIFICATION AND APPEARANCES

Background retinopathy
- Microaneurysms.
- Dot and blot haemorrhages.
- Hard exudates.
- Cotton wool spots.

Preproliferative retinopathy
- All of the above plus venous beading and looping and larger haemorrhages.

Proliferative retinopathy
- New vessels at the disc or in the periphery.
- Increased fibrosis.
- Retinal detachment.

Maculopathy
- Ischaemia or oedema of the macula area.

SCREENING AND PREVENTION

Prevention of diabetic blindness is possible in most people as long as treatment is initiated early. As the initial features of retinopathy are symptomless, screening is worthwhile and effective at detecting this and should be started from the age of 12 years (Scottish Intercollegiate Guidelines Network (SIGN) 55 2001). In Diana's case, she had not had any eye screening for at least 8 years and it was fortunate that only background retinopathy was found.

Impaired vision is an early feature of maculopathy and can develop before any retinal changes are evident on ophthalmoscopic examination. A fall in visual acuity is therefore the first sign of serious maculopathy developing. By contrast, people with proliferative retinopathy will be unaware of any eye problem until a vitreous haemorrhage occurs, which causes a sudden loss of vision. By this stage retinopathy will be advanced and difficult to treat effectively. It is evident therefore that any screening programme must include both the routine measurement of visual acuity and fundoscopy or retinal photography (SIGN 2001).

VISUAL ACUITY

Distance vision is measured with a well illuminated Snellen chart at 6 metres. Each eye is tested separately, while the other eye is covered with a card. Visual acuity is quoted as the smallest letters that can be read. Thus, if a person can only read at 6 metres letters that should normally be read at 24 metres, visual acuity is recorded as 6/24. Normal vision is 6/6 but those with long sight and young people can often manage 6/5 or 6/4. Vision deteriorates with age and 6/9 vision is not necessarily abnormal in the elderly. If no letters can be read, the ability to count fingers (CF), identify hand movements (HM) or perceive light (PL), should be tested and recorded. Vision should be tested with the person wearing glasses if these are normally used for distance. If vision is impaired, the test should be repeated viewing the chart through a hole punched in a card (a pinhole). This partially corrects refractive errors. The best acuity measurement for each eye should be recorded.

Tests of reading ability using cards with varying sizes of script test central vision and are therefore particularly sensitive to macula changes.

FUNDAL EXAMINATION

Fundoscopy should be carried out only by doctors with training and experience of looking at the eyes of people with diabetes. For this reason, most GPs prefer to send individuals with diabetes to an ophthalmology clinic for retinal examination. In some areas of the UK, local opticians have been trained in assessing diabetic fundi and are used in screening programmes.

To obtain full and clear views of the retina, it is necessary for the pupils to be dilated by using mydriatic drops. Tropicamide (0.5% or 1%) one drop in each eye with phenylephrine hydrochloride 2.5% one drop in each eye (added after to maximise dilatation) are the most suitable agents because they act rapidly and wear off within 6 hours. There is little to be gained from reversing the dilatation using pilocarpine after the consultation. Drops are usually initiated by nursing staff, who should first check that the person does not suffer from glaucoma. The person should be advised previously that an eye examination will happen and warned that his or her vision may remain blurred and/or sensitive to light for up to 6 hours after the examination. Individuals might need to wear dark glasses and driving during this period is not recommended.

The examination should take place in a suitably darkened room using an ophthalmoscope with a fully charged battery providing adequate illumination.

In the UK a national retinal screening program is underway using non-mydriatic digital retinal cameras. Administrative call and recall procedures link diabetes registers to the precess where trained screeners and graders offer a quality assured service.

RETINAL PHOTOGRAPHY

Retinal screening by ophthalmoscopy should be considered the bare minimum standard of screening. Retinal photography as part of a local or regional scheme should be accessible to most people with diabetes. The National Service Frameworks for Diabetes recommended that retinal screening programmes be put into place throughout the UK by 2006. Leese et al (2005) found that robust screening resulted in more appropriate referrals to ophthalmologists. Digital retinopathy with assessment and a grading is likely to become the gold standard in most areas. This has the advantage of being able to store and compare images with successive assessments. Digital photographs can also be used for telemedicine in remote and rural areas where there is robust quality assurance it is practical and advantageous (Schneider et al 2005). Criteria for referral to ophthalmologist are detailed in Box 9.1.

GENERAL MEASURES FOR PREVENTION AND TREATMENT

As for all microvascular and macrovascular complications, improving clinical and lifestyle factors will help prevent the onset and deterioration of diabetes complications (Diabetes Control and Complications Trial (DCCT) 1993):

- tight glycaemic control
- tight blood pressure control
- tight lipid control
- smoking cessation.

SPECIFIC TREATMENT

Photocoagulation

Laser photocoagulation is particularly effective in preventing visual loss due to new vessel formation. To be effective it must be given early. In 90% of people the new vessels disappear or become insignificant. In ischaemic maculopathy, treatment is less effective. However, in clinically significant macula oedema, laser treatment has

---

Box 9.1
Criteria for referral to an ophthalmologist

Routine referral

- Cataract
- Non-proliferative retinopathy

Early referral

- Preproliferative changes
- Retinal haemorrhages and perimacular hard exudates
- Decreasing visual acuity (because this might indicate maculopathy)

Urgent referral

- New vessels
- Rubeosis iridis

Immediate referral

- Vitreous haemorrhage
- Neovascular glaucoma
- Advanced diabetic eye disease including retinal detachment

been show to be beneficial (SIGN 2001). For proliferative retinopathy, photocoagulation is applied to a larger area of the retina (pan retinal photocoagulation). This can involve between 1500 and 7000 separate burns and can be performed over several sessions of outpatient treatment, following the application of topical local anaesthetic drops. Some people experience mild discomfort with this procedure. If severe discomfort is experienced, retrobulbar local anaesthetic can be given. The underlying principle of photocoagulation is that it halts deterioration; it might not lead to improved visual acuity.

WHAT IT ALL MEANS TO THE INDIVIDUAL WITH DIABETES

Whereas healthcare professionals seek to detect and treat diabetic retinopathy at various stages, the reality of diabetic eye disease occurs when the persons' visual acuity starts to deteriorate. This has an increased significance for self-management because good visual acuity is required to undertake self blood glucose monitoring, inject insulin and to inspect a person's own feet. A number of services within the UK are available for people with poor visual acuity (Box 9.2):

- Talking books are available from the Royal National Institute for the Blind (RNIB).
- British Talking Book Service for the Blind.
- Royal National Library for the Blind.
- Talking newspapers, available from the Talking Newspaper Association.
- Library services: most libraries have large print books and tapes.
- Residential establishments, courses, holiday homes and caravans for the blind organised by the RNIB.
- Talking meter (see Chapter 7).

BLIND REGISTRATION

In the UK, blind registration is available for people with a visual acuity of less than 3/60 in their better eye. Individuals with a visual acuity of less than 6/60 in the better eye can be registered as partially sighted. These processes are undertaken by a consultant ophthalmologist.

Box 9.2
Useful addresses

- Action for Blind People: 14–16 Verney Road, London SE16 3DX tel: 0207 7328771
- Partially Sighted Society: Queens Road, Doncaster DN1 2NX tel: 01302 323132
- Royal National Institute for the Blind (RNIB), 224 Great Portland Street, London W1N 6AA tel: 0207 3881266

Blind registration gives access to tuition in Braille that will help to maintain some independence. Insulin click pens are also a valuable resource for the visually impaired.

DIABETIC NEPHROPATHY

THE FACTS

- The natural history of nephropathy in type 1 diabetes and type 2 diabetes is different.
- About 30% of people with type 1 diabetes will develop nephropathy.
- About 10% of people with type 2 diabetes will develop nephropathy.
- Many people with diabetes die from macrovascular disease before the nephropathy progresses.
- Nephropathy is associated with an increased risk of retinopathy and an increased risk of coronary artery disease (Gross et al 2005). The incidence of nephropathy in both type 1 and type 2 diabetes is falling due to earlier detection and improved methods of treatment for glycaemic control and blood pressure (DCCT 1993, SIGN 2001, UK Prospective Diabetes Study (UKPDS) 33 1998).

MICROALBUMINURIA

Microalbuminuria precedes the development of nephropathy and is characterised by an albumin excretion rate of 30–300 mg/day. Microalbuminuria is detectable by radioimmunoassay and by highly sensitive urine dipstick tests such as Micral Test©. Alternatively, a urinary albumin : creatinine ratio (ACR) can be measured from an early-morning specimen.

Diabetic nephropathy is characterised by persistent albuminuria (an albumin excretion rate greater than 300 mg per 24 hours). This is the equivalent of a 24-hour urinary protein excretion of 500 mg (Fig. 9.2).

Type 1 diabetes

In type 1 diabetes, it is unusual to detect microalbuminuria within 5 years of diagnosis (Gross et al 2005). Thereafter, the incidence increases such that after 15 years from diagnosis, 50–60% of people will have microalbuminuria; the incidence is higher in men. About 35% of people will progress to nephropathy.

Type 2 diabetes

Many people with type 2 diabetes have microalbuminuria or even proteinuria at diagnosis and this is associated with the co-existence of hypertension. People of Afro-Caribbean and Asian descent have a higher prevalence of nephropathy (Wu et al 2005); 50% of people who develop end-stage renal disease in Britain have type 2 diabetes.

Fig. 9.2
Normoalbuminuria,
microalbuminuria and
macroalbuminuria.
Reproduced, with
thanks, from Williams &
Pickup (1998)

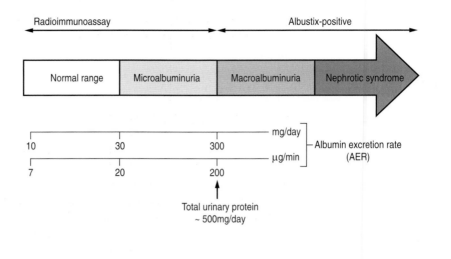

PROGRESSION OF NEPHROPATHY

As nephropathy progresses, the glomerular filtration rate (GFR) progressively decreases. Serum creatinine levels start to rise and once these exceed 20 μmol/L progression to end-stage renal failure is relentless. Blood pressure also rises progressively. In many people with type 2 diabetes, the blood pressure is already elevated at the time that albuminuria is detected.

Case study 9.2

Eric was diagnosed with type 2 diabetes at the age of 35. He takes 850 mg metformin twice a day. Five years later at his annual review for complication screening, he was found to be hypertensive with a blood pressure of 160/95 mmHg; his glycated haemoglobin had deteriorated to 9%. His lipid profile had also deteriorated, showing an increased LDL and decreased HDL. He complains of pins and needles and a burning sensation in both feet that was worse at night. His biochemistry profile showed a rise in serum creatinine but still within the normal range. His glomerular filtration rate (GFR) was decreasing and he had a persistent albuminuria greater than 300 mg in 24 hours. His ACR measured at 25 mg/mmol.

Eric had a previous history of background retinopathy and, as is often the case with renal complications, it is very possible that his diabetic eye disease has also progressed. Urgent screening for diabetic eye disease would be recommended if this was not already due.

CLINICAL SIGNS OF NEPHROPATHY

There are few clinical signs in the early stages of nephropathy. Anaemia develops as the disease progresses and in the later stages oedema and breathlessness will develop. People with type 2 diabetes have often developed severe cardiovascular disease by this point. Neuropathic and ischaemic foot ulceration is also more common in those people with nephropathy and hyperlipidaemia commonly co-exists (see Chapter 10).

SCREENING AND EARLY DETECTION

Urinary screening for microalbuminuria and proteinuria should be performed in all people with diabetes at least annually. Those with type 1 diabetes should have this done from 5 years after diagnosis (Gross et al 2005). In those with type 2 diabetes, it should be done from diagnosis (Gross et al 2005). Screening elderly people is problematic because errors are common due to urinary tract infections and prostate disease, and also because the benefits of screening and early treatment take several years to accrue. If the individual is found to have albuminuria on two separate early-morning urine specimens, further investigation should be undertaken to exclude other renal disease. These investigations would include a midstream specimen of urine (MSU), possible renal ultrasonography and a 24-hour urine protein collection.

If the individual's urinalysis is albustix negative, screening for microalbuminuria should be undertaken. This can be done by microalbuminuria testing strips or by ACR. The ACR value should be less than 2.5 mg/mmol in men and less than 3.5 mg/mmol in women. If the screen is positive, an MSU test should be undertaken. If this is negative, timed overnight urine collections should be performed. It might be necessary to repeat this investigation on two or three occasions.

Confounding factors

The following can cause false-positive results in microalbuminuria testing:

- urinary tract infection
- exercise
- prostatic disease
- heart failure
- day-to-day variation.

MANAGEMENT

Eric's long-term health is seriously under threat not only from microvascular complications but also from macrovascular complications. Several issues need to be addressed:

- In Eric's situation the first parameter to address would be to encourage him to improve his glycaemic control. The UKPDS 33 (1998) and the DCCT (1993) both showed that tight glycaemic control in people with diabetes reduces the progression of renal disease. Eric might require a change or addition to his treatment regimen. Depending on the extent of his nephropathy, he might need to reduce or stop metformin.

■ Eric's elevated blood pressure requires aggressive management. This can reduce the progression from microalbuminuria through albuminuria to end-stage renal failure. His blood pressure should be reduced to 135/85 mmHg. Diuretics, beta-blockers and calcium channel blockers have all shown to be effective in managing hypertension associated with diabetic renal disease. However, angiotensin-converting enzyme inhibitors (ACE) and angiotensin-II receptor antagonists have been shown to have an extra effect on progression of microalbuminuria over and above their antihypertensive effect. Those with type 1 diabetes with microalbuminuria should be started on an ACE inhibitor regardless of the level of blood pressure (SIGN 2001). Those with type 2 diabetes with microalbuminuria should also be started on an ACE inhibitor with the aim of reducing blood pressure to 130/80 or 120/70 mmHg in the face of established disease (see Chapter 8 for further details on blood pressure management).

■ Eric also requires lipid-lowering agents. People with diabetic renal disease will almost certainly have dyslipidaemia and require aggressive treatment to reduce cardiovascular risk. This is addressed in Chapter 8.

■ There is minimal evidence that the decline in GFR is reduced by limiting protein intake (Williams & Pickup 2004).

■ If appropriate, Eric would be referred to discuss smoking cessation (see Chapter 11).

■ Low-dose aspirin therapy should be started.

These measures are advocated mainly in relation to their role in the management of cardiovascular risk, which in this case, is high.

RENAL FAILURE

Those with progressing diabetic renal disease should be referred to a nephrologist once the serum creatinine exceeds 150 µmol/L (SIGN 2001).

Options for managing end stage renal failure include:

■ Haemodialysis.

■ Continuous ambulatory peritoneal dialysis (CAPD).

■ Renal transplantation: the 5-year survival rate after renal transplantation in people with type 1 diabetes has recently been reported as being better following a combined pancreas and kidney transplantation (82%) than after kidney transplantation alone (60%) (Orsenigo et al 2004).

■ Palliative care.

DIABETIC NEUROPATHY

THE FACTS

■ Eric displays typical symptoms of a painful peripheral neuropathy and will need treatment for this debilitating problem. Around 25% of persons with diabetes however have an asymptomatic neuropathy and are thus prone to foot problems (see Chapter 10).

- Neuropathy is rare in people newly diagnosed with type 1 diabetes but is often present at the time of diagnosis in people with type 2 diabetes. However, there might be symptoms of painful peripheral neuritis in both type 1 diabetes and type 2 diabetes. These can resolve in a matter of weeks with improved glycaemic control.
- Neuropathy can seriously affect mental health in people with diabetes, and depression and anxiety are prevalent (Vileikyte et al 2005).
- Acute neuropathies can be related to poor glycaemic control and can respond well to improvement. Chronic neuropathies are more difficult to manage and treatment can be difficult.
- Whereas neuropathy is more often evident in the lower limbs, it can affect any nerve in the body. Hence there are a variety of neuropathies including cranial nerve palsies, foot drop, amyotrophy and autonomic neuropathy.

CLASSIFICATION AND OUTCOMES

Chronic distal sensory neuropathy

This is the most common form of neuropathy in people with diabetes. The onset is insidious, usually with numbness starting in the toes and soles of the feet and spreading proximally in a symmetrical 'stocking' distribution. Clinical examination will reveal reduced sensitivity to fine touch, vibration and temperature sensation. The ankle reflexes are often absent.

The significance of this condition is that the individual with reduced sensation is more likely to experience undetected injury from ill fitting shoes, foreign objects in shoes and from burns due to hot water bottles and electric fires. This predisposes the individual to foot ulceration and its appalling consequences. For this reason people who are found to have distal sensory loss should be referred to a foot clinic for appropriate education and management (see Chapter 10).

Painful neuropathy

In this situation, the person can complain of a variety of sensory symptoms of a severe nature, usually in the lower aspects of the legs. The pain might be burning, shooting or tingling and is characteristically worse at nights when in contact with bed clothing. It is usually associated with poor glycaemic control and rectification of this or stabilisation of blood glucose profiles leads to recovery over several months or even up to 2 years.

Various treatments are available. It is essential to improve diabetic control. For quality of life, it is important to give adequate pain control, predominantly through membrane stabilisation drugs (Barbano et al 2003) (Box 9.3).

Diabetic amyotrophy

This painful condition usually affects people with type 2 diabetes over the age of 50 (Simmons & Feldman 2002). Affected individuals usually report severe pain,

Box 9.3
Treatments for painful
neuropathy

- Tricyclic antidepressants and antiepileptic drugs have been shown to be beneficial, particularly gabapentin, carbamazepine and phenytoin
- Capsaicin cream 0.075% applied topically can have some benefit in painful neuropathy but involves prolonged treatment and might initially cause a burning sensation when applied
- A role for aldose reductase inhibitors has been postulated

normally in the upper legs, that has developed over weeks and months. There is also severe muscle wasting of the quadriceps muscles and people might struggle to rise from a chair unaided. The upper limbs can also be affected. The individual might report some weight loss.

This condition appears to resolve without active treatment about 2–9 months after the onset (Simmons & Feldman 2002). People with this would be treated symptomatically for pain and physiologically for blood glucose control. Most people with diabetic amyotrophy experience resolution of their pain and some motor recovery of their muscles; however, this latter aspect might not be complete. Even after 1–2 years, people may still struggle with daily functions like climbing stairs or getting in and out of bed. This condition is rare and members of the primary healthcare team will not normally be asked to manage this condition but need to be aware of the affects it has on the lives of individuals.

Focal neuropathies

- Carpal tunnel syndrome.
- Third cranial nerve palsy.
- Sixth cranial nerve palsy.
- Peripheral mononeuropathies, such as common peroneal nerve.

Some of these neuropathies are due to nerve entrapment or pressure or to vascular damage, i.e. they are not related to the level of glycaemic control, and might respond to surgical intervention. Some of these neuropathies resolve spontaneously (Fig. 9.3).

ASSESSMENT

As neuropathy can be insidious, neurological examination is mandatory at diagnosis and at least annually thereafter. Simple clinical examination can be undertaken (see Chapter 10).

REFERRAL

Everyone presenting with newly diagnosed neuropathy affecting their feet should be referred to a podiatrist for specialist advice (Chapter 10). People who appear not to receive relief from normal treatment might benefit from referral to a pain clinic.

Fig. 9.3

Clinical patterns of diabetic peripheral neuropathy. Reproduced, with thanks, from Williams & Pickup (1998)

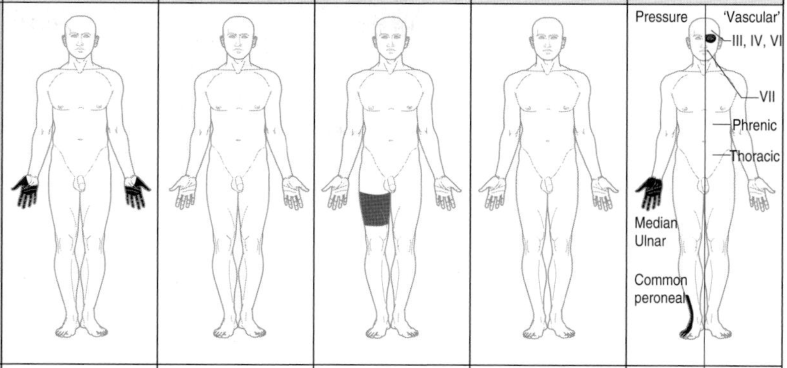

Syndrome	Chronic insidious sensory neuropathy	Acute painful neuropathy	Proximal motor neuropathy	Diffuse motor neuropathy	Focal nerve palsies	
Pattern					Pressure 'Vascular'—III, IV, VI —VII —Phrenic —Thoracic Median Ulnar Common peroneal	
Sensory loss	$+ \rightarrow ++$	$+$	0	$0 \rightarrow +$	$++$	$++$
Pain	$0 \rightarrow +++$	$+++$	$+ \rightarrow +++$	0	$++$	$0 \rightarrow ++$
Tendon reflexes	$\downarrow$	$\downarrow$	$\downarrow$	$\downarrow$	$+$	$+$
Muscle wasting and weakness	$0 \rightarrow ++$	$+ \rightarrow ++$	$+++$	$++ \rightarrow +++$	$+ \rightarrow ++$	$0 \rightarrow ++$
Autonomic features	$+ \rightarrow ++$	May be present	May be present	May be present	May be present	May be present
Prevalence and relationship to glycaemia	Common; usually unrelated to glycaemia	Relatively rare; onset often during hyperglycaemia	Relatively rare; onset often during hyperglycaemia	Relatively rare; generally unrelated to hyperglycaemia	Relatively rare; usually unrelated to hyper-glycaemia	Relatively rare; sometimes related to hyper-glycaemia

AUTONOMIC NEUROPATHY

THE FACTS

Autonomic neuropathy is relatively uncommon. It is due to damage to the sympathetic and parasympathetic nerves and is usually associated with peripheral neuropathy. The symptoms that people present with can be intermittent.

ASSESSMENT OF AUTONOMIC NEUROPATHY

Simple tests for autonomic neuropathy can be undertaken in a community care setting:

- lying and standing blood pressure: record lying blood pressure then stand the person up and record blood pressure 2 minutes later; a fall of more than 30 mmHg is expected
- pupillary reflexes: these are often abnormal
- heart rate variation after deep breathing: this would normally be greater than 15 beats per minute.

More complicated assessment involves the use of the Valsalva manoeuvre.

CLINICAL FEATURES AND TREATMENT

Postural hypotension

Postural hypotension can cause dizziness and faintness, particularly on rising from sitting or lying. The fall in blood pressure is usually > 30 mmHg. Assessment involves reviewing medication, as certain drugs can aggravate the hypotension, including antidepressants and diuretics. Elevation of the head of the bed when sleeping can be helpful, elastic support stockings can also be of benefit. Therapeutic measures include the use of fludrocortisone.

Gastroparesis

This is due to delayed gastric emptying and might be associated with vomiting. Treatment options include metoclopramide and domperidone. Erythromycin can increase gastric emptying but is of limited use. In extreme situations surgery is necessary.

Diarrhoea and constipation

Diarrhoea is one of the more common autonomic disturbances. The individual complains of explosive diarrhoea, which is often worse at night. Other causes of diarrhoea should be excluded by investigation. Treatment is with loperamide or codeine phosphate.

Some people complain of constipation, which can be managed by bulking agents and laxatives.

Urinary tract

People can suffer from urinary retention and overflow incontinence. Treatment is by regular toileting but, ultimately, self-catheterisation could be required.

Gustatory sweating

This occurs when eating and can lead to excessive sweat production from the face, neck and chest. Treatment is by anticholinergic drugs or glycopyrronium powder.

Anhidrosis

There can be absence of sweating, particularly on the lower limbs, which poses an additional risk factor for the development of diabetic foot conditions. Emollient creams are recommended.

ERECTILE DYSFUNCTION

Erectile dysfunction is defined as the inability to achieve or maintain an erection sufficient for satisfactory sexual intercourse. Of the numerous clinical problems affecting persons with diabetes mellitus, erectile failure is one of the most common but is probably the least talked about – by the person, his partner and the attending healthcare professionals.

Case study 9.3

Fred is 64 years old and has had type 2 diabetes for 15 years. He took early retirement from his job 9 years ago and lives a full life. He and his wife have been married for 40 years and have two children and five grandchildren, of whom they are very proud. Fred is a local councillor and considered to be a pillar in the community. He is active in fighting for play areas for children and traffic-calming measures. He frequently writes articles for the local paper on issues affecting the community.

Fred comes to see the GP and appears to be very awkward in his conversation. He eventually admits that he has 'men's problems'. After encouragement to discuss his problem, Fred admits that he has impotence, which has occurred fairly recently. He feels it is beginning to cause a strain between himself and his wife and it was at his wife's insistence that he attended the GP.

Healthcare professionals in such situations must always be alert to problems of a sexual nature and ensure that they adopt an accepting, open approach to encourage the person to discuss their problem. Fred would be reassured of the confidential nature of any appointment with a healthcare professional and advised that there are several options to explore. Fred would first be informed of the facts.

THE FACTS

- Erectile dysfunction is common: it can affect up to 40% of men with diabetes.
- The aetiology can be complex, involving many physical factors.
- Other diseases interfere with physiological mechanisms (Saenz de Tejada et al 2005).
- Psychological factors in men with diabetes should not be ignored.
- The parasympathetic nervous system mediates erection; the sympathetic nervous system mediates ejaculation.
- Erectile dysfunction is independently associated with cardiovascular disease, increasing fasting glucose levels, diabetes and future coronary risk (Grover et al 2006).

CAUSES OF ERECTILE DYSFUNCTION

Common

- Diabetic neuropathy.
- Peripheral vascular disease.
- Drugs such as antihypertensives, diuretics and anti-depressants.
- Psychological factors.
- Alcohol.

Less commonly

- Trauma.
- Penile abnormalities.
- Endocrine causes such as hypogonadism.

ASSESSMENT

The first stage in any clinical situation is to undertake a detailed assessment. Fred's assessment would include a clear history to determine whether there is a lack of erections or whether the problem is more complicated and includes disorders of libido or ejaculation. The absence of nocturnal or morning erections, together with a gradual onset of symptoms, favours an organic cause.

A physical examination would be undertaken to detect signs of peripheral and autonomic neuropathy, vascular disease, penile disorders and endocrine disturbance. Investigations should include an assessment of overall glycaemic control, thyroid function tests, liver function tests, serum lipids and, if appropriate, serum testosterone, prolactin and ferratin.

Psychological aspects of erectile dysfunction must be considered. These would include anxiety about sexual performance, psychological affects of trauma or abuse and depression. Relationship problems can also cause erectile dysfunction. Eliciting facts around this require the healthcare professional to be sensitive to Fred's feelings and it might take a few visits before a full picture of any psychological trauma emerges.

MANAGEMENT

The management of erectile dysfunction should always include sympathetic enquiry and counselling. The introduction of oral treatments for this problem prompted a lot of media interest, and as a result, individuals might be more comfortable in discussing their problems. It is often helpful to invite the partner to be present and in this instance Fred and his wife were asked to attend all appointments. There is now a wealth of information in the form of leaflets, tapes and videos, which can be helpful and is available from pharmaceutical companies. Diabetes UK offers advice and information from its website (www.diabetes.org.uk).

Oral therapies

The management of erectile dysfunction has been revolutionised by the introduction of phosphodiesterase type 5 inhibitors. These drugs prevent the degradation of the smooth muscle relaxant cyclic GMP, thereby increasing blood flow to the penis. Sildenafil was the first to be introduced and one study on 188 men with type 1 diabetes demonstrated that it was an effective treatment and well tolerated (Stuckey et al 2003). Tadalafil and vardenafil are also now available on the NHS in the UK. They should be taken 30–60 minutes before sexual activity and work only in the presence of sexual stimulation. Tadalafil claims that the efficacy can persist for up to 36 hours. These drugs are contraindicated in the presence of cardiac disease, recent myocardial infarction and unstable angina. They should not be taken with nitrates.

Apomorphine hydrochloride is a selective dopamine agonist. Taken sublingually, it produces an erection within 20 minutes.

Transurethral alprostadil

Transurethral alprostadil is prostaglandin E1 that is introduced into the urethra by a special device.

Intracavernosal alprostadil

Individuals are taught how to self-inject alprostadil into the base of the penis. This is used less frequently now that oral therapies are available.

Vacuum devices

A cylinder fitted over the penis enables a vacuum to be created, which results in penis engorgement. The erection is maintained by a construction ring at the base of the penis.

Penile prosthesis

These semi-rigid or inflatable devices can be implanted in the penis when other treatments have failed.

Thus Fred and his wife could be reassured by the range of treatment options and encouraged to try appropriate ones until they found one that was mutually satisfying.

CONCLUSION

Microvascular disease is a major cause of morbidity in people with diabetes. Screening plays an important part in the early detection of clinical changes as often, by the time people complain of clinical signs and symptoms, irreparable damage has been done. Early detection can ensure that the appropriate treatment is initiated to reduce or delay the onset of microvascular disease in people with diabetes.

REFERENCES

Barbano R, Hart-Gouleau S, Pennella-Vaughan J, Dworkin RH 2003 Pharmacotherapy of painful diabetic neuropathy. Current Pain & Headache Reports. 7(3):169–177

Cormack TG, Grant B, Macdonald MJ et al 2001 Incidence of blindness due to diabetic eye disease in Fife 1990–9. British Journal of Ophthalmology 85(3):354–356

Diabetes Control and Complications Trial (DCCT) Research Group 1993 The effect of intensive treatment of diabetes on the development and progression of long-term complications in insulin-dependent diabetes mellitus. New England Journal of Medicine 329:977–986

Gross JL, de Azevedo MJ, Silveiro SP et al 2005 Diabetic nephropathy: diagnosis, prevention, and treatment. Diabetes Care 28(1):164–176

Grover SA, Lowensteyn I, Kaouache M et al 2006 The prevalence of erectile dysfunction in the primary care setting: importance of risk factors for diabetes and vascular disease. Archives of Internal Medicine 166(2):213–219

Icks A, Trautner C, Haastert B et al 1997 Blindness due to diabetes: population-based age- and sex-specific incidence rates. Diabetic Medicine 14(7):571–575

Kenny C 2004 Primary diabetes care: yesterday, today and tomorrow. Practical Diabetes International 21(2):65–68

Leese GP, Morris AD, Swaminathan K et al 2005 Implementation of national diabetes retinal screening programme is associated with a lower proportion of patients referred to ophthalmology. Diabetic Medicine 22(8):1112–1115

Orsenigo E, Fiorina P, Cristallo M et al 2004 Long-term survival after kidney and kidney-pancreas transplantation in diabetic patients. Transplantation Proceedings 36(4): 1072–1075

Saenz de Tejada I, Angulo J, Cellek S et al 2005 Pathophysiology of erectile dysfunction. Consensus Development Conference. Journal of Sexual Medicine 2(1):26–39

Schneider S, Aldington SJ, Kohner EM et al 2005 Quality assurance for diabetic retinopathy telescreening. Diabetic Medicine 22(6):794–802

Scottish Intercollegiate Guidelines Network (SIGN) 2001 SIGN 55: management of diabetes. SIGN, Edinburgh

Simmons Z, Feldman EL 2002 Update on diabetic neuropathy. Neurology 15(5):595–603

Stuckey BG, Jadzinsky MN, Murphy LJ et al 2003 Sildenafil citrate for treatment of erectile dysfunction in men with type 1 diabetes: results of a randomized controlled trial. Diabetes Care 26(2):279–284

UK Prospective Diabetes Study (UKPDS) Group 1998 Intensive blood-glucose control with sulphonylureas or insulin compared with conventional treatment and risk of complications in patients with type 2 diabetes (UKPDS 33). Lancet 352:837–853

Vileikyte L, Leventhal H, Gonzalez JS et al 2005 Diabetic peripheral neuropathy and depressive symptoms: the association revisited. Diabetes Care 28(10):2378–2383

Williams G, Pickup JC 1998 Handbook of diabetes, 2nd edn. Blackwell Science, Oxford

Williams G, Pickup JC 2004 Handbook of diabetes, 3rd edn. Blackwell Science, Oxford

Wu AY, Kong NC, de Leon FA et al 2005 An alarmingly high prevalence of diabetic nephropathy in Asian type 2 diabetic patients: the MicroAlbuminuria Prevalence (MAP) Study. Diabetologia 48(1):17–26

CHAPTER 10

Foot care

Christine Skinner

INTRODUCTION

The foot is a complex structure that is not only responsible for locomotion but is also designed to withstand the stresses of body weight while walking and standing. These stresses can result in microtrauma, which can lead to foot lesions. Foot problems are still the most common cause of hospital admissions for people with diabetes in the UK (Young et al 1994) and the length of stay is greater than for any other diabetic complication (Williams 1985). Foot disease remains one of the most common and devastating of diabetic complications, being responsible for a considerable amount of healthcare resource in the UK (Scottish Intercollegiate Guidelines Network (SIGN) 55 2001). The estimated cost for ulceration and amputation in the UK in 2001 was £244 million (Shearer et al 2003). Diabetic foot disease often arises as a result of neuropathy, ischaemia, structural deformity or a combination of two or all of these factors.

Overall 20–40% of people with diabetes have neuropathy and 20–40% have peripheral vascular disease (Hutchinson et al 2000). Neuropathy and peripheral vascular disease develop as a result of poor blood glucose control and adverse risk factors such as smoking and dyslipidaemia (Hutchinson et al 2000). People with diabetes must also be aware of the influence of good glycaemic control, as hyperglycaemia can affect the microvascular status (UK Prospective Diabetes Study (UKPDS) 1998).

Any minor trauma occurring in the foot can easily become infected and, if not managed correctly, can lead to the development of cellulitis, osteomyelitis and ultimately amputation. Of those people with diabetes, 5–7 % will develop a foot ulcer at some time in their life (SIGN 2001).

As complications associated with the diabetic foot have been described as a 'major medical, social and economical problem' of global proportions (Boulton &

Vileikyte 2000), it is imperative that all those involved in the care of the people with diabetes are familiar with aspects of care in the diabetic foot.

Foot complications can be associated with social deprivation, poor vision, disability, foot deformity and absence of professional foot care (Hutchinson et al 2000). All of these factors can influence the person's ability to practise good foot care; however, there are two key aspects of foot care:

1   assessing the foot
2   treating foot lesions.

The management of the person should always have a multidisciplinary approach with close liaison between podiatrist, diabetologist, general practitioner, diabetes nurse specialist, the primary and community care nurse and orthotist.

Treatment by a podiatrist is free to all those with diabetes within the UK. The podiatrist should be involved in the care of the person with diabetes soon after diagnosis and thereafter as the individual is referred to them. It is recommended that people with diabetes only attend those podiatrists in the UK who are registered with the Health Professions Council.

FOOT HEALTH EDUCATION

Foot health education plays an important part in any successful management strategy. People who have had diabetes for many years may be unaware of the potential problems that can affect their feet. It must be remembered that whereas individuals with diabetes should be aware of these problems, it is important that they are not caused unnecessary alarm. It is essential, therefore, to gain the individual's confidence and trust and to establish a rapport. In so doing, the practitioner will be able to gauge the levels of knowledge and understanding the person might have. Reassurance is essential to minimise the individual's anxiety and re-enforcement of foot health education optimises self management.

ASSESSING THE DIABETIC FOOT

The multidisciplinary team must be aware of the guidelines published by National Collaborating Centre for Primary Care (National Institute for Health and Clinical Excellence (NICE) 2004) and of the Scottish Intercollegiate Guideline 55 (SIGN 2001) in caring for the feet of a person with diabetes.

Primary care nurses might be involved in assessing the foot for diabetic complications as part of the annual screening visit or as part of their everyday care for these individuals. GPs might also be involved in assessing the feet at the screening clinic. It is important to record the outcome of findings to allow subsequent monitoring of the person's feet.

Before examining the feet, certain facts should be ascertained:

- duration of diabetes
- does the person have type 1 or type 2 diabetes?
- present level of glycaemic control
- do they experience pain or cramping in their legs when walking?
- do they have a numbness or tingling sensation in their feet?
- Is there a history of foot ulceration?
- does the person smoke?
- Is there any visual handicap?

Foot assessment requires some skills and experience in examining and interpretation. Examination of the foot involves assessment of soft tissues, structural deformities, vascular and neurological status and it is essential to assess and compare both lower limbs and feet.

SOFT TISSUE ASSESSMENT

This involves assessing both the skin and the nails.

Skin

When assessing the colour of the skin a comparison of the feet should be made. The colour and temperature of the skin are indicative of the blood flow through the foot. The skin of a foot with a good blood flow will be pale pink and warm to touch. If there is impaired blood flow the skin will be cold and pale. Cyanosis indicates a poor oxygen content and therefore poor blood supply. The appearance of a cold, hyperaemic (bright red) foot demonstrates ischaemia to the peripheral tissues and should be considered as a potential problem. The skin of an ischaemic foot is shiny, stretched, hairless and cool to touch.

The foot should be examined for the presence of soft tissue lesions such as callus, corns and any abrasions or indications of trauma. The interdigital spaces are often macerated and are a potential site for fungal infection and should not be overlooked.

People with autonomic neuropathy in their feet will have decreased sweating which results in dry, devitalised skin. The plantar aspect of the foot and the heel area are often affected, with the posterior aspect of the heel liable to fissuring providing a potential site for infection to develop.

Nails

The nails can vary in appearance depending on the vascular state of the foot. In the ischaemic foot the nails may be thickened and slow growing. If they are infected by fungi they will appear thickened, discoloured and have a 'musty' smell (Fig.10.1). The nail grooves should also be examined to ensure that no callus or small spike of nail has penetrated the soft tissues of the groove, which can lead to an infected ingrowing toenail (Fig. 10.2). Nails that have been cut inappropriately can cause damage to the adjacent toe.

Fig. 10.1
The diabetic foot:
nails thickened and
discoloured by fungal
infection

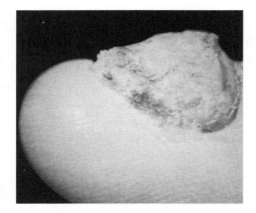

STRUCTURAL DEFORMITIES

Structural deformities as a complication of diabetes act as a potential site for ulceration because the area is subjected to abnormal stresses. The combination of sensory neuropathy and increased pressure on the plantar aspect of the metatarsal heads may result in ulceration (Pham et al 2000).

The toes are often in a clawed position as a result of motor neuropathy, which causes wasting of the small intrinsic muscles and allows the long flexors to have an unopposed action (Fig. 10.3). The metatarsal heads therefore become much more prominent on the plantar surface and are subjected to greater stress during walking leading to the formation of hyperkeratosis. The dorsal aspect and tips of the toes are also liable to develop corns.

Structural deformities might also be present in the diabetic foot as a result of changes from Charcot neuropathic joints (Armstrong et al 1997). In the Charcot foot, pain perception and the ability to sense the position of the joints in the foot are severely impaired or lost, and muscles lose their ability to support the joint(s)

Fig. 10.2
Infected in-growing
toenail

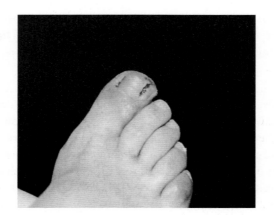

Fig. 10.3
Clawing of the toes as a result of motor neuropathy: long flexor muscles have unopposed action because small intrinsic muscles are wasted

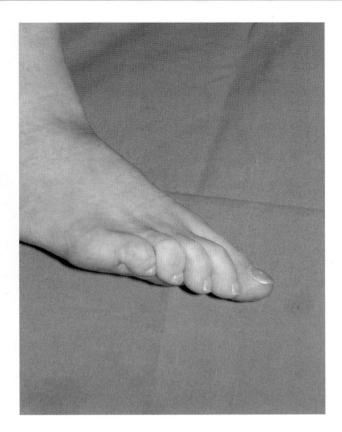

properly. Loss of these motor and sensory nerve functions allow minor traumas such as sprains and stress fractures to go undetected and untreated leading to ligament laxity, joint dislocation, bone erosion, cartilage damage, and deformity of the foot. The bones most often affected are the metatarsals and the mid-foot (Fig. 10.4).

VASCULAR ASSESSMENT

The diabetic foot can be affected by both macrovascular and microvascular disease. Both have significant influences on the clinical appearance and the subsequent management of the foot. Symptoms of vascular insufficiency should be elicited from the individual. If the person complains of intermittent claudication, its severity can be assessed by determining how far the individual can walk before symptoms develop. It is also necessary to determine if the person suffers from pain when at rest, which is an indication of severe ischaemia.

It is essential to distinguish the pain of ischaemia from that of neuropathy, which often presents as a burning sensation.

Clinical assessment of the vascular state can be carried out routinely by performing a variety of physical tests. All members of the healthcare team, after

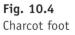

Fig. 10.4
Charcot foot

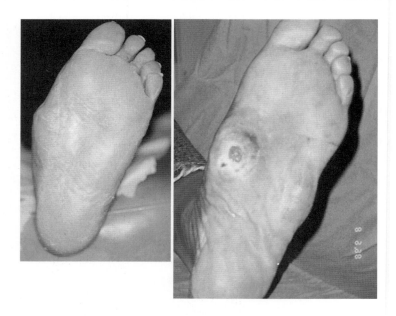

suitable training, should be able perform these tests. To meet national guidelines, assessment must be carried out annually. People who are identified as 'at risk' following a vascular assessment should be referred for a more detailed peripheral arterial assessment (Stuart et al 2004, Watkins 2003).

PHYSICAL TESTS

Palpation of pulses

Peripheral circulation can be assessed by palpation of pedal pulses (Fig. 10.5):

- The dorsalis pedis artery is a continuation of the anterior tibial artery. The pulse can be palpated on the dorsal aspect of the foot in the region of the intermediate cuneiform.

Fig. 10.5
Palpation of pedal pulses

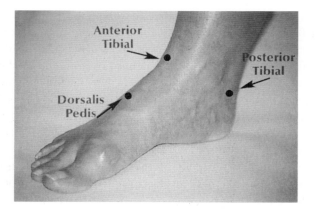

- The anterior tibial pulse can be palpated on the front of the ankle mid-way between the two malleoli.
- The posterior tibial pulse can be palpated immediately behind the medial malleolus.

Confidence is essential in palpating pedal pulses, and such confidence is only acquired through practice. All members of the healthcare team need to be encouraged to develop this skill with normal, healthy people before progressing to people with known vascular complications. A hand-held Doppler can also be used.

It should be noted that arteriovenous shunts will develop due to autonomic neuropathy and, as a result, blood flow bypasses the capillary bed. Thus people might have bounding arterial pulses but have poor blood supply to the surrounding tissues. This is responsible for the venous engorgement often seen on the dorsum of the foot (Ward & Boulton 1987).

Temperature gradient

The temperature gradient can be assessed by gently running the back of the hand from below the knee distally to the toes. If there are any obvious changes intra- and interlimb, these should be noted.

Capillary refill

This is assessed by gently pressing the plantar aspect of the hallux until it blanches. Pressure is removed and the tissues allowed to reperfuse. Normal capillary refill should be 3 seconds.

Presence or absence of oedema

The presence of oedema can prevent the palpation of pedal pulses. If present, the affected sites should be noted.

Presence or absence of varicose veins

Varicose veins can lead to oedema of the ankle or dorsum of the foot and create a problem with socks and shoes. Any varicose veins should also be noted.

NEUROLOGICAL ASSESSMENT

Neuropathy is a major contributory factor in the development of ulceration in the diabetic foot (Thomson et al 1991). Neuropathy can affect sensory, motor or autonomic function. The most common diffuse neuropathy affecting people with diabetes is distal symmetric sensorimotor polyneuropathy (Boulton 2000). Some people with diabetes present with painful neuropathic symptoms; alternatively, this can develop over the following years. The person suffering from neuropathy can present with varying symptoms. He or she might complain of pain, which can be burning, sharp shooting or lancinating; paraesthesia; numbness with loss of pain; hot or cold sensations or irritation from bedclothes. Other unusual sensations might also be experienced and individuals might complain of the 'feeling of cotton wool under their toes' or 'walking on hot sand'. If the person complains of pain it is important to distinguish the pain from that of ischaemia by assessing the quality of the pain and by examining the peripheral circulation.

If there is neuropathy present then a thorough structural assessment must be performed. This determines areas of pressure that might result in the development of callus and corns and eventually ulcers (Pham et al 2000).

Neuropathy might also result in damage to the soft tissue of the foot because, having lost sensation, the individual is unaware of trauma to the foot. Hence people are advised not to walk around on bare feet (Boxes 10.1 and 10.2). Prior to the neurological assessment being undertaken it is essential what is involved is explained to the person with diabetes. It is also useful to let the person experience the perceived sensation on an area where there is no sensory loss.

Box 10.1
Foot health education for the person with healthy feet

- Never walk barefoot
- Change hosiery daily
- Wash feet daily, dry carefully in between the toes
- Apply a cream to the soles and heels
- Inspect feet daily for corns/callosities/plantar warts/athlete's foot
- If any of the above is present, they should only be treated by a registered podiatrist
- With the slightest abrasion or infection in your feet, contact your GP, community nurse, diabetic nurse specialist, diabetic consultant or podiatrist
- Never use proprietary treatments for callus or corns, as they contain acids
- Cut toenails straight across
- Buy new shoes from a shop that measures your feet and fits the shoes for you
- Never wear new shoes for a long period of time
- Stop smoking
- Only attend a podiatrist registered by the Health Professions Council

---

Box 10.2
Foot health education for the person with an 'at risk' foot

- All of Box 10.1 plus:
- Do not cut your own toenails
- Inspect feet daily for any open lesions, cracking, dryness, change in colour, swelling, corn, callus, blisters, warts or signs of infection
- Use a mirror to inspect the soles of your feet or ask someone to look for you
- Only use a hot water bottle to heat your bed: never place it next to your feet
- Never sit close to the fire or heater
- Check inside shoes for foreign objects
- Wear shoes with soft uppers, preferably lacing
- Never wear garters to hold up stockings or socks

Light touch

This can be assessed using a piece of cotton wool. The person's foot is gently touched with the cotton wool and sites identified where it can/cannot be appreciated. This commences distally and moves proximally, thereby moving from a potentially numb area to a normal area. It is easier to identify the boundary of sensory loss when moving from a numb area to an area of normal sensation. The person should have his or her eyes closed during this examination. Ensure that there is minimal variation in the pressure of application of the cotton wool. Note that the cotton wool should not be run across the tissues as people with paraesthesia can experience discomfort and pain.

Sharp and blunt sensation

A Neurotip can be used to identify if sharp and blunt sensation is present or absent. Again, the person's eyes should be closed during this examination and the assessor should commence distally and work proximally.

Pressure

Pressure can effectively be assessed using a 10-g Semmes–Weinstein monofilament in predicting the risk of foot ulceration (Abbott et al 1998). Monofilaments are cheap and easy to use, making them an ideal screening tool. The sites tested are usually defined by local protocols but are generally agreed to be plantar aspects of the hallux, first, third and fifth metatarsal heads, heel and apices of the fourth and/or fifth digits; these are the most common sites for ulceration to develop. The monofilament is calibrated to buckle when a force of 10 g is exerted and if the person cannot feel the pressure the foot is considered to be insensate. The greater the number of negative responses identified, the greater the risk (Baker et al 2005).

It is important to ensure that any areas of hyperkeratosis are removed before carrying out this test (Fig. 10.6).

Vibration

Vibration perception can be assessed using a standard 128-Hz tuning fork or a Reydell Sieffer tuning fork with a graduated scale, which will give a recordable measurement. Sites that should be assessed are the ankle, first metatarso-phalangeal

Fig. 10.6
Monofilament

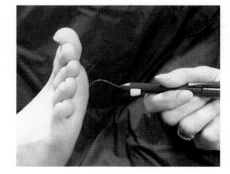

joint and the plantar of the hallux. The person should have his or her eyes closed for this assessment. He or she should experience a buzzing sensation and indicate when this can no longer be felt. A neurothesiometer can also be used and will give a quantifiable reading but this is an expensive piece of equipment not available to many practitioners.

Autonomic neuropathy

Individuals with autonomic neuropathy usually have dry and flaky skin on their feet, and sometimes fissuring in the heel area. This can be a potential site for bacterial infection, which might result in ulceration.

Other tests, which require specialised equipment, can be used to enhance the examination of the diabetic foot. These are usually carried out by the podiatrist. The purpose of assessing the diabetic foot under the various parameters outlined above is to determine the foot which is 'at risk' and undertake a management strategy according to SIGN (2001).

The 'at risk' foot may, therefore, be defined as the foot which has any one of the clinical signs detailed in Box 10.3.

Further detailed instructions in foot health care (see Box 10.2) should be given if the person is assessed as having an 'at risk' foot. Patient education in the prevention of foot problems is the first line of defence. The individual's ability to understand the importance of foot health education should be assessed. The person should also receive regular podiatry care and be made aware of a system for seeking immediate medical attention if a foot problem arises. All healthcare professionals must continually reinforce appropriate foot health education.

TREATMENT AND MANAGEMENT OF FOOT LESIONS

People can present with a wide range of foot problems. Some people require only routine nail cutting and simple advice on foot care (see Box 10.1). Others will have nail problems, callus, corns or even ulceration and will require more intensive care and education (see Box 10.2).

Box 10.3
The 'at risk' foot has any one of these clinical signs

- Ischaemia
- Numbness
- Structural deformities
- Callus and/or corn
- Absence of pedal pulses
- A capillary refill time in excess of 3 seconds
- Limb pain and/or paraesthesia
- Intermittent claudication
- History of foot ulcers
- Loss of sensation of light touch, sharp and blunt touch

NAIL REDUCTION

Toenail cutting in people with diabetes is a matter of great debate, and whether individuals receive this care routinely very often depends on local health board protocols. The task can be one that a nurse, carer or other practitioner can undertake if they have been taught appropriately and deemed to be competent. Many people with healthy feet can undertake safe practice in nail care themselves. However, those 'at risk' must attend a podiatrist regularly for nail routine.

Nails should be cut straight across without cutting down into the corners. Check that there are no ragged edges or sharp corners, which could irritate either the soft tissues of the sulcus of the nail or the adjacent toe. Small spurs of nail may penetrate the soft tissues of the sulcus and an in-growing toenail can develop (see Fig. 10.2).

If the nail is excessively curved, a light pack of sterile cotton wool or chamois can be used under the lateral edge of the nail to prevent it irritating the soft tissues of the sulcus (Fig. 10.7).

The person should be referred to a podiatrist if the nails are thickened as a result of trauma or peripheral vascular disease.

CALLUS AND CORNS

People with diabetes are advised never to treat callus or corns with proprietary medication. 'Corn pads' contain salicylic acid, which can cause chemical trauma to the foot. This is undesirable, especially if the person has neuropathy. These lesions should only be treated by a registered podiatrist.

MECHANICAL THERAPY

In the presence of callus or corns, the podiatrist will reduce these to minimise the pressure being exerted onto the area, and provide mechanical therapy to either redistribute abnormal pressure or cushion the area.

Fig. 10.7
Nail reduction: sterile cotton wool used under lateral edge of the nail to prevent irritation

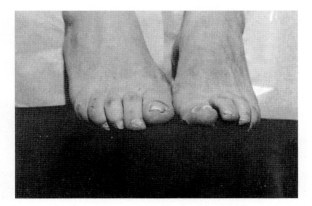

Footwear

Ill-fitting footwear can contribute to foot problems such as ulceration in the person with diabetes (Thomson et al 1991). Footwear should be adequate to accommodate the shape of the foot. People with healthy feet and no lesions can be advised to purchase shoes from a reputable retailer where their feet will be measured and shoes fitted prior to purchase.

Footwear should also be appropriate to the lifestyle of the individual. Good-quality training shoes are ideal for the person who is involved in walking a great deal, as this type of footwear has a deep toe box and thick cushioned sole.

Women with diabetes should be advised on the limited use of court shoes that constrict the toes and have no retaining strap. The height of the heel results in the weight being concentrated onto the forefoot.

People with foot deformities such as hallux valgus, hammer or claw toes require shoes that are wider and deeper than normal. These can be provided from a number of specialist footwear suppliers and are available from the NHS (Fig. 10.8). People with gross foot deformities will require custom-made shoes, which can be authorised by their GP, orthopaedic surgeon or diabetes physician. Some people will require insoles to alleviate abnormal pressures in the foot. Again, the podiatrist can facilitate and supervise these.

INFECTION

People whose glycaemic control is poor are more susceptible to infections and, if ulceration is present, are likely to have delayed healing.

FUNGAL INFECTION

The most common site on the foot for fungal infection is the interdigital spaces. The skin in the affected area may be white, macerated and peeling. The person will

Fig. 10.8
Footwear for people with foot deformities

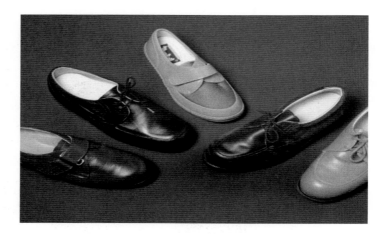

complain of itching and there is the danger of scratching the area and spreading the infection on to the dorsum of the foot. Treatment is usually easy when the fungus responsible has been identified and antifungal agents commenced. However, as with non-diabetic people, fungal infections tend to recur.

When dealing with this type of infection it is important to stress to the person the need for good foot hygiene and that they avoid scratching as this may break the skin allowing a secondary bacterial infection to develop. The person should be referred to their GP for consideration of antibiotic therapy should this occur.

BACTERIAL INFECTION

Secondary infection can be a common problem following tissue breakdown in the diabetic foot. The most common organisms responsible are staphylococci, beta-haemolytic streptococci, aerobic Gram-negative bacilli and anaerobic bacteria (Edmonds et al 1986). When the person presents with a discharging lesion, a swab of the pus should be taken and sent to bacteriology. The individual should be referred immediately to their GP for consideration of antibiotic therapy. Localised treatment involves cleansing the wound with sterile, tepid, saline and dressing with an appropriate dressing (Fig. 10.9) as well as providing protection and pressure

Fig. 10.9
Diabetic foot ulcer protocol

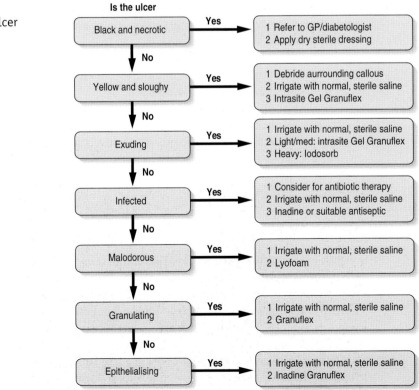

Is the ulcer		
Black and necrotic	Yes	1 Refer to GP/diabetologist 2 Apply dry sterile dressing
Yellow and sloughy	Yes	1 Debride aurrounding callous 2 Irrigate with normal, sterile saline 3 Intrasite Gel Granuflex
Exuding	Yes	1 Irrigate with normal, sterile saline 2 Light/med: intrasite Gel Granuflex 3 Heavy: Iodosorb
Infected	Yes	1 Consider for antibiotic therapy 2 Irrigate with normal, sterile saline 3 Inadine or suitable antiseptic
Malodorous	Yes	1 Irrigate with normal, sterile saline 2 Lyofoam
Granulating	Yes	1 Irrigate with normal, sterile saline 2 Granuflex
Epithelialising	Yes	1 Irrigate with normal, sterile saline 2 Inadine Granuflex

relief to the area. The area is monitored for signs of cellulitis and lymphangitis. X-ray of the foot is important to exclude gas gangrene or osteomyelitis.

Close liaison with all those involved in the treatment of the person with a bacterial infection should enable a satisfactory outcome. This is important as infection in the foot, usually as a result of ulceration, still remains one of the major final pathways to lower limb amputations in people with diabetes (Apelqvist & Larsson 2000).

ULCERATION

Diabetic foot ulceration is a major management problem and prevention of the occurrence and recurrence of such lesions is challenging for all members of the multidisciplinary team.

Abnormal foot pressures are a contributory factor in the development of ulceration in the diabetic foot (Masson et al 1989). Clinical evaluation identifies structural abnormalities creating areas of abnormally high pressure, which might result in the development of corn and callus. There is an increased risk of ulceration developing if callus is not reduced, if pressure persists or if the foot has diminished sensation.

The most common sites are the plantar aspect of the metatarsal heads and the dorsum of the toes if they are clawed. This clinical evaluation is particularly important if there is neuropathy or vascular disease present (see Box 10.3).

Ulceration can also develop in the diabetic foot as a result of constant pressure, e.g. poorly fitting shoes or a foreign object in the shoe. A person affected by peripheral neuropathy causing loss of sensation will allow the pressure to continue for many hours, unaware of tissue damage.

The clinical appearance of the ulcerated area must be recorded to allow objective assessment of healing, by serial measurement of ulcer size. Using a ruler, trace the area and surrounding tissue. Alternatively a photograph of the area and surrounding tissue is more desirable. The person should be referred to the diabetes physician for guidance on antibiotic therapy if an ulcer is present.

RELIEVING PRESSURE ON AN ULCER

To assist in the healing process, the wound must not be subjected to any unnecessary trauma or excessive, abnormal weight-bearing stresses. Complete bed rest is often desirable but not always practical or acceptable to the individual concerned. Therefore, alternative regimes should be considered. The podiatrist can advise on various techniques which can play an important role in this aspect of management of diabetic ulceration.

There are various examples of boots available on the market that can provide pressure relief at the ulcerated site either in the forefoot or heel area (Fig. 10.10)

Fig. 10.10
The IPOS Boot

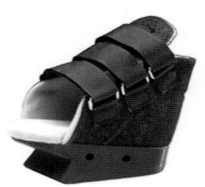

but still allow easy access to the wound for dressing and assessment. These boots are usually acceptable to the individual and encourage compliance. An alternative is a total contact cast that relieves pressure on the affected area but still allows the person to remain mobile (Pollard & Le Quesne 1983). Another alternative is an aircast boot (Fig. 10.11), although some people find these cumbersome. They are contraindicated if severe infection is present or if there is peripheral ischaemia.

When the ulcer has healed it is important to reduce the risk of recurrence at the site and the person should be provided with either a simple insole or a moulded insole (Fig. 10.12).

People must be advised on suitable footwear, which should be sufficiently wide and deep to accommodate any foot deformity. It should also have a retaining medium, such as laces or a 'T' bar, and no stitching or seams on the upper, which may cause unnecessary trauma.

Fig. 10.11
The total contact cast

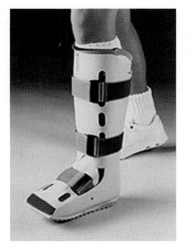

Fig. 10.12
A moulded insole to prevent excessive pressure on a foot ulcer

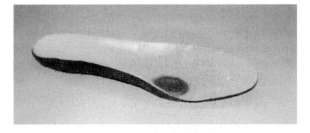

CLINICAL APPEARANCE OF ULCERS

Neuropathic ulcers

A remarkably accurate description of a neuropathic ulcer was first given as long ago as the early nineteenth century (Mott 1818):

> *A round ulcer in the sole of the foot surrounded by a remarkably rough hardening of thick cuticle, characterised by a great degree of insensitivity.*

Neuropathic ulcers characteristically develop on areas of abnormal pressure, such as the plantar aspect of the metatarsal heads. Ulceration can also develop on the medial side of the first metatarsal or lateral side of the fifth metatarsal as a result of pressure from shoes.

The ulcer often has a 'punched out' appearance and consists of a central cavity, usually much larger than the opening into it, surrounded by a hard thick plaque of hyperkeratotic tissue. The ulcer may have slough present on the base or have an infected pus discharge with or without surrounding cellulitis. It may be necessary to X-ray the foot to exclude for osteomyelitis.

Characteristically, the ulcer is painless; often, a moist discharge on hosiery alerts the person to the lesion. The foot is often warm, pink and dry with palpable pedal pulses. The neuropathic foot is also at risk of ulceration from direct trauma, e.g. standing on sharp objects; thermal trauma, e.g. hot water bottles; chemical trauma, e.g. 'corn pads' that contain salicylic acid. The latter being the reason why the person with diabetes is advised never to use these products.

Case study 10.1

Mary is a 64-year-old woman who has had type 2 diabetes for 10 years. She has been meticulous about her diet and blood glucose control since diagnosis. She attends the diabetic clinic for annual review and regularly attends the podiatrist to have her nails cut, having no other

Case study 10.1
Continued

foot problems. On a routine visit to the clinic she complains of numbness in her right foot.

On closer inspection of her foot there is a small ulcer under the second metatarsal head and evidence of leakage on her tights. Mary is adamant that she never walks barefooted and only ever wears the lacing shoe she had with her. The shoe is examined and reveals a drawing pin sticking through the sole of her right shoe. It was unclear how long it had been there as Mary stated that she had not checked the inside of her shoe for several days.

From the development of this lesion and the history it was obvious that Mary had peripheral neuropathy. Tests were carried out by the podiatrist to determine its extent. As on all visits, Mary's circulation was assessed by checking pedal pulses, colour, capillary refill and temperature gradient. These latter tests were satisfactory. The findings of the assessment were recorded.

With Mary's permission, the podiatrist proceeded to dress the ulcer. The foot was cleansed with antiseptic solution and the ulcer was debrided using a scalpel. All dressings should be considered as sterile dressings, whether done in a clinic setting or in the person's home. An assessment of the ulcer was made regarding size and condition of the base. As there was a discharge and surrounding inflammation, a swab was taken of the exudate and sent for bacterial culture and sensitivity. As the wound was showing signs of infection and there was slough at the base, an appropriate dressing was selected (see Fig. 10.9). The ulcer was irrigated with tepid, sterile, normal saline and surrounding tissues gently dried using sterile gauze. The area was dressed with an appropriate dressing and a deflective felt pad applied.

The drawing pin was removed from Mary's shoe and her GP was contacted to inform him of the situation and to consider antibiotic therapy. A further appointment was made for Mary to attend the podiatrist the next day and she was advised to elevate her foot meantime. To minimise weight bearing at the site, Mary was given an Ipos shoe (see Fig 10.10).

As Mary had now developed peripheral neuropathy she required further foot health education, which could be provided by the podiatrist.

On the subsequent visit the dressing to Mary's ulcer was removed and the area assessed. There was evidence of discharge. The area was irrigated with sterile, normal saline. The base of the ulcer was cleaner but there was still evidence of slough. A further dressing was applied and Mary was again asked to return the next day. Thereafter, Mary was closely monitored until the ulcer healed. Her diabetes physician was kept informed of the developments in her condition.

The long-term management of Mary would be to re-educate her in foot health and continue to see her at the clinic at regular intervals.

Ischaemic ulcers

Ischaemic ulcers can develop on the foot of a person with diabetes suffering from peripheral vascular disease. These ulcers can develop on the dorsum or apices of the toes, or on the outer borders of the foot. This is particularly so if hallux valgus is present, the forefoot is broad and the person wears tight-fitting shoes.

Ischaemic necrosis of the tissue can develop as a result of pressure of the footwear obliterating the capillary flow to the area, or as a result of a blockage in the vessel to the area.

The area is usually dry and has a definite line of demarcation which is characteristic of gangrene. If the blockage has been acute, oedema and infection will occur giving a wet gangrene. The person will complain of severe pain and there is usually a history of intermittent claudication and rest pain.

Case study 10.2

Bob is a 70-year-old man who has had type 1 diabetes for 45 years. His diabetes is well controlled. He is retired and leads a relatively inactive life and smoked 25 cigarettes a day until 3 years ago. He regularly attends the podiatrist for the reduction of a corn on his left foot and to have his toenails cut. Bob is aware of the importance of these visits as his circulation has deteriorated over the past 10 years. There has been a history of intermittent claudication, with his walking distance decreasing, and rest pain. Previous assessment by the vascular surgeon showed a blockage at the popliteal fossa. Bob presents at the clinic complaining of a small discoloured area at the tip of his left second toe and another on his 'bunion', which had appeared when he was on holiday. On examination of his feet, they are pale and cold to touch.

Bob's second toe of the left foot is dusky purple at the metatarsal phalangeal joint and gets progressively darker towards the tip, where it is black. An area of necrosis is also present on the medial aspect of his left 1st metatarsal phalangeal joint. Both areas are dry and show no sign of any exudate. Bob complains of severe pain, which prevents him from sleeping at night and also makes him feel nauseous.

With Bob's permission, the area is swabbed with sterile, normal saline and a dry, sterile dressing applied. The podiatrist, in consultation with the diabetes physician, agrees to refer Bob to the vascular surgeon for investigation of his main limb arteries to ascertain if any surgical intervention is feasible.

Bob is given an Ipos shoe to relieve any pressure on the area and prescribed pain relief. His GP is informed of the development in his condition. Twice-weekly visits were arranged for Bob to allow the podiatrist to monitor his condition. After 2 weeks his foot was showing signs of deterioration: the pain had increased and his quality of life had deteriorated. Multiprofessional review indicated that no reconstructive surgery could be carried out. Unfortunately, Bob needed a below-knee amputation.

CURRENT RECOMMENDATIONS FOR WOUND DRESSINGS

There is great variation and debate in the treatment of both ischaemic and neuropathic ulceration with regard to topical dressing and antibiotic therapy. Treatment therefore depends on the local expertise and protocols on the use of the currently available dressings. Consultation with tissue viability nurses is useful when dealing with diabetic ulceration.

Assessment of the wound for dressing

A greater understanding of the science of wound management and the importance of providing the best environment for wound healing has led to a significant improvement in the range of treatments available. The selection process of the dressing is dependent on the assessment of the wound initially. On examination of the wound it is essential to determine which features are present (Box 10.4).

The wound might have more than one of these features. The dressing of choice should address the most prominent or serious factor.

If infection is suspected, a swab must be sent for bacterial culture and antibiotic sensitivity with the person commenced on antibiotic therapy. In people with diabetes, such antibiotic therapy is often of a much longer duration than in the normal population and cover for periods of several weeks is not unusual.

Wound cleansing is essential before applying any dressing and tepid, sterile, normal saline is the one of choice. The use of chlorinated solutions such as Milton or Eusol are no longer recommended for cleansing wounds as they have been found to be toxic to tissues and cells involved in the healing process. They can be irritants to surrounding healthy tissue and have been known to cause bleeding. Hydrogen peroxide is no longer recommended for irrigation of wounds as it can cause irritation to the tissues, stinging and a burning sensation (Leaper 1986). However, a number of wound dressings are currently available that have been used with a degree of success depending on the stage of ulceration.

The use of more traditional dressings, such as gauze with antiseptics, is less favoured because fibres from the gauze can remain on the surface, acting as an irritant and delaying healing. Discharge from the wound can cause adherence of the dressing to the wound surface. Removal of the dressing can further traumatise the healing wound, damaging the granulating tissue. Care should also be taken

Box 10.4
Features that can be present when assessing the wound for a dressing

- Necrosis
- Epithelialisation
- Infection
- Depth
- Slough
- Exudate
- Granulation
- Malodour

when dealing with thin, friable skin because the repeated application and removal of adhesive dressings and tapes can cause tissue damage (Dykes et al 2001).

Interactive dressings

Interactive dressings provide the optimum conditions for wound healing by maintaining a moist environment at the wound surface. They also allow gaseous exchange of oxygen, carbon dioxide and water vapour but are impermeable to the passage of bacteria.

There has been a great deal of controversy as to the use of totally occlusive dressings, preventing the passage of oxygen to the wound. Some research has found that there is rapid formation of capillaries and granulation tissue with an anaerobic environment and as a result of the occlusion, prostaglandin synthesis is inhibited and therefore pain is reduced (Morgan 1990a).

When dealing with diabetic ulceration, however, a great deal of consideration must be given before selecting or applying an occlusive dressing. This should not be used if microvascular disease is present or if anaerobic bacteria infect the wound (Morgan 1990b).

Thermal insulation also aids in the healing process, so dressings should provide insulation and the person should be encouraged to choose suitable footwear.

Environmental dressings

These dressings tend to be more expensive than the traditional dressings. They can be cost-effective, however, because they may be left in situ for several days if the wound is clean. This reduces the need to redress a foot on a daily basis, thus decreasing the costs of both materials and time for the podiatrist or primary care team.

There are many types of environmental dressings from which to select. The groups are listed in Box 10.5.

It is essential that the appropriate dressing is chosen depending on the characteristics of the wound. Each group will be considered in turn to allow the reader the opportunity to compare and contrast the advantages and disadvantages of each.

Box 10.5
Classification of environmental dressings

- Hydrogel
- Hydrofibre
- Hydrocellular foam
- Alginate
- Hydrocolloid
- Semi-permeable films
- Silver antimicrobial

Semi-permeable polymeric films

These are cheap, permeable to water vapour and gases and act as a barrier to external contamination. They can be left in situ for up to 7 days. However, there is sometimes a problem with sizing for smaller wounds and, because they are non-absorbent, they cannot be used if there is a heavy exudate. Care should be exercised with thin, fragile but intact skin. Semi-permeable polymeric films are recommended for shallow ulcers with little exudate.

- *Example:* Dermafilm, Dermoclude, Ensure-it, Omiderm, Opsite, Polyskin, Tegaderm.
- *Features:* sterile, thin, transparent, hypoallergenic, adhesive film.
- *Uses:* shallow ulcers with little exudate.
- *Contraindications:* heavily exuding wounds, as they may trap the exudate.
- *Requirements:* top dressing to protect and insulate the wound.

Hydrocolloids

These dressings are adhesive, flexible and occlusive. They consist of two layers: an outer protective waterproof layer is bonded to an inner layer of hydrocolloid particles and a hydrophobic polymer.

The inner layer of these dressings absorbs the exudate, swells, liquefies and forms a soft moist yellow gel over the wound surface. *Note*: it is important that this feature is not confused with slough. When removed, the gel separates causing no trauma to the tissues. However, care should be taken when removing the dressings because they can damage fragile skin. They encourage formation of granulation tissue but might be malodorous. They are easy to use and allow rapid debridement and, as they are waterproof, allow the person to bathe while wearing the dressing. Hydrocolloids should not be used where anaerobic activity is suspected due to the occlusive properties of the dressing as anaerobic activity may be encouraged.

- *Examples:* Granuflex, Duoderm, Tegasorb.
- *Uses:* wound requiring debridement of necrotic tissue; moderate exudate.
- *Contraindications:* anaerobic bacteria are present in the wound.

Hydrogels

This dressing consists of a pale yellow transparent gel containing starch copolymer. It is usually available in a small plastic dispenser and is used where hydration of necrotic slough within the wound is required. Dressings must be changed daily if slough is present but they can be left for 3 days in clean wounds. The gel is easy to apply and can reduce pain. However, it could be considered wasteful as the remainder of the dispenser must be discarded. If the gel is difficult to remove, a soak of sterile, tepid saline solution should be used. Care should also be taken not to macerate the edges of the wound by overloading it with the gel.

- *Examples:* Intrasite Gel, Purilon.
- *Indications:* sloughy wounds (deep or shallow), granulating wounds, sinuses.
- *Contraindications:* do not use with iodine or povidone iodine preparations.

One stated aim of the St Vincent Declaration is:

> *...to raise an awareness in the population and among health care professionals of present opportunities and the future needs for prevention of the complications of diabetes and of diabetes itself, and to reduce the number of amputations for diabetic gangrene in Europe by 50%. (Diabetes Care and Research in Europe 1990)*

A multidisciplinary approach will facilitate the achievement of this goal.

REFERENCES

Abbott CA, Vileikyte L, Williamson S et al 1998 Multicentre study of the incidence of and predictive risk factors for diabetic neuropathic foot ulceration. Diabetes Care 21(7):1071–1075

Apelqvist J, Larsson J 2000 What is the most effective way to reduce incidence of amputation in the diabetic foot? Diabetes and Metabolism 1:75–83

Armstrong DG, Todd WF, Lavery LA et al 1997 The natural history of acute Charcot's arthropathy in a diabetic foot speciality clinic. Journal of the American Podiatric Medical Association 87:272–278

Baker N, Murali-Krishnan S, Rayman G 2005 A user's guide to foot screening. Part 1: peripheral neuropathy. Diabetic Foot 8(1):28–37

Boulton A, Vileikyte L 2000 The diabetic foot: the scope of the problem. Journal of Family Practice 49:S3–S8

Boulton AJ 2000 The pathway to ulceration; aetiopathogenesis. In: Boulton AJ, Connor H, Cavanagh PR (eds) The foot in diabetes, 3rd edn. John Wiley, Chichester

Courtney M, Church J, Ryan T 2000 Larvae therapy in wound management. Journal of the Royal Society of Medicine 93(Feb):72–74

Diabetes Care and Research in Europe 1990 The Saint Vincent Declaration. Diabetic Medicine 7(4):360

Dykes PJ, Heggie R, Hill SA 2001 Effects of adhesive dressings on the stratum corneum of the skin. Journal of Wound Care 10:2

Edmonds ME, Blundell MP, Morris HE et al 1986 Improved survival of the diabetic foot: the role of the specialised foot clinic. Quarterly Journal of Medicine 60:763–771

Evans P 2002 Larvae therapy and venous leg ulcers: reducing the 'yuk factor' Journal of Wound Care 11(10):407–408

Hobson R 1931 On an enzyme from blow-fly larvae (*Lucillia sericata*) which digests collagen in alkaline solution. Biochemistry 25:1458–1463

Hutchinson A, McIntosh A, Feder G et al 2000 Clinical guidelines for type 2 diabetes: Prevention and management of foot problems. Royal College of General Practitioners, London

Lansdown A 2004 A review of the use of silver in wound care: facts of fallacies? British Journal of Nursing 13(6 suppl):6–17

Leaper D 1986 Antiseptics and their effect on healing tissue. Nursing Times 82(22):45–47

Masson EA, Hay EM, Stockley I et al 1989 Abnormal foot pressures alone may not cause ulceration. Diabetic Medicine 6:426–428

Morgan D 1990a Development of a wound management policy: part 1. Pharmaceutical Journal March:295–297

Morgan D 1990b Development of a wound management policy: part 2. Pharmaceutical Journal March:358–359

Mott VA 1818 A cause of circular callous ulcer in the bottom of the foot. Medical Surgical Register New York 1:129

National Institute for Health and Clinical Excellence (NICE) 2004 Type 2 diabetes: prevention and management of foot problems. NICE, London

Pham H, Armstrong DG, Harvey C et al 2000 Screening techniques to identify people at high risk for diabetic foot ulceration: a prospective multicentre trial. Diabetes Care 23:606–611

Pollard JP, Le Quense LP 1983 Method of healing diabetic forefoot ulcers. British Medical Journal 286:436–437

Scottish Intercollegiate Guidelines (SIGN) 2001 No. 55: management of diabetes. SIGN, Edinburgh

Shearer A, Scuffham P, Gordois A, Oglesby A 2003 Predicted costs and outcomes of reduced vibration detection in the UK. Diabetic Foot 6(1):30–37

Sherman RA 2003 Maggot therapy for treating diabetic foot ulcers unresponsive to conventional therapy. Diabetes Care 26(2):446–451

Stuart L, Wiles P, Chadwick P, Smith P 2004 Improving peripheral arterial assessment of people with diabetes. Diabetic Foot 7(4):183–186

Thomas S, Andrews A, Hay NP, Bourgoise S, 1999 The anti-microbial activity of maggot secretions: results of a preliminary study. Journal of Tissue Viability 9(4):127–132

Thomson FJ, Veves A, Ashe H et al 1991 A team approach to diabetic foot care – the Manchester experience. The Foot 1(2):75–82

United Kingdom Prospective Diabetes Study (UKPDS) 1998 Intensive blood glucose control with sulphonylureas or insulin compared with conventional treatment and risk of complications in patients with type 2 diabetes. Lancet 352:837–853

Ward JD, Boulton AJM 1987 Peripheral vascular abnormalities and diabetic neuropathy. In Dyck PJ et al (eds) Diabetic neuropathy. Saunders, Philadelphia

Watkins PJ 2003 The diabetic foot. ABC of diabetes BMJ Publishing Group, London p 59–64

Wayman J, Nirojogi V, Walker A et al 2000 The cost effectiveness of larval therapy in venous ulcers. Journal of Tissue Viability 10(3):91–94

Williams DRR 1985 Hospital admissions of diabetic patients: information from hospital activity analysis. Diabetic Medicine 2:27–32

Young MJ, Breddy JL, Veves A, Boulton AJ 1994 The prediction of diabetic neuropathic foot ulceration using vibration perception thresholds. A prospective study Diabetes Care 17:557–560

Education for life

Vivien Coates and David Chaney

INTRODUCTION

Education has always been fundamental to caring for people with diabetes. Over the last 20 years the process of educating people with diabetes has evolved, moving from a perspective in which education was often a case of 'telling' the person certain facts to a more structured and complex activity. Traditionally, people with diabetes assumed a passive role, receiving information that might or might not have been individualised to their lifestyle. Currently, a more active role on the part of the person with diabetes is advocated, in which choice and participation is promoted. In addition to offering information, education should help people to acquire psychomotor and problem-solving skills to enable them to self-manage their diabetes alongside all the other demands of daily living. Diabetes education is a major challenge for healthcare professionals as the number of people with diabetes and the complexity of self-management continues to increase.

This chapter considers the development of diabetes education, from provision of information to a more complex activity in which the individual's capability to actively self-manage a difficult chronic condition. The process of providing education will be discussed, as will a range of topics that are to be covered when providing a comprehensive education programme to enable people to successfully self-manage their diabetes.

THE EVOLVING NATURE OF DIABETES EDUCATION

During the last 20 years, great changes have occurred in the provision of diabetes services. The delivery of care has moved to being based predominantly in primary rather than secondary care, the diabetes teams have extended and become more specialised and the role and number of diabetes nurse specialists and practice nurses has radically altered the composition of the diabetes work force. Furthermore, the incidence of diabetes has increased and the treatment and management regimens are much more complex.

In view of such changes it is not surprising that diabetes education has also progressed. Lucas and Walker (2004) reviewed the changing modes of diabetes education over the last 20 years and noted that during the 1980s and early 1990s education was usually delivered during a routine hospital outpatient clinic. It was likely that the education was largely didactic in nature, conventionally the healthcare professional would give advice and information to the individual in the expectation that the advice would be followed. This approach did not allow individuals to balance diabetes self-management with the exigencies of daily living, for example, not having time to make a healthy meal, being unable to eat at an ideal time or not being able to take exercise despite knowing that this would benefit blood glucose levels. Individuals need to know how to manage these situations and such problems cannot be left to be successfully resolved at the next clinic visit. Didactic teaching did not help people to develop skills in which trade-off and compromise were acceptable.

As it was realised that an *ad hoc* approach to education was not ideal, more structured approaches were required. In addition, programmes that fostered decision making and problem solving, as well as providing the baseline information for diabetes self-management, were required. The expansion in the numbers of people presenting with diabetes and the increasing complexity of management regimens necessitated a greater involvement of all healthcare professionals in diabetes care. Of particular importance is the increase in the numbers of specialist dieticians, specialist podiatrists, diabetes nurse specialists, practice nurses, nurse practitioners and community nurses, who all play a major part in the development and delivery of diabetes education programmes.

WHY EDUCATE PEOPLE WITH DIABETES?

It is generally accepted that people need knowledge and skills, and the motivation to use these, to begin self-management of diabetes. According to the European Diabetes Policy Group Guidelines (International Diabetes Federation (IDF) Europe 1999a) for those with type 1 diabetes:

The aims of education and training are to provide information in an acceptable form, in order that people with diabetes develop the knowledge to self-manage their diabetes and empower them to make informed choices in their life. (p. 255)

Similarly, for those with type 2 diabetes:

It is the responsibility of the diabetes team to ensure that the person with diabetes can follow the life-style of their educated choice, achieved through the three elements of empowerment: knowledge, behavioural skills and self-responsibility. (IDF 1999b, p. 719)

These quotations plot out the scope of education and immediately indicate that knowledge alone is not the goal. Knowledge is essential, but on its own is not enough, to enable effective self-management of diabetes (Snoek 2003). If educating people was simply about remedying an information deficit then the task would be easier. When psychomotor skills and psychological attributes such as empowerment and self-responsibility are added in, the whole endeavour becomes more challenging.

The definitions and guidelines from the IDF were designed to ensure that diabetes strategies were consistent at a European level, however, the sentiments are also endorsed at more local levels. For example, the National Service Framework (NSF) for Diabetes (Department of Health (DH) 2001a) published 12 standards, the third of which emphasised the need for a broad reaching view of educating people with diabetes. The aim of Standard 3 was:

To ensure that people with diabetes are empowered to enhance their personal control over the day-to-day management of their diabetes in a way that enables them to experience the best possible quality of life.

The accompanying standard is set as follows:

All children, young people and adults with diabetes will receive a service which encourages partnership in decision-making, supports them in managing their diabetes and helps them to adopt and maintain a healthy lifestyle. This will be reflected in an agreed and shared care plan in an appropriate format and language. Where appropriate, parents and carers should be fully engaged in this process.

When the details of the standard are considered in greater detail it can be seen that education is at its core. The range of the standard covers much more than an understanding of diabetes as a medical condition. To experience the best possible quality of life might also involve, for example, symptom management, access to social and other services, managing work and the resources of employment services and developing strategies to deal with the psychological consequences of illness.

DIABETES SELF-MANAGEMENT

Successful diabetes self-management is notoriously difficult to achieve. Research relating to diabetes self-management confirms that people with diabetes are often unable to manage their condition as fully as might be desired by themselves and by healthcare professionals (Donnan et al 2002, Reed et al 2003, Vermeire et al 2003). Suboptimal self-management can translate into poor metabolic and psychological outcomes, although as DeVries et al (2004) point out, the causes of suboptimal glycaemic control are multifactorial. Furthermore, developing educational interventions to help improve self-management is also difficult (Hampson et al 2001, Norris et al 2001).

STRUCTURED DIABETES EDUCATION

Although a robust case can be made for the need for education, the way in which it is best provided is not clear. For example, the National Institute for Health and Clinical Excellence (NICE 2003) conducted a systematic review of the available evidence to inform the provision of educational programmes. As a result of the review it was not possible to advocate any particular educational programme. However, it was possible to recommend that a programme of structured diabetes education covering all major aspects of diabetes self-care should be made available to all people with diabetes shortly after diagnosis and then on an agreed continuing basis.

The provision of education is a complex intervention and, as such, it is a difficult area to research. Despite the wealth of papers dealing with education of people with diabetes the quality of research on this subject has often been criticised (Brown 1992, Ellis et al 2004, Griffin et al 1998). Cooper et al (2001) explored the effects of education by analysing 12 meta-analyses based on research into education for people with a chronic disease where behaviour modification is a part of the treatment regimen. While this review was broader than diabetes, they found that the methodological rigour of the research was often poor; therefore, despite a large volume of work being conducted, it was not of good-enough quality to enable it to be used as evidence on which to base practice. Nonetheless, the authors were able to recommend that 'practitioners use theoretically based teaching strategies which include behaviour change tactics that affect feelings and attitudes' (Cooper et al 2001, p. 107).

Healthcare professionals are therefore often in a situation where they must provide education programmes for people with diabetes but there is a dearth of information to inform their practice. This is an area that is now receiving greater attention. For example, if the Diabetes UK website is consulted (www.diabetes.org.uk), a range of studies evaluating education programmes can be viewed.

The NICE Health Technology Appraisal mentioned above (NICE 2003), described structured education as:

> *A planned and graded programme that is comprehensive in scope, flexible in content, responsive to an individual's clinical and psychological needs and adaptable to his or her educational and cultural background.*

In response to the NICE report, the Department of Health and Diabetes UK established the Patient Education Working Group in May 2004, which reported in 2005 (DH & Diabetes UK 2005). The working group established a set of criteria with recommendations that implementation of the criteria would ensure a high-quality, structured diabetes education programme. These are:

- have a stated philosophy
- to have a structured, written programme
- to have trained educators
- to be quality assured
- to be audited.

Three of the most widely cited structured education programmes that fulfil these criteria are: the Diabetes Education for Self-Management for Ongoing and Newly Diagnosed programme (DESMOND see: www.diabetes.org.uk and www.desmond-project.org.uk); the Dose Adjustment For Normal Eating (DAFNE Study Group 2002) and the Diabetes X-PERT Programme. These will be considered in turn.

DIABETES EDUCATION AND SELF-MANAGEMENT FOR ONGOING AND NEWLY DIAGNOSED

Whereas DAFNE is designed for people with type 1 diabetes, the Diabetes Education and Self-Management for Ongoing and Newly Diagnosed (DESMOND) programme provides structured self-management group education to individuals who are newly diagnosed with type 2 diabetes. The DESMOND programme was based on chronic disease management programmes in the USA and European models of care that included structured diabetes education. At the time of writing, the programme is being evaluated according to the Medical Research Council Framework for evaluating complex interventions (Campbell et al 2000).

A randomised controlled trial, the largest of its kind in newly diagnosed adults with type 2 diabetes, is in progress and is due to report in 2007.

The programme can be offered as a 1-day 6-hour programme or in two half-day sessions or three 2-hour sessions. Groups consist of between five and ten individuals and are facilitated by two trained educators. Part of the programme involves personal goal setting and action planning to achieve goal outcomes. Goal setting and action planning increases self-efficacy and this has been shown to lead to improved biomedical and psychosocial outcomes (Bodenheimer et al 2002, see Chapter 3).

Meanwhile in the UK and, following NICE guidance mentioned above, the DESMOND programme is being rolled out to primary care services with the backing of the DH. It is considered to be the only widely available programme that currently fulfils the criteria for structured diabetes education for people with type 2 diabetes.

There are other examples of structured diabetes education programmes (Everett et al 2003, Sumner & Dyson 2004) and research in which structured diabetes education has been evaluated (Anderson et al 1995, Cooper et al 2003, Griffin et al 1998, Hampson et al 2001, Norris et al 2001, Trento et al 2002). All this work is contributing to an evidence base to guide this area of practice and in so doing is slowly making up for a long-recognised deficit in this aspect of care.

DOSE ADJUSTMENT FOR NORMAL EATING

One programme that has been specifically applied to diabetes is the Dose Adjustment For Normal Eating (DAFNE) project. This programme, which is jointly funded by the DH and Diabetes UK, involves structured training in intensive insulin therapy and self-management. The main principles of the course are:

- that individuals learn the skills required to adjust insulin to match the free choice of carbohydrates eaten during a meal
- to promote self-management and independence from the diabetes care team
- to do this using the principles of adult education in a group setting.

The programme is based on a well established and evaluated inpatient model pioneered in Düsseldorf (Muhlhauser et al 1987). The objective of the programme was to evaluate whether such a training programme could lead to improved glycaemic control and quality of life (DAFNE Study Group 2002). Further details can be obtained from www.dafne.uk.com.

Sue, (case Study 11.1) to complete the DAFNE programme would have participated in 5 days of outpatient training. The overall aim was to enable Sue to enhance her self-management abilities and gain confidence and, subsequently, independence from her diabetes team. She would have been in a group of six to eight people in which three main topics are covered: (1) nutrition, (2) dose

Case study 11.1

Sue had lived with type 1 diabetes for 29 years. She had been on a multiple injection regimen of insulin for the past 10 years and regularly monitored her blood glucose levels. She had been frustrated because despite doing her best she found that adjusting her insulin doses was a bit 'hit and miss' and she often ended up with too high or too low readings. She felt angry much of the time, and burdened – as if diabetes ruled her life. She attended a DAFNE training programme and learned (or in her case relearned) about carbohydrate counting. She also learned a more precise method of working out exactly how much insulin she needed for the amount of carbohydrate she ate. By following this regimen she managed to reduce her insulin dose and yet be more flexible with her diet in terms of quality and quantity. Her glycaemic control improved, she had less hypoglycaemia and she managed to lose some weight. She described her new knowledge and skills as 'liberating'.

adjustment of insulin and (3) preventing and managing hypoglycaemia and hyperglycaemia and managing special circumstances such as exercise. To be able to attend the DAFNE course, Sue would have needed to attend an approved hospital diabetes centre that met specific criteria. To be an approved site, the diabetes centre staff would have completed a DAFNE Educator Programme and be registered as DAFNE educators. It is preferable that at least four members of staff are trained and registered to deliver the DAFNE programme. Another criterion required for approval is that the whole diabetes team must be committed to the philosophy of DAFNE. This philosophy states that the culture of the diabetes centre must be supportive of autonomous, knowledgeable people with diabetes. It is essential that the whole team commits to this and not just the registered educators.

Hence, Sue would remain on her multiple injection regimen as this will maximise her opportunities for dose adjustment. Sue would learn how to use quick-acting insulin according to the amount of carbohydrate that she had eaten. During the DAFNE programme, she would have worked out how many units of quick-acting insulin she needed for each 10 g of carbohydrate that she ate. This ratio of insulin units : carbohydrates varies from person to person and sometimes at different times of the day. During the DAFNE programme, Sue had worked out that her insulin units : carbohydrate portion ratio was as follows:

- Breakfast: 2 units of quick-acting insulin per 10 g of carbohydrate.
- Lunch: 1 unit of quick-acting insulin per 10 g of carbohydrate.
- Evening meal: 1 unit of quick-acting insulin per 10 g of carbohydrate.

As part of the DAFNE programme, blood glucose targets are agreed between the person with diabetes and the DAFNE team. Targets are agreed for fasting levels of blood glucose, pre-meal and bedtime. The actual ratio of insulin dose to carbohydrate portion is explained during the programme and individualised to each person. The above ratios are presented as an example only and will differ from person to person.

DIABETES X-PERT PROGRAMME

A more locally based structured education programme, which has been evaluated by a randomised controlled trial, is the Diabetes X-PERT programme. This is based on the theories of empowerment and discovery learning for adults. Results were positive in the biomedical and psychosocial outcomes of the programme. This programme offers training and quality assurance for healthcare professionals. Further details can be found on www.xpert-diabetes.org.uk. (Department of Health (DH) 2001b).

PLANNING EDUCATION

Education can be facilitated on a one-to-one basis, in small groups or in a more formal seminar or discussion group. However, adults learn best when the principles of adult education are used (NICE 2003). Education can take place in a person's home, at a health centre or at a diabetes centre, in the community or in hospital. While it is crucial that a structured programme is the foundation of education, casual and opportunistic education will also occur in relation to episodes, such as illness, that demand new or revised knowledge and skills. Much has been written about group education versus individual education (Cooper et al 2002, Griffin et al 1998, Sumner et al 2001) and the balance will depend on circumstances, such as numbers of people requiring education and staff resources. Whereas education for those with newly diagnosed type 1 diabetes is usually delivered on an individual basis, increasing numbers of people newly diagnosed with type 2 diabetes are lending themselves to group education. As yet, there is little evidence to inform the relative merits of which approach is best employed, with which type of person and in which circumstances. However, group education should also be seen as an opportunity for individuals to share experiences and offer each other mutual support.

VISUAL AIDS

Materials used for education will include audiovisual and computer-based material, posters, leaflets, diagrams and practical equipment such as food models. Visual aids should encourage interaction between educator and the person with diabetes (Llahana et al 2001). Materials are very important to assist with the educational process and must be of the highest standards of accuracy as well as comprehensible, relevant and culturally specific.

Healthcare professionals using literature to support their education sessions should be aware of the problems of readability and literacy status of the material that they use. These problems are compounded where English is not a person's first language. There is, therefore, a considerable need for educational materials which are culturally specific. Diabetes UK has made a determined effort to provide educational material suitable for a wide range of individuals, cultures and topics (see www.diabetes.org.uk).

TIMING OF EDUCATION

At diagnosis, the person newly diagnosed with diabetes is usually anxious and although appearing keen to learn, is not necessarily in the most receptive frame of mind to acquire new knowledge. An education programme must therefore be planned and staged to take into account the person's ability to assimilate information (Coates 1999).

The first stage of education commences at the time of diagnosis. The person will require emotional support and might want to ask questions regarding diagnosis, cause and implications of diabetes. This is a time when the educator will learn about the physical, psychological, spiritual and cultural needs of the individual and what is important to him or her. For example, the newly diagnosed individual might be terrified that the diagnosis will impact negatively on work or relationships, or on his or her abilities to be a parent or indeed to become a parent. A needs assessment will inform the educational content of immediate and ongoing education. The educational programme should be structured to provide the person with essential facts based on what questions he or she is asking and what he or she needs to know to be safe.

When commencing education with the individual concerned, it is important to determine first how much the individual already knows about diabetes and to discuss any misconceptions that he or she might have. It is common for people to be aware of the worst complications of diabetes, such as amputation or blindness, and many believe that these are inevitable.

The second stage requires a learning plan that has more detailed education on aspects of diabetes that address both the individual's agenda and that of the educator (Box 11.3). Although the healthcare team has its own agenda for education, individuals determine which area they want to learn about next. Educational material must be presented in small, bite-sized chunks to enable the person assimilate it. Inviting questions, reiterating and encouraging the person to verbally reflect what has been said will assist the individual to make sense of his or her new knowledge and relate it to his or her own circumstances. Reinforcement with written material will help the individual to remember new facts but should not be a substitute for face-to-face collaborative education (Ellis et al 2004). It is good practice to review what the person understands of the content covered at a previous session prior to moving on to the next topic. This helps to secure the knowledge and skills acquired and give an opportunity to discuss how these have been implemented into the real world of living with diabetes. Collaborative goal setting will help the individual to ground his or her new-found knowledge into his or her unique circumstances.

For education to be effective, it must be reinforced and the person motivated in self-management. This is the third stage in education. A multitude of evidence demonstrates that educational interventions work for a limited period of time only. Stressful periods (see Chapter 3) get in the way of the hard work that optimal self-management requires. Hence, education becomes a lifelong process and includes facilitating individuals in problem solving to manage new situations.

DEVELOPING EDUCATIONAL PROGRAMMES

According to the NICE report (NICE 2003), there are no trials specifically concerned with the content of initial education for those with type 1 diabetes. However, there is a reasonable consensus of professional opinion of the important issues that should be included in diabetes education programmes (Audit Commission 2000, IDF Europe 1999a, 1999b, NICE 2003). As education is delivered by a multidisciplinary team it is vital that the content of education is agreed to avoid conflicting information. All members of the team will be involved in educational care from time to time as the need arises. When developing programmes, people with diabetes should be involved to help determine content as it is known that healthcare professionals and individuals with chronic diseases have differences of opinion regarding the content of educational programmes (Clark & Hampson 2003, Woodcock & Kinmonth 2001).

PEOPLE WITH TYPE 2 DIABETES

For most people, the diagnosis and management of type 2 diabetes starts in general practice. At the first visit after diagnosis, the person might well be bewildered and hence not very receptive to education. However, some 'first aid' measures are appropriate until the next appointment. These would include a simple explanation of diabetes, simple adjustments to diet following the taking of a dietary history and, for some, the commencement of monitoring might be appropriate (Box 11.1). The person should be advised regarding contact numbers should there be a problem.

Box 11.1

Suggested staged approach to the education of the person with type 2 diabetes

First clinic visit

- answer person's questions
- simple explanation of diabetes
- dietary history and some adjustments
- choice of monitoring and how to undertake it (if advocated)
- screening for complications, e.g. blood pressure, neuropathy, feet, eyes, proteinuria/microalbuminuria
- assess smoking status and offer cessation advice if necessary
- contact numbers

Second clinic visit

- answer person's questions
- dietary reinforcement and encouragement
- assessment of monitoring, review results
- explanation as to what affects glucose levels
- simple explanation of benefits of good diabetic control
- foot health education
- prescription exemption (if relevant)
- Department of Social Security benefits (if relevant)
- driving
- related insurances
- carry identification that the person has diabetes
- Diabetes UK

Third clinic visit

- answer person's questions
- dietary reinforcement and encouragement
- review monitoring and explain meaning of results
- explain the benefits of clinic attendance
- simple explanation of diabetic complications and benefits of using the healthcare team to screen for these
- benefits of exercise
- enabling appropriate self-management during illness or any new problem
- progressive nature of diabetes
- lifestyle modifications
- potential impact on employment
- subsequent visits might include education regarding oral hypoglycaemic agents, travel and holidays and hypoglycaemia

As far as possible, the family and friends of the individual should be included. Engaging social support has been shown to improve glycaemic and psychosocial outcomes in diabetes self-management (Van Dam et al 2005). At a further visit, the individual's questions regarding diabetes would first be addressed.

Monitoring technique would be assessed and the results discussed. From the outset the person with diabetes should be encouraged to make sense of monitoring results with help from the clinician rather than have the clinician immediately offering explanations about reasons for results. As diet is the mainstay of management for the person with type 2 diabetes, more detailed and tailored dietary advice from the dietician would be appropriate (see Chapter 6).

If the person has already started oral hypoglycaemic therapy, it would be appropriate to advise that prescriptions can be obtained free in the UK by completing a FP92A form. This is not available to people who are treated by diet alone.

Education should take into account that people with type 2 diabetes have multiple risk factors contributing to premature cardiovascular disease. Subsequent visits would include education about the personal risk factors for the individual. The person with diabetes then has the knowledge to make decisions about what he or she would like to do to improve his or her risk factors. The individual can identify his or her own personal goals for self-management and an action plan to operationalise goal achievement is put into place. Goals might be to do with taking exercise, dietary changes or finding strategies to take medication regularly. Goals need to be realistic and achievable (see Chapter 3).

Diabetes education will include foot care, the clinic attendance that includes screening for complications and the associated cardiovascular risk factors and the need for exercise. The progressive nature of diabetes, the potential impact on employment, driving and insurance also need to be discussed. Thereafter, all visits are opportunities for revising education and educating people as their management alters or complications develop and progress.

People with type 2 diabetes requiring insulin therapy

In the UK, until recently, most people with type 2 diabetes who required insulin therapy were referred to the local hospital clinic and consequently education was initiated and maintained by the secondary care diabetes specialist nurse (DSN). However, this situation is changing as more practice nurses and community nurses are developing expertise in diabetes care and striving to keep people with type 2 diabetes in their own environment in primary care. The involvement of family and friends is encouraged to dispel some of the myths about diabetes and to promote a positive approach to the individual concerned (Van Dam et al 2005).

One of the main issues for someone with type 2 diabetes starting insulin therapy is weight gain. The nature of type 2 diabetes means that many people are already overweight and might struggle with healthy eating. Insulin therapy in type 2 diabetes can lead to weight gain and associated increasing insulin resistance with limited improvement in glycaemia (UKPDS 1998). Subsequently, insulin doses increase, weight increases and the vicious cycle continues. It is important that the person with diabetes approaching insulin therapy understands why insulin therapy is the optimal treatment. The best way to make sense of this is through blood glucose monitoring. People might also want an opportunity to maximise healthy eating and exercise and observe the impact of this through blood glucose monitoring. If there is no change in results then it will help the individual to know that, despite best efforts, insulin therapy is the only alternative. If there are improvements then, depending on the level of improvement, the individual might need to make a decision about whether these lifestyle options are realistic and sustainable in the long-term.

PEOPLE WITH TYPE 1 DIABETES

The individual with newly diagnosed type 1 diabetes would be referred to secondary care services as assessment is required as to whether or not he or she is suffering from diabetic ketoacidosis, which would result in admission to hospital.

Subcutaneous insulin is commenced immediately if the person does not have diabetic ketoacidosis. This is usually done by the DSN in secondary care but as an outpatient or in the person's own home. The individual is usually in a state of shock at the time of diagnosis. Many of the questions a newly diagnosed person has at this time are around how this could have happened and whether he or she has caused it. In terms of education, people usually respond well to undertaking practical procedures but will not necessarily retain much factual information. Hence, at the first visit, blood glucose monitoring and how to inject insulin will be taught (Box 11.2). When starting insulin therapy, the person will usually be seen at least daily for a few days and thereafter followed up as necessary with telephone contact being maintained by way of further support. Again, a staged approach is required, with more detailed explanations in response to the individual's questions being introduced over a period of about 6 weeks. As people with type 1 diabetes tend to be seen more frequently, reinforcement of education is easier and individuals have greater opportunities to ask pertinent questions.

TOPICS THAT REQUIRE EDUCATIONAL INPUT

Many topics need to be covered in an education programme, as illustrated in Box 11.3. The subjects that follow are not intended to indicate the entire range of topics rather they reflect important areas which have not yet been discussed.

Box 11.2
Suggested staged approach to the education of the person with type 1 diabetes

First clinic visit

- answer person's questions
- simple explanation of diabetes and the actions of insulin
- dietary history and some adjustments
- initiate home blood glucose monitoring
- initiate insulin injections
- assess smoking status and offer cessation advice if necessary
- identification of diagnosis of diabetes

Box 11.2
Continued

Within the first week

- answer person's questions
- full dietary assessment and adjustments
- how to acquire necessary equipment for injecting and monitoring
- prescription exemption
- Department of Social Security benefits (if relevant)
- discuss goals for blood glucose levels using a staged approach
- assessment of monitoring technique and review results
- explanation of what affects glucose levels
- employer
- hypoglycaemia
- driving
- insurances
- Diabetes UK telephone number and address

Within the second/third week

- answer person's questions
- insulin dose adjustment
- foot health education
- alcohol
- advantages of good diabetic control
- the benefits of clinic attendance
- explanation of the complications of diabetes and benefits of screening for diabetic complications
- benefits and effects of exercise

Within the first month

- answer person's questions
- hyperglycaemia
- what to do if person is unwell
- subsequent visits may include education regarding travel and holidays, sexual health matters, stress related problems

---

Box 11.3
Checklist detailing recording of topics in diabetes education programme

Alcohol

Contact numbers

- surgery
- community nurse
- hospital clinic
- diabetes nurse specialist

Complications

- annual review
- eyes (blurred vision at diagnosis)
- kidneys

- feet
- blood pressure/coronary heart disease
- sexual health

Diabetes UK

Department of Social Security benefits

Diet

- seen by dietician
- date to see dietician
- current weight, body mass index and waist size
- importance of regular meals (people with type 1 diabetes especially)
- diabetic foods
- alcohol
- special occasions
- what to do when unwell

Driving

- DVLA
- insurance
- planning a long journey
- what to do if hypoglycaemic (not relevant if controlled by diet or a biguanide)

Employment

- informing employer
- shift work
- can register disabled

Exercise

- benefits of exercise
- forms of exercise
- adjusting insulin (if relevant)
- adjusting diet

Hypoglycaemia (if relevant)

- what causes it
- how to recognise it
- how to treat it
- what happens if you do not recognise or treat it
- telling your family and friends
- telling employers
- exercise
- driving
- nocturnal hypoglycaemic episodes
- use of glucagon

Hyperglycaemia

- what does it feel like
- what causes it

Box 11.3
Continued

- how to recognise it
- how to treat it
- what happens if you do not recognise or treat it
- when to call for help

Identification

- carry identification of diagnosis of diabetes

Insulin (only if relevant)

- how it works
- how to inject (including mixing insulins if necessary)
- when to inject
- where to inject and rotation of sites
- storage of insulin and equipment
- disposal of equipment
- availability of equipment
- can relatives inject person?
- never omit insulin
- how to manage missed injections
- insulin dose adjustment

Insurance

- car insurance
- life insurance

Monitoring

- blood glucose/urinary glucose
- when to test
- recording results
- explanation of results
- goals to aim for
- urinary/blood ketone testing (if relevant)
- glycated haemoglobin

Oral hypoglycaemic agents

- when to take
- expected side-effects
- what to do if unwell

Podiatrist

- referred to podiatrist
- seen by podiatrist
- foot health education

Prescription exemption (not relevant if controlled by diet alone)

Sexual health

- contraception
- planned pregnancies and why

- impotence
- menopause

Smoking

- help to stop

Stress

Travel and holidays

- lying in
- adjusting therapy

What is diabetes?

What to do if unwell?

HYPERGLYCAEMIA

The person newly diagnosed with type 1 diabetes or type 2 diabetes will be informed that their blood glucose levels are high. All those with type 1 diabetes will be well aware of the symptoms that took them to see their doctor and these include thirst, polyuria, lethargy and probably a dramatic weight loss (Box 11.4). They might also have experienced *Candida*, cramps, painful peripheral neuritis and blurring of vision, which are all a consequence of hyperglycaemia (see Chapter 1). If the individual was acidotic then he or she might also have had nausea and/or vomiting and have been breathless. Those with type 2 diabetes might also have had all or some of these symptoms but possibly over a longer period of time and less intensely. Some people will have rationalised their symptoms and decided that they were tired because they were working too hard, or that they were thirsty because the weather had been hot. In helping to make sense of diabetes it is important to explain how the different symptoms relate to the physiology of diabetes and that if these symptoms return then it means that some aspect of treatment and/or self-management needs to be reviewed. Self-referral should be encouraged especially as it has been shown that type 2 diabetes requires progressively increasing treatment over time (UKPDS 1998).

Some people with type 2 diabetes might not have experience of hyperglycaemic symptoms if their diabetes had been diagnosed through a screening procedure at work or at a clinic. It can make the diagnosis more difficult to come to terms with if this is the case and blood glucose or urine monitoring can help to accept the reality of having diabetes.

Hyperglycaemia can be due to any one of several factors (Box 11.5). People with diabetes might be anxious about finding that their blood glucose levels are above target levels but can be reassured that they have time on their side to adjust their treatment or to seek advice. Left untreated, metabolic decompensation progresses to a hyperosmolar hyperglycaemic syndrome in the person with type 2 diabetes or diabetic ketoacidosis (DKA) in the person dependent on insulin (see Chapter 5).

Box 11.4
Symptoms and Signs of hyperglycaemia

Symptoms of hyperglycaemia

Polydipsia
Polyuria
Abdominal pain especially in children
Weight loss
General tiredness
Blurring of vision
Itching and skin
Pain and paraesthesia in the feet and limbs
Nausea and vomiting

Signs of hyperglycaemia

Hypovolaemia
Glycosuria
Tachycardia
Dehydration
Acidotic breath
Deep rapid breathing
Skin infections
Confusion and restlessness

Box 11.5
Factors that affect blood glucose levels

Hyperglycaemia

- not enough insulin
- not enough exercise
- too much food
- any other illness
- stress
- erratic absorption of insulin

Hypoglycaemia

- too much insulin
- unplanned exercise
- not enough food, delaying or missing a meal
- recovering from an illness
- alcohol
- erratic absorption of insulin

WHAT TO DO IF UNWELL

Self management during an acute illness has always been an educational challenge because the elements of diabetes self-management during illness might have been taught early on but the individual with diabetes might not experience illness for many years and will have completely forgotten 'the rules'. The most important advice to be given here is to seek help and to seek it quickly (Box 11.6). People who are unwell lose their appetite and tend to stop their drugs or insulin therapy because they fear hypoglycaemia; however, metabolic control can rapidly deteriorate under these circumstances. Food substitutes are presented in Box 11.6.

When a person is unwell, in most situations, the blood glucose will rise due to the hormones of stress even if the appetite has been suppressed (see Chapter 1). This means that the individual should not reduce his or her insulin or hypoglycaemic agents but in fact might need to increase the doses. Hence, people who are ill need to increase their monitoring to four times daily.

People with type 1 diabetes need to test their blood or urine for ketones and, if present, should self-refer to their GP, nurse or local accident and emergency centre for assessment. If all else is forgotten, people should be encouraged to remember the golden rule 'Never stop taking insulin'. Vomiting might be a sign of diabetic ketoacidosis and the individual needs to seek urgent medical help, if not from the GP then again at his or her local accident and emergency centre.

People with type 2 diabetes who are unwell are also encouraged to increase self-monitoring as treatment might need to be started for those controlling their diabetes by diet alone, or treatment adjusted if already on oral hypoglycaemic agents or insulin. People taking metformin should continue with treatment if possible but as metformin needs to be taken with food this may be problematic. Alternative treatment might be required if the illness is prolonged.

Those people who are taking a sulphonylurea (e.g. gliclazide) and/or a thiazolidinedione (pioglitazone or rosiglitazone) need to continue with these but, again, adjustment of the sulphonylurea might be required in prolonged illness. Advice must be sought if there are any elevated blood glucose levels and ketonuria or evidence of raised blood ketones.

Box 11.6
What to do if unwell

- *Do not* stop taking medication or insulin
- If unable to eat food, take small, frequent amounts of semi-solids. Examples of 10 g of carbohydrate are:
  - 50 g scoop ice cream
  - 200 mL milk
  - 200 mL tomato soup
  - 50 mL Lucozade
- half a small carton of fruit yoghurt
- Drink about 3 litres of water or sugar-free fluids per day to prevent dehydration
- Increase self-monitoring to twice a day if urine testing and four times a day if blood testing
- If facilities are available, test urine for ketones if there is a 2% glycosuria or if blood glucose levels are above 15 mmol/L
- Contact the GP or nurse if any of the following apply:
  - the presence of ketonuria
  - vomiting
  - abdominal pain
  - elevated temperature
  - the illness has lasted longer than 24 hours

The exception to becoming hyperglycaemic during illness is if the person is suffering from a gastrointestinal illness causing diarrhoea but is not affected systemically. In this case, the person might become hypoglycaemic and, should this happen, he or she needs to seek advice. Oral hypoglycaemic medication might need to be stopped for the duration of the diarrhoea and insulin, in people with type 1 diabetes and type 2 diabetes, might need to be reduced. However, insulin in type 1 diabetes can never be stopped (see Box 11.6).

Case study 11.2

Bill is 38 years old and has had type 1 diabetes for the last 15 years. He has remained fit and well during this time and has been fortunate enough to avoid any serious illnesses since diagnosis. The previous evening, after being out with friends, he began to feel very nauseous. He had a disturbed night during which he vomited and developed abdominal cramps. In the morning he measured his blood glucose level, as was his usual routine, and was a little surprised that it was 15 mmol/L. He could not face any fluids or breakfast and decided to crawl back into bed and take the day off work. As he was not having breakfast he thought he should miss his morning insulin in case he became hypoglycaemic while asleep. By mid-morning he was still nauseated and feeling very thirsty. He called his GP and then went back to bed. His GP visited him and took his temperature, blood pressure, examined his abdomen and then tested his urine and blood glucose. Bill was astonished to learn that his blood glucose was now 24 mmol/L, despite no food, and that he had a large amount of ketones in his urine. The GP arranged for him to be admitted to hospital where his blood glucose levels were brought under control using intravenous fluids and insulin.

Before discharge a nurse discussed with Bill his rationale for missing his insulin. Bill learned the hard way that missing his insulin had resulted in this medically dangerous situation. The nurse helped Bill to make sense of what had happened and he was reminded that he should never stop taking his insulin, even if he cannot take his usual meals. In such circumstances he might even require more insulin depending on his blood glucose levels.

The reasons and significance of why ketones must be monitored if the blood glucose exceeds 10 mmol/L were discussed Even during illness the target blood glucose levels should remain in the 4.0–7.0 mmol/L range. The actual adjustment of insulin will vary according to individual needs.

It emerged that whereas Bill had always attended his clinic appointments he had never faced this situation before so he had never thought to check up on what to do when unwell. This is a common example of the importance of continuing education for people with diabetes.

HYPOGLYCAEMIA

Education about hypoglycaemia features prominently in caring for people with diabetes. Hypoglycaemia is the most common side effect of insulin therapy or sulphonylurea treatment. Individuals are frightened of hypoglycaemia and so may deliberately keep their blood glucose levels high. People must be taught how to achieve healthy glucose profiles and prevent, recognise and treat hypoglycaemia.

Case study 11.3

> John is a 54-year-old man who was diagnosed with type 2 diabetes 10 years ago. John was controlled on oral medication for the first 8 years following diagnosis. Two years before, despite maximum dose oral therapy and lifestyle changes, John was started on a regimen of a fixed mixture of insulin. John's current body mass index is $29\,kg/m^2$ and until recently was achieving optimal blood glucose control. At his recent clinic visit John expressed concern about some hypoglycaemic episodes he had been experiencing.

Every year, about 25–30% of insulin-treated people with diabetes suffer one or more severe hypoglycaemic episodes requiring the assistance of others (Williams & Pickup 2004). Symptoms such as hunger, pallor, tremors, palpitations, anxiety and confusion in association with a blood glucose level of less than 4 mmol/L is diagnostic of a hypoglycaemic episode.

The concern expressed by John is both common and well founded, given that hypoglycaemia can lead to both recurrent physical morbidity and to recurrent or persistent psychosocial morbidity and sometimes even death (Cryer 1997).

The issue of hypoglycaemia within type 2 diabetes has received more attention since the reporting of the UKPDS (1998), in which it was noted that 11.2% of people with type 2 diabetes using insulin experienced major hypoglycaemia for which hospital admission was required. More recent studies suggest that this might be an underestimate (Donnelly et al 2005, Leese et al 2003). It is therefore necessary to review the education John received when diagnosed with type 2 diabetes and when he started on insulin therapy. There might be clinical reasons why John has started to become hypoglycaemic and these must be considered. The possible causes of these hypoglycaemic episodes should be discussed (see Box 11.5).

Each of these issues should be discussed in a session with John. On reflection, he might thereafter understand what has caused his hypoglycaemia and also how to prevent it recurring. Sometimes, however, the cause is not obvious and clinical causes should be considered. These include:

- Weight loss leading to reduced insulin or sulphonylurea requirements.
- Renal impairment causing delayed excretion of insulin or sulphonlyurea.
- Rarely, other physical causes such as Addison's disease or insulinoma.

In the event of no cause being found then insulin needs to be reduced and John is encouraged to learn and become confident in adjusting his insulin.

Treatment should be discussed with John and his family/friends as overcorrection can lead to rebound hyperglycaemia and undercorrection can lead to recurrence of the hypoglycaemic episode within a short space of time. Hypoglycaemia can be treated with:

- 10–20 g rapidly absorbing carbohydrate, such as between three and six Dextroenergy glucose sweets, 50–100 mL Lucozade or two to four teaspoons sugar dissolved in water.
- This should be backed up with a meal, if it is due, or a snack if the hypoglycaemic episode has occurred between meals. The snack should contain carbohydrate and could consist of two or three biscuits, fruit, crackers or a sandwich.

John should be encouraged to carry fast-acting carbohydrate with him at all times. He should also have a card or equivalent that identifies him as having diabetes in case he should have a severe hypoglycaemic episode that requires external help.

Symptoms of hypoglycaemia vary from person to person and most people experience only one or two of a number of possible symptoms (McAuley et al 2001). John is already clear that his symptoms include tremor and profuse sweating and this wakes him up at night. However, it has been shown that people can sleep through overnight hypoglycaemia and wake up in the morning none the wiser (Diabetes Control and Complications Trial (DCCT) 1993). A history of headache or feeling 'hungover' might be a clue to overnight hypoglycaemia. A nocturnal hypoglycaemic episode is frightening for the individual and their bedfellow! People who require reassurance about this are advised to check their blood glucose level before going to bed at night and, if below 6 mmol/L, to consume extra carbohydrate before sleeping. It might be necessary to reduce the overnight basal insulin; however, the use of a short-acting insulin analogue with evening meal or within a fixed mixture of insulin has also been shown to reduce the incidence of night-time hypoglycaemia (Hermansen et al 2001).

Hypoglycaemic symptoms can be experienced at glucose levels greater than 4 mmol/L. If John's blood glucose levels had been running consistently high for a period of time then, when the blood glucose falls, John might experience hypoglycaemic symptoms but not be at risk of impaired consciousness. The experience of hypoglycaemia is still very unpleasant and needs to be treated in the same way; however, as John improves his glycaemic control then his symptoms of hypoglycaemia would occur at a lower level.

John is right to be concerned about hypoglycaemia because there is a possibility if he continues to have episodes regularly his warning symptoms will become impaired or lost. If this happens then John would be asked to reduce his insulin doses and run his blood glucose levels at a higher level, completely avoiding all hypoglycaemia for a period of about 3 months. Thereafter, his insulin dose could be increased gradually to optimise glycaemic control and he should then find that his warning symptoms have returned. In a few people, warning symptoms do not return and specialist advice should be sought.

Hypoglycaemia is normally classified as mild (self-recognised and self-treated), moderate (usually conscious and able to self-treat or be treated with help from another person but without emergency intervention) and severe (requires the assistance of a third party and normally emergency intervention). Treatment of hypoglycaemia depends on the individual's level of consciousness and should preferably be administered after confirmation of blood glucose. If the individual needs help from another (apart from medical help) then there are two treatments that can be administered by others.

Glucose in the form of a viscous gel ('Hypostop' now known as 'Glucagel') can be squeezed into the mouth if the person is uncooperative and is of particular value in children but should not be used if a person is unconscious.

Left untreated, the person would eventually lapse into a hypoglycaemic coma and would require assistance from someone for treatment. In this situation, relatives and friends can be taught how to administer glucagon 1 mg intramuscularly. Glucagon (known as 'Glucagen') is available in convenient packs containing 1 mg of the dried form of the agent and 1 mL diluting solution. The expiry date needs to be checked regularly and another prescription obtained before the current vial expires. Glucagon can be rapidly dissolved and injected subcutaneously or intramuscularly by another adult. A competent healthcare professional can give glucagon intravenously. The person should recover within 10 minutes then be encouraged to consume at least 20 g oral carbohydrate to replace glucose stores.

It is not unusual if a person is in a hypoglycaemic coma for emergency attention to be sought even though relatives or carers administer glucagon. Likewise, it should be sought calmly and quickly in the event of a person's inability to swallow or loss of consciousness. While glucagon can bring a person out of a comatose state, it is not without its problems. One problem with glucagon is that it can cause nausea and vomiting, so although the person becomes more responsive, he or she may be resistant to eating or drinking. It is, however, necessary for the individual to eat in addition to receiving the glucagon injection to replenish liver glycogen stores and prevent secondary hypoglycaemia.

Glucagon is less effective when the person has been unconscious for a prolonged period of time (Cryer et al 2003). Under these circumstances, an intravenous injection of 50% dextrose is preferred and this is usually carried out in the hospital emergency care department. People can experience a severe headache for up to 24 hours after a prolonged episode of hypoglycaemia. Remember that although used in type 1 diabetes, glucagon is less useful in type 2 diabetes as hypoglycaemia, when induced by sulphonylureas, is often prolonged and a rise in glucose will stimulate a further rise in insulin secretion (Cryer et al 2003).

In the elderly, hypoglycaemia might simulate a transient ischaemic attack or a cerebral vascular accident. It is therefore important to check a blood glucose level in any elderly person who presents with neurological signs. Although these might appear to be of a minor nature, all such individuals should be admitted to hospital for a minimum of 24 hours for observation.

EXERCISE

Exercise has many physical and psychological benefits especially for people with diabetes. A moderate to high level of exercise in people with type 2 diabetes has been shown to reduce the risk of cardiovascular mortality (Hu et al 2005). In another study, regular exercise was associated with reduced development of metabolic risk factors for cardiovascular disease, fewer exercise-induced cardiac abnormalities and reduced comorbidity (Petrella et al 2005). Exercise promotes a feeling of well-being and also improves the tissue sensitivity to insulin, thus decreasing insulin resistance. It is recommended that all people should be advised to maintain at least moderate levels of physical activity on a regular basis (SIGN 2001). The recommended form of exercise builds on what a person currently does rather than commence some new strenuous form of exercise. An example of this would be to increase the distance they walked each day for example, by walking to a further bus stop rather than using the closest one. When discussing exercise with people it is worth mentioning that physical activity such as gardening and housework can be regarded as a form of exercise, and not only those activities associated with recreational exercise. However, for those people with type 2 diabetes who wish to pursue a new form of exercise, a medical examination by their GP is advisable to ensure that there are no contraindications. Warm-up and cool-down exercises are recommended to avoid undue physical stresses to muscles and joints.

Exercise and hypoglycaemia

The person who is taking a sulphonylurea or insulin therapy might be at risk of hypoglycaemia in relation to exercise.

For the person taking insulin, hypoglycaemia can be prevented by reducing the relevant insulin 'vigorously' and consume extra carbohydrate during the exercise (Gallen 2005, and see Chapter 6). If the person is overweight, then reduction in insulin/sulphonylurea would be the best option as extra carbohydrate might negate any weight loss intended by the individual. The reduction in insulin dose depends on the intensity and length of time the exercise takes. People are also advised to inject their insulin into their abdomen and so avoid injecting into their 'active' limbs, which will increase their absorption of insulin (Frier 1999). People should also avoid exercising at the peak time when their insulin is working. Carbo-loading before exercise to increase blood glucose will impair exercise performance and so normal intake with reduction in insulin is more effective both in preventing hyperglycaemia and hypoglycaemia. Taking rapidly absorbed carbohydrate in the form of a sport drink will provide the energy needed as well as the fluid intake required (Gallen 2005). People are advised to discuss this fine-tuning of their self-management with the healthcare team prior to undertaking exercise.

To achieve optimal self-management, the individual should use blood glucose monitoring prior to exercise, immediately afterwards and for several hours thereafter. If a person's blood glucose is above 17 mmol/L, they should avoid exercise, especially if they also have ketosis (Frier 1999, page 278). On the basis of these results and by a system of trial and error, people can learn by how much their insulin should be altered in response to differing amounts of exercise. The prevention of exercise-induced hypoglycaemia partly depends on the type of exercise, its frequency and intensity.

People's perception of exercise varies markedly. A person who frequently walks his or her children to school might be very active but does not consider this as exercise, whereas a person who works out on an exercise bicycle at home for 10 minutes might believe that he or she is taking sufficient exercise. It is important to determine each individual person's normal lifestyle so that advice can be tailored.

It should also be remembered that hypoglycaemia can occur several hours after exercise has ceased. Hence, the person who goes swimming is unlikely to become hypoglycaemic in the pool but is more likely to feel hypoglycaemic a few hours later and insulin may need to be reduced.

The intensity of the exercise will affect the rate at which hypoglycaemia develops. Thus walking might gradually reduce the blood glucose level, resulting in hypoglycaemia several hours later, whereas half an hour on a squash court will rapidly reduce a blood glucose level. People should be guided and advised regarding their own requirements on an individual basis.

It is recommended that if the individual has experienced a severe hypoglycaemic episode within the previous 24 hours then exercise should be avoided as the counter-regulatory hormone response to hypoglycaemia is reduced and the likelihood of hypoglycaemia would be increased (Gallen 2005). Further information regarding managing diabetes during exercise can be found at www.runsweet.com.

IDENTIFICATION

Everyone with diabetes is advised to carry some form of identification to inform others that they have diabetes. This may be a card, a Medical Alert bracelet or a similar locket. Most pharmaceutical companies produce identification cards and there are advertisements in the *Balance* magazine of Diabetes UK for these products.

SMOKING

The combination of smoking and diabetes has been shown to escalate coronary heart disease, arterial disease (UKPDS 1998) and renal disease (Biesenbach et al 1997). Hence, the person who smokes is at greater risk of having heart disease, a cerebrovascular accident or developing peripheral vascular disease. People might not be aware of the increased risks due to both conditions and every effort must be made to strongly encourage those who smoke to stop. Those people wishing to stop should be referred to the smoking cessation support in primary care or increasingly at local pharmacies. There are various methods recommended to help people stop smoking (SIGN 2001). These include the use of nicotine patches, group or individual counselling and hypnosis. A recent study showed that cigarette smokers with diabetes had poor awareness, knowledge and uptake of smoking cessation treatments and concluded that this is a neglected area of diabetes education (Gill et al 2005).

STRESS

Stress, both physical and psychological, can have adverse effects on an individual's blood glucose levels. This is important because suboptimal glycaemic control can be a symptom of stress and diabetes education would include assessment as to whether there were physical or emotional barriers to self-management. This holistic approach to care views the individual as a whole person and not just the sum of the parts (see Chapter 3).

ALCOHOL

Healthy drinking limits are the same for all whether or not they have diabetes. The recommended limits are 14 units of alcohol per week for women and 21 units of alcohol per week for men. People who are trying to lose weight should restrict their alcohol intake further (see Chapter 6). Alcohol taken with food seldom causes problems unless drunk to excess. When excessive alcohol is taken, hypoglycaemia can result. Others might wrongly assume that the person is drunk and not appreciate that the person needs glucose. People should be advised not to drink on an empty stomach but to consume food as well. Specific guidance is required for those who are trying to follow a calorie-restricted diet, and they should be referred to the dietician for this (see Chapter 6). It is difficult to manage diabetes if the person concerned has problems with excessive alcohol intake. People should be advised that there might be a greater lowering of their blood glucose if they undertake exercise after consuming alcohol (SIGN 2001). Both sulphonylureas and insulin can cause profound hypoglycaemia in the presence of excess alcohol. Under these circumstances, relaxing of glycaemic control is necessary if there is concern about excessive alcohol intake. The person should be encouraged to eat while drinking alcohol and to consume a carbohydrate-rich snack before going to bed.

DRIVING

A recent, large, multicentre study showed that people with type 1 diabetes were more likely to have driving mishaps due to hypoglycaemia than people with type 2 diabetes. However, it was found that half of those with type 1 diabetes and three-quarters of those with type 2 diabetes had never discussed hypoglycaemia and driving with their physicians (Cox et al 2003). This is clearly an important and neglected area of diabetes education.

In the UK, only those on oral hypoglycaemic agents or insulin therapy are required to inform the Driving and Vehicle Licensing Authority (DVLA). The responsibility for informing the DVLA lies with the individual. The primary healthcare team must ensure that the person is aware of this obligation. Once the DVLA has been informed then those on insulin therapy have a driving licence that is issued for 3 years and renewed at 3-yearly intervals thereafter, provided there is a satisfactory medical report. Those on oral hypoglycaemic agents will be given information and invited to inform the DVLA if there is any change in their treatment. They must also inform the DVLA if there is any other diabetes-related reason that might impair their ability to drive, i.e. diabetic eye disease. Once the person reaches 70 years of age the driving licence is renewed annually subject to a satisfactory medical report. This report is usually obtained from the GP or hospital specialist.

By contrast, in Northern Ireland the regulations state that every person with diabetes must inform the DVLA for Northern Ireland, regardless of their treatment. It is anticipated that this will change in the near future and will be brought into line with the DVLA in the rest of the UK. Those people who are controlled by diet or diet and tablets are issued with a licence for 10 years. Those individuals requiring insulin are issued with a licence for 1–3 years (Deegan 1995).

The great risk to the person and others is of hypoglycaemia while driving. For this reason, people who are taking a sulphonylurea or insulin are usually prohibited from driving any form of public service transport or heavy goods vehicle. Indeed, it is currently against the law for a Large Goods Vehicle licence or a Passenger Carrying Vehicle licence to be issued to a person requiring insulin therapy. As the UK becomes more involved in the European Union, this discretionary basis is likely to disappear. Helpful details can be downloaded from the Diabetes UK website (www.diabetes.org.uk).

Prevention of hypoglycaemia when driving is paramount. Any journey must be planned, especially a long journey. A blood glucose measurement must be taken before commencing any journey and carbohydrate consumed if below 5 mmol/L as driving becomes impaired when blood glucose is at 3.6 mmol/L (Cox et al 2003). Thereafter, blood glucose should be monitored at intervals on long journeys. A journey should not be undertaken when the person has injected insulin without having eaten. The person must allow for stops for food and to monitor blood glucose levels every 2 hours. Both rapidly absorbed carbohydrate and more substantial carbohydrate should be kept in a car in case of breakdown or delays in traffic, which could cause circumstances leading to hypoglycaemia.

Glucose must be kept in the car within easy access. If the person should feel hypoglycaemic, he or she should stop the car (using the hard shoulder on a motorway if needs be), switch off the engine, get out of the driver's seat and take glucose to correct the hypoglycaemia. All this is required because the person could legally be charged with being in control of a vehicle while under the influence of drugs (Frier 1999). It is recommended that the journey is not resumed until 45 minutes after the hypoglycaemic episode so that cognitive function is fully resumed (Frier 1999).

All people with diabetes who are drivers should be advised to have their eyesight checked regularly and not to drive if their vision deteriorates suddenly or if their visual acuity with glasses is less than 6/12 in both eyes. Any eyesight changes must be notified to the DVLA.

EMPLOYMENT

It is illegal for employers to discriminate against people with diabetes except when there is substantial risk. Therefore people who are in employment are strongly advised to inform their employer of their diabetes. For those who have type 2 diabetes treated with diet and/or metformin there is not usually any problem with this. People who have type 1 diabetes or type 2 diabetes on sulphonylureas or insulin may find that certain aspects of their job are restricted because of the risk of hypoglycaemia.

There are, however, some forms of employment which are prohibited to any person who has type 1 diabetes (Box 11.7). Diabetes UK has lobbied hard to reduce the use of a 'blanket ban' on recruitment and is pressing hard for individual assessment (Diabetes UK 2005). Any employment where hypoglycaemia might not only endanger the life of the individual but also the lives of others is either prohibited or will require careful individual assessment. Those people who are currently employed in jobs that are classed as high risk and who then acquire type 1 diabetes might be allowed to continue in employment but in a less demanding post. Some forms of employment could be considered as inadvisable for a person with type 1 diabetes to pursue, again because of the risk of hypoglycaemia (Box 11.7).

While it is possible for people with type 1 diabetes to undertake shift work, they will need advice regarding insulin doses and the balancing of food intake to accommodate this. Where this is relevant, the person would be advised to visit his or her diabetes specialist nurse for detailed, personal advice.

Diabetes is a condition for which a person can register as disabled within the UK. However, people should be warned of the employment consequences of being thus labelled. They should also be advised that, once registered as disabled, they cannot request removal from the register at a later date. The Disability Discrimination

Box 11.7
Prohibited and inadvisable employment

Occupations prohibited to people with type 1 diabetes

- Airline pilot
- Train driver or working track-side
- Armed forces
- A job that needs a large goods vehicle (over 7.5 tonnes) or any large passenger-carrying licence
- Cab or taxi licences: some local authorities still operate a blanket ban

Types of occupation that would be inadvisable for people with type 1 diabetes

- Deep-sea diver
- Steeplejack
- Blast furnaceman

Act (1995) introduced new laws to reduce discrimination against disabled people and this should help people with diabetes seeking some types of work from which they were previously excluded, such as in the emergency services. For further information see the Diabetes UK website (www.diabetes.org.uk).

BENEFITS

As mentioned earlier, those people whose diabetes is controlled by the use of oral hypoglycaemic agents or insulin are eligible for prescription exemption within the UK. Previously, individuals controlled by diet were also exempt but this is no longer the case as the 'diabetic diet' is now regarded as healthy eating and not a 'special diet' (see Chapter 6). To apply for prescription exemption, the person must complete a FP92A form, which is available from the local social security office, some GP surgeries and local pharmacists. The person's GP, who is required to complete part of the form, will then send it to the Family Health Services Authority (FHSA). The FHSA issues the exemption certificate and on its presentation, the person has exemption from paying for any items which are available on prescription. Prescription exemption can make a financial saving for those individuals who have multiple comorbidities requiring several different medications.

There are other benefits to which people with diabetes may be entitled within the UK. Further advice can be obtained by contacting the local Citizens' Advice Bureau, the welfare rights adviser or social services department. Although several social security benefits are available, not everyone with diabetes is eligible for them. All people with diabetes are eligible for a free NHS eye test. However, only those on a low income are eligible for NHS vouchers for glasses. All these areas of policy are subject to change and if required the Citizens' Advice Bureau webpage and advice guide can be consulted (www.citizensadvice.org.uk, www.adviceguide.org.uk).

INSURANCE

People should be advised to inform all the insurance companies from which they have relevant policies once they are diagnosed as having diabetes. The responsibility for informing the various companies rests with the individual; this includes driving insurance. Failure to do so might jeopardise future claims. Some companies confer an additional premium for people with diabetes. The Disability Discrimination Act (1995) has not led to a reduced premium for life assurance or health-related policies as there is proof of higher risk for people with certain conditions, including diabetes. It is therefore important to shop around and receive quotations from several different companies. Diabetes UK has special arrangements with various insurance companies for people with diabetes. Advice can be given on motor insurance, life assurance and travel insurance. People should be encouraged to contact their regional Diabetes UK office for further information.

DIABETES UK

Diabetes UK, formerly known as the British Diabetic Association, is a charitable organisation, set up in 1934 by Dr R D Lawrence and the author H G Wells, both of whom had diabetes. Diabetes UK was the first patient organisation in the UK and promotes quality care for people with diabetes through campaigning, providing information, support and also funding research. It has an Advisory Council of people with diabetes and healthcare professionals to provide guidance on policy and care issues. Under the auspices of Diabetes UK, there are over 400 active local groups which are run entirely by volunteers. These groups offer support and companionship to people with diabetes and their carers. There are also a number of support events, such as adult and family weekends, children's holidays and diabetes for life conferences throughout the UK. In addition, there is a network of regional offices to support and promote the work of Diabetes UK at a regional and national level across the UK. A careline (0845 1202 8960) is also available for professionals and people who wish to seek support and advice.

Those who join Diabetes UK receive a copy of *Balance* magazine bimonthly, updates on local or UK work and information on local Diabetes UK groups. The *Balance* magazine is for people with diabetes and is a welcome resource on current issues in diabetes management. Voluntary groups play an important part in caring for people with diabetes and people should be encouraged to link up with their local group.

For the healthcare professional, Diabetes UK is a valuable resource centre, which offers help and advice on a wide variety of topics. Healthcare professionals also have the opportunity to join Diabetes UK, which offers information and supplies professional journals.

PREPREGNANCY COUNSELLING AND SEXUAL HEALTH

Females

Some women with type 1 diabetes might require an alteration in insulin requirement around the time of menstruation (Steel 1991); some find that they require an increase in the insulin dose for a few days whereas others need to decrease the dose. Each woman has to be considered individually. Women with optimal glycaemic control have similar fertility to non-diabetic women. Hence, it is important that contraceptive advice is offered. Ideally, optimal glucose control should be achieved before conception and most women of child-bearing age should be encouraged to self-refer if they are considering pregnancy.

All forms of contraception currently available can be used by women with diabetes. The combined oral contraceptive pill is acceptable, especially with lower doses of oestrogen (Price 2003). Mechanical devices, intrauterine devices, caps and condoms have a fairly high failure rate, unless they are used very carefully, within the population as a whole. They are therefore not recommended where pregnancy is contraindicated. The intrauterine device was initially thought to increase pelvic inflammatory disease but this concern has now been resolved (Price 2003). Sterilisation is a suitable method of contraception for both men and women with diabetes once they are sure that their families are completed.

Planning for pregnancy is of vital importance for a healthy outcome of both mother and baby. Suboptimal glycaemic control at the time of conception and during the first trimester is associated with an increased risk of fetal malformation and mortality (Girling & Dornhorst 2003). It is, therefore, important that all women of childbearing age are made aware of this fact and encouraged to achieve optimal glycaemic control before stopping contraception. The majority of women of child-bearing age with diabetes will have type 1 diabetes, although there are an increasing number of women with type 2 diabetes now becoming pregnant as the age of those diagnosed with type 2 diabetes continues to decrease. Those people on oral hypoglycaemic agents should be changed to insulin regimens prior to conception.

Hormone Replacement Therapy is suitable for women requiring symptomatic relief.

Males

Erectile dysfunction (ED) is usually under-reported by men with diabetes. The causes are multifactorial (see Chapter 9). Erectile dysfunction that is due to psychogenic causes might respond to psychosexual counselling. Men with diabetes should be informed of this potential complication and encouraged to report it if it is present and causing problems. The treatment options for those with erectile dysfunction have increased greatly over the last 10 years and include oral treatments such as phosphodiesterase 5 (PDE 5) inhibitors such as sildenafil (Viagra), intracavernosal injection therapy, transurethral administration of a vasoactive agent (e.g. alprostadil) (MUSE) and vacuum therapy. For a minority of men, surgery might also be required. Price (2003) suggests considerable advantages to erectile dysfunction being treated in primary care and, as no specialised equipment is required, there is no reason why GPs with an interest in diabetes and the management of erectile dysfunction should not effectively treat the majority of men with this problem.

DIABETES AND TRAVEL

Case study 11.4

> Samantha is a 32-year-old woman who was diagnosed with type 1 diabetes at the age of 23. Since diagnosis she has maintained excellent control and is very meticulous about her diabetes care. She is married with two children and is planning a foreign holiday this year with her husband and family. This is her first holiday abroad and she is worried about how she will maintain control of her diabetes as she is flying to New York and so will enter a new time zone.

Travel abroad is no longer an aspiration but a reality for many. Overseas travel can pose special problems but these can be minimised by taking a few simple steps prior to departure. Samantha will need a consultation with her diabetes care team to discuss insulin adjustment in relation to the times of her flights, meals taken and time change experienced. She should contact the travel agent or airline involved and request anticipated mealtimes and flight duration. This information, along with departure and arrival times, and time zone differences, should be made available to the diabetes team so that Samantha can be advised on insulin adjustment. Although not necessary in Samantha's case, it must be remembered that all immunisations should be completed 1 month before travel to allow time to recover from side effects.

Before travelling, Samantha should be advised to pack extra insulin, two insulin pens and/or syringes, a blood glucose monitoring device, lancets and test strips and prescription medicines such as glucagon where needed. These should be packed in hand luggage. A travelling companion, in this instance her husband, should carry extra supplies in case hand luggage is lost. Samantha should also have supplies of both simple and complex carbohydrate sources, such as glucose tablets and biscuits in case of hypoglycaemia, identification such as an identity card, insurance papers and medication for diarrhoea (Chandran & Edelman 2003, Diabetes UK 2002). Before departure she should obtain a doctor's letter containing a list of medication and any medical devices that she must carry. The letter should also include any allergies or medications to which Samantha is sensitive. As she is travelling by air, this letter should be presented to airline staff at check-in. All medication, especially insulin, should be carried in Samantha's hand luggage and must not be stored within the cargo hold of the aircraft as this will be subject to temperature extremes and so the medication might be damaged. For up to date information on air travel contact the Diabetes UK website.

Special diabetic airline meals are available but tend to be low in carbohydrates. A standard airline meal, supplemented with extra bread, fresh fruit or beverages where necessary is recommended. Samantha should wait until she receives her meal on the plane before taking her insulin in case of delay in eating or low carbohydrate content of the meal. For those on oral agents, such as sulphonylureas, it might be easier to skip a dose and have slight hyperglycaemia for 6–8 hours than to take two doses too close together (Chandran & Edelman 2003).

Having arrived at her destination, Samantha will store her insulin in a thermal insulated bag or refrigerator, if available, as insulin vials maintain their potency at room temperature but not in temperatures that are either too warm or freezing. She should be advised that blood glucose meters generally perform best between 15 and 35°C, when outside these temperatures she should always check her meter with a control solution. If Samantha has problems with peripheral neuropathy or arteriopathy then she will need to be aware of foot-care guidelines, including avoiding going barefoot in case of foot injury. In the event of illness, injury or loss of medication, a list of English-speaking doctors practising abroad can be obtained from the International Association for Medical Assistance to Travellers at www.iamat.org. Samantha should be advised that insulin might be named differently in other countries and might come in different strengths, thus she should always double-check and ask about prescriptions when uncertain.

Travelling is an opportunity to revise what to do if unwell (Box 11.6). There is no reason why people with diabetes should avoid travel; early planning considering diabetes needs should ensure a happy and successful journey.

CONCLUSION

In the UK, diabetes education is considered an integral aspect of diabetes care and self-management. People with diabetes need to understand how to manage their condition on a day-to-day basis if optimal physical outcomes and quality of life are to be achieved and maintained. Although self-management of diabetes is widely advocated, research shows that individuals find this an onerous and difficult task. Healthcare professionals should be able to support people with diabetes to make autonomous informed decisions about how to integrate self-care strategies into their lives with diabetes. Effective education is time-consuming and its effects on an individual's lifestyle and quality of life can be difficult to measure although it is acknowledged that this should be part of a multidisciplinary lifestyle-intervention programme (SIGN 2001). In diabetes the trend has moved from informal *ad hoc* education towards a more structured approach delivered over time. More diabetes education is taking place in community settings as opposed to hospital settings. While for many years there was a dearth of high-quality research on the process and outcomes of diabetes education this situation is changing and as the rigor of the research improves, so the evidence base for practice is also increasing.

REFERENCES

Anderson RM, Funnell MM, Butler P et al 1995 Patient empowerment: results of a randomised controlled trial. Diabetes Care 18:943–949

Audit Commission 2000 Testing times. Audit Commission, London

Biesenbach G, Grafinger P, Janko O, Zazgornik J 1997 Influence of cigarette smoking on the progression of clinical diabetic retinopathy in type 2 diabetic patients. Clinical Nephropathy 48:146–150

Bodenheimer T, Lorig K, Holman H, Grumbach K 2002 Patient self-management of chronic disease in primary care. Journal of the American Medical Association 288(19):2469–2475

Brown SA 1992 Meta-analysis of diabetes patient education research: variations in intervention effects across studies. Research Nursing Health 15:409–419

Campbell M, Fitzpatrick R, Haines A et al 2000 Framework for design and evaluation of complex interventions to improve health. British Medical Journal 321(7262): 694–696

Chandran M, Edelman SV 2003 Have insulin, will fly: diabetes management during air travel and time zone adjustment strategies. Clinical Diabetes 21(2):82–85

Clark M, Hampson SE 2003 Comparison of patients' and healthcare professionals' beliefs and attitudes towards type 2 diabetes. Diabetic Medicine 20:152–154

Coates VE 1999 Education for patients and clients. Routledge, London

Cooper H, Booth K, Gill G 2002 Diabetes education: the patient's perspective. Journal of Diabetes Nursing 6(3):91–95

Cooper H, Booth K, Gill G 2003 Using combined research methods for exploring diabetes patient education. Patient Education and Counseling 51:45–52

Cooper H, Booth K, Fear S, Gill G 2001 Chronic disease patient education: lessons from meta-analyses. Patient Education & Counseling 44:107–117

Cox DJ, Penberthy JK, Zrebiec J et al 2003 Diabetes and driving mishaps: frequency and correlations from a multinational survey. Diabetes Care 26(8):2329–2334

Cryer PE 1997 Hypoglycaemia pathophysiology, diagnosis and treatment. Oxford University Press, New York

Cryer PE, Davis SN, Shamoon H 2003 Hypoglycaemia in diabetes. Diabetes Care 26(6):1902–1912

DAFNE Study Group 2002 Training in flexible, intensive insulin management to enable dietary freedom in people with type 1 diabetes: dose adjustment for normal eating (DAFNE) randomised controlled trial. British Medical Journal 325:726

Deegan G 1995 Medical Q and As. Balance 144:36

Department of Health (DH) and Diabetes UK 2005 Structured patient education in diabetes: Report from the Patient Education Working Group. DH, London

Department of Health (DH) 2001a, National Service Framework for Diabetes, DH, London

Department of Health (DH) 2001b, The expert patient: a new approach to chronic disease management for the 21st century. DH, London

DeVries JH, Snoek FJ, Heine RJ 2004 Persistent poor glycaemic control in adult type 1 diabetes. A closer look at the problem. Diabetic Medicine 21:1263–1268

Diabetes Control and Complications Trial (DCCT) Research Group 1993 The effect of intensive treatment of diabetes on the development and progression of long-term complications in insulin-dependent diabetes mellitus. The New England Journal of Medicine 329(14):977–986

Diabetes UK 2002 Air travel and insulin. Online. Available: www.diabetes.org.uk/infocentre/inform/airtravel.htm [accessed 6 February 2005]

Diabetes UK 2005 Information for health care professionals/structured education. Online. Available: www.diabetes.org.uk [accessed 31 January 2005]

Donnan PT, MacDonald TM, Morris AD 2002 Adherence to prescribed oral hyperglycaemic medication in a population of patients with type 2 diabetes: a retrospective cohort study. Diabetes Medicine 19:279–284

Donnelly LA, Morris AD, Frier BM et al DARTS/MEMO Collaboration 2005 Frequency and predictors of hypoglycaemia in type 1 and insulin-treated type 2 diabetes: a population-based study. Diabetic Medicine 22(6):749–755

Ellis SE, Speroff T, Dittus RS et al 2004 Diabetes patient education: a meta-analysis and meta-regression Patient Education and Counseling 52(1):97–105

Everett J, Jenkins E, Kerr D, Cavan DA 2003 Implementation of an effective outpatient intensive education programme for patients with type 1 diabetes. Practical Diabetes International 20(2):51–55

Frier BM 1999 Living with hypoglycaemia. In Frier BM, Fisher BM (eds) Hypoglycaemia in clinical diabetes. John Wiley, Chichester

Gallen I 2005 The management of insulin treated diabetes and sport. Practical Diabetes International 22(8):307–312

Gill GV, Morgan C, MacFarlane IA 2005 Awareness and use of smoking cessation treatments among diabetic patients. Diabetic Medicine 22:658–660

Girling J, Dornhorst A 2003 Pregnancy and diabetes. In Pickup JC, Williams G (eds) Textbook of diabetes, 3rd edn. Section 16:65.1. Blackwell Scientific, Oxford

Griffin S, Kinmonth AL, Skinner C, Kelly J 1998 Educational and psychosocial interventions for adults with diabetes. British Diabetic Association, London

Hampson SE, Skinner TC, Hart J et al 2001 Effects of educational and psychosocial interventions for adolescents with diabetes mellitus: a systematic review. Health Technology Assessment 5:1–79

Hermansen K, Madsbad S, Perrild H et al 2001 Comparison of the soluble basal insulin analog and insulin detemir with NPH insulin. Diabetes Care 24:296–301

Hu G, Jousilahti P, Barengo NC et al 2005 Physical activity, cardiovascular risk factors and mortality among Finnish adults with diabetes. Diabetes Care 28(4):799–805

International Diabetes Federation (IDF) Europe 1999a A desktop guide to type 1 (insulin-dependent) diabetes mellitus. Diabetic Medicine 16(3):253–266

International Diabetes Federation (IDF) Europe 1999b A desktop guide to type 2 diabetes mellitus. Diabetic Medicine 16(9):716–730

Leese GP, Wang J, Broomhall J et al. DARTS/MEMO Collaboration. 2003 Frequency of severe hypoglycemia requiring emergency treatment in type 1 and type 2 diabetes: a population-based study of health service resource use. Diabetes Care 26(4):1176–1180

Llahana SV, Poulton BC, Coates VE 2001 The paediatric diabetes specialist nurse and diabetes education in childhood. Journal of Advanced Nursing 33(3):296–306

Lucas S, Walker R 2004 An overview of diabetes education in the United Kingdom: past, present and future. Practical Diabetes International 21(2):61–64

McAulay V, Deary IJ, Frier BM 2001 Symptoms of hypoglycaemia in people with diabetes. Diabetic Medicine 18:690–705

Muhlhauser I, Bruckner I, Berger M et al 1987 Evaluation of an intensified insulin treatment and teaching programme as routine management of type 1 (insulin-dependent) diabetes. The Bucharest-Dusseldorf Study. Diabetologia 30(9):681–690

National Institute for Health and Clinical Excellence (NICE) 2003 Guidance of the use of patient education models for diabetes. Technology appraisal 60. NICE, London

Norris SL, Engelgau MM, Narayan KMV 2001 Effectiveness of self-management training in type 2 diabetes: a systematic review of randomized controlled trials. Diabetes Care 24:561–587

Petrella RJ, Lattanzio CN, Demeray A et al 2005 Can adoption of regular exercise later in life prevent metabolic risk for cardiovascular disease? Diabetes Care 28(3):694–701

Price D 2003 Sexual function in diabetic men and women. In Pickup JC, Williams G (eds) Textbook of diabetes, 3rd edn. Section 15: 58.1, 58.10–12. Blackwell Scientific, Oxford

Reed JA, Ashton H, Lawrence JM et al 2003 Diabetes self-management: how are we doing? Practical Diabetes International. 20(9):318–322

Scottish Intercollegiate Guidelines Network (SIGN) 2001 SIGN 55: management of diabetes. SIGN, Edinburgh

Snoek FJ 2003 Improving quality of life in diabetes: how effective is education? Patient Education and Counseling 51:1–3

Steel JM 1991 Sexual function in diabetic women. In: Pickup JC, Williams G (eds) 1991 Textbook of diabetes. Blackwell Science, Oxford

Sumner J, Dyson PA 2004 An intensive education programme for people with type 1 diabetes. Nursing Times 100(16):20–26, 51–53

Sumner J, Gillet M, Harper J 2001 Audit of group education for patients converting to insulin. Journal of Diabetes Nursing 5(5):137–140

Trento M, Passera P, Bajardi M et al 2002 Lifestyle intervention by group care prevents deterioration of type II diabetes: a 4-year randomized controlled clinical trial. Diabetologia 45(9):1231–1239

UK Prospective Diabetes Study (UKPDS) Group 1998 Effect of intensive blood-glucose control with metformin on complications in overweight patients with type 2 diabetes (UKPDS 34). Lancet 352:854–865

Van Dam HA, van der Horst FG, Knoops L et al 2005 Social support in diabetes : a systematic review of controlled intervention studies. Patient Education and Counselling 59:1–12

Vermeire E, Van Royen P, Coenen S et al 2003 The adherence of type 2 diabetes patients to their therapeutic regimens: a qualitative study from the patient's perspective. Practical Diabetes International 20(6):209–214

Williams G, Pickup JC (eds) 2004 Handbook diabetes, 3rd edn. Blackwell Science, Oxford

Woodcock A, Kinmonth AL 2001 Patient concerns in their first year with type 2 diabetes: patient and practice nurse views. Patient Education and Counseling 42:257–270

Improving care

Joan McDowell and Derek Gordon

INTRODUCTION

ORGANISATION OF CARE

People with diabetes require support to manage their own condition; this must be provided by the right people, at the right time, in the right place and with the right care. As health care in the UK is funded from public taxes, there is a public responsibility to ensure that money is used appropriately to ensure the most effective use of resources. Within the UK, the NHS facilitates equity in service provision, although its translation at national level might vary according to the unique health needs of the four nations.

The UK, and Scotland in particular, are taken as the template for this chapter. However, it is acknowledged that some of the principles outlined here are of relevance to healthcare settings in different countries across the world. It is also acknowledged that the funding for health care in different countries will drive the manner in which care is provided and hence there will be variations of practice due to economic factors (Bakker & Bilo 2004, Pedrosa 2004, Urbancic & Koselj 2004).

THE RIGHT PEOPLE

People with diabetes need access to a wide variety of people to support them in their diabetes care. In the first instance, general practitioners are the gate-keepers to specialist expertise. People who are not registered with GPs are therefore denied this point of contact.

The current delivery of care within the UK determines that most people with type 2 diabetes can receive satisfactory care within the primary care setting where structured support is offered (Griffin & Kinmonth 2005). GPs in the UK work as independent practitioners and hence hold a separate contract with the government for delivery of services. The General Medical Services Contract has introduced a new method of funding primary care practitioners with financial incentives offered to GPs who deliver diabetes care and meet national quality standards. These include annual screening for diabetes complications and percentage of people with diabetes whose cholesterol is below government targets (Kenny 2004). This is one example of government policy directly impacting on practice delivery. A Cochrane systematic review was undertaken on interventions to improve the management of diabetes in primary care, outpatient and community settings. This concluded that interventions that were targeted at healthcare professionals and organisational interventions increased the continuity of care. The effect on outcomes for people with diabetes was less clear (Renders et al 2005).

People with type 1 diabetes or those requiring specialist support around different parameters of their care, e.g. pregnancy, the use of an infusion pump or complications of diabetes, normally require specialist services in secondary care. People with complex needs, e.g. renal dialysis, also require specialist support. For the individual with diabetes, regardless of the care setting, a multidisciplinary team including doctors, nurses, podiatrists and dieticians is there to provide care.

At times, it is carers who require support. All members of the healthcare team are encouraged to involve carers in all their communications as they have a central role in supporting the person with diabetes. As diabetes affects an individual's whole lifestyle, it is important that his or her family and friends are aware of what the person is going through, the support available and what they can contribute to the person's care.

COMMUNICATION BETWEEN PEOPLE

It is essential that all professionals who are involved in the care of those with diabetes communicate effectively with individuals with diabetes, their carers and also with each other. The use of information technology has greatly facilitated this process. The development of primary care and hospital information technology systems with a common data set has resulted in the development of SCI-DC (Scottish Care Information Diabetes Collaboration, see: www.show.scot.nhs.uk/crag/topics/diabetes/diabit/Q&A.doc). This allows the flow of clinical information between different members of the team without the normal delay met through more routine channels.

PROFESSIONAL'S KNOWLEDGE

All members of the healthcare team need to be up to date in their knowledge base of diabetes to provide evidence-based care to individuals. Although post-registration education is developing as a norm within the UK (Scottish Executive 2002) it is not yet mandatory. The Scottish Executive Health Department has set up an advisory committee on diabetes education that addresses the education of professionals. In America, The Declaration of the Americas (DOTA) has set up an education task group which has established the norms for diabetes education programmes for people with diabetes in the Americas (www.paho.org). This addresses organisational issues, the educational programme for people and the professional characteristics required.

VOLUNTARY ORGANISATIONS

Voluntary organisations have a major role to play in supporting people with diabetes. The mission of the American Diabetes Association (ADA) is to 'prevent and cure diabetes and to improve the lives of all people affected by diabetes'. Through their auspices, people with diabetes can be linked with peers or professionals as required. The ADA is a non-profit-making organisation that funds research and provides information and other services to people with diabetes, their families, professionals and the public. The association also advocates for the rights of people with diabetes. It is, therefore, very similar to Diabetes UK, which was discussed in Chapter 11.

The Scottish Executive aims to ensure that the NHS meets the needs and wishes of people receiving care and treatment and that services were designed for this purpose (www.scotland.gov.uk/library3/health/pfpi-00.asp). One consequence of this was that, under the auspices of The Scottish Diabetes Group, the Patient Focus Public Involvement Group was set up. The aim of this group is to 'drive forward the implementation of the patient focus elements of the Scottish Diabetes Framework (Scottish Executive 2002) and to support the development of patient-centred diabetes services throughout NHS Scotland' (www.diabetesinscotland.org/ diabetes). Hence, within Scotland, there is a voluntary patient group that directly impacts on health service delivery for people with diabetes.

THE RIGHT TIME

People with diabetes need to access care when they determine that it is needed. This care can take the form of advice or an intervention. For this, the role of NHS 24 in Scotland, or NHS Direct in England, is crucial as an advice call centre. Diabetes UK also provides advice and a help line that can be accessed at its website (www.diabetes.org.uk). Most specialist diabetes centres offer telephone access to individuals. Both primary and secondary care normally offer drop-in clinics for individuals who want to use them.

Knowledge is power and to ensure that people with diabetes are empowered to take control of their lives, education plays an important part. Differing educational models are offered at different times within the person's journey with diabetes.

Professionals working in countries who do not necessarily have the same resources for educational programmes can still offer some form of information days for people with diabetes provided the multidisciplinary team work together to plan and shape the programme (Pender 2005).

Within the UK, Diabetes UK has taken a lead in several initiatives and their website is a ready source of material (www.diabetes.org.uk). The Welsh Assembly has supported a grant for Diabetes UK that has enabled them to compile a database of resources for people whose first language is not English. This database is to assist health professionals and covers 33 languages (www.diabetes.org.uk/health/patient/cymru.htm). Although this is not an exhaustive list, it is an excellent starting point when caring for people with different cultural backgrounds.

Information technology can also aid in the dissemination of information and can ensure that it is immediately available during consultations. SCI-DC is one example of a system that supports this for professionals. The internet has revolutionised global communications and access to information. People can access websites at a time that is most convenient to them to answer their questions or to link with others. There are thousands of websites that address aspects of diabetes care. Professionals and lay people are cautioned to access only those that are of a reputable organisation as the quality of websites is not always assured.

The web has added benefits for people with diabetes and professionals as they can all access current research through e-journals. The NHS Education for Scotland e-library (www.elib.scot.nhs.uk) aims to manage a knowledge-base to support people with diabetes. This is considered essential to ensure high-quality person-centred care. Within the e-library there is a diabetes portal that, as well as managing the many databases of books and journals, allows for ongoing discussion around topical issues in diabetes care from people with diabetes, carers, Diabetes UK and professionals. People need an Athens login address before entering the e-library. Relevant web addresses have been interspersed throughout chapters in this book, although these are not exhaustive. Two readily accessible search engines for locating professional material on the web are PubMed and Google Scholar.

THE RIGHT PLACE

To support people with diabetes, advice and interventions need to be accessible to individuals. People with type 2 diabetes are more frequently offered such services within primary care, which is usually nearer to them geographically. Those with type 1 diabetes are usually offered care within their local specialist care setting. It is acknowledged, however, that within the UK, boat, train or plane journeys might be required to access specialist care facilities.

There are particular challenges to delivering care to people who are not in a position to autonomously access care. People who live in an institutionalised setting are not usually mobile enough to attend any care settings. Those residing in nursing homes or in long-term care are dependent on others to meet their health needs, which can be complex (Benbow et al 1997). People who are housebound might not have access to some services. Community nurses in particular are uniquely placed to provide support for those who are unable to access care within a GP's practice (Forbes et al 2002, Harris 2005).

Prisoners with diabetes also have difficulty in accessing the same level of service as those living in the community (Meakin 2004). Given that the Department of Health in the UK aims to provide prisoners with the same level of care as those outside the prison, it would appear that there is still a lot of work to be done in this area (*Balance* 2005).

People who have other complex problems might also be reliant on others taking the lead role to ensure they receive the appropriate care. Those who have learning difficulties, other disease entities, or an addiction to alcohol or drugs might all experience problems in accessing care due to situations beyond their control.

We live in times of globalisation and most Westernised cities are multicultural in population groups. It is therefore essential that care is offered in a culturally sensitive way and in a culturally appropriate place. It might be necessary to hold clinics in a mosque or social club to meet the needs of particular population groups.

THE RIGHT CARE

INTERNATIONAL PERSPECTIVE

The World Health Organization (WHO) has developed a variety of documents detailing the standard and level of care that people with diabetes should expect (www.who.int/topics/diabetes_mellitus/en/) within an international framework. An international group of experts has also presented recommendations on quality indicators for diabetes care (Greenfield et al 2004). This demonstrates global collaboration to ensure that the right care is being made available for people with diabetes.

To improve care for people with diabetes requires several factors. There must first be a political will, nationally and internationally, to invest in making changes. There needs to be ongoing investment in health care, both for prevention and treatment, because of the projected pandemic of type 2 diabetes with its associated morbidity and mortality. For people with diabetes, early prevention of its complications has many cost-effective benefits. As well as enhancing people's quality of life, prevention of complications ensures a person's contribution to society is maintained.

There has also recently been a united call for a diabetes framework across Europe that would build on the UK Diabetes Frameworks mentioned below. This call has come from Diabetes UK, the International Diabetes Federation-European Region and the Federation of European Nurses in Diabetes (*Diabetes Update* 2004).

UK PERSPECTIVE

Throughout the 1990s there were many changes in the UK organisation of diabetes care (Gordon & McDowell 1996) that aims to ensure that the right care is offered to people with diabetes. In the late 1990s, the UK Government launched a programme of National Service Frameworks (NSF) for Diabetes. These NSFs span the four countries of the UK: Scotland, Northern Ireland, England and Wales.

The aim of these NSFs was to set national minimum standards of diabetes care through raising the quality of health services and reducing geographical variations in the delivery of care. The scope of the NSFs includes prevention, diagnosing and management of diabetes and its complications long term. The progress of the four NSFs has been variable but in due course they have all produced strategic implementation plans:

- Scottish Executive (2002): Scottish Diabetes Framework
- Department of Health (2003): National Service Framework for Diabetes Delivery Strategy
- Department of Health (2002): National Service Framework for Diabetes Standards in Wales
- Diabetes UK and Clinical Resource Efficiency Support Team (CREST) (2001): Northern Ireland Task Force on Diabetes.

The implementation of the plans is the responsibility of local health boards, which have devolved these to professional groups who comprise a managed clinical network.

Previously, the UK health service operated with a hierarchical structure and an internal market. With the change in government at the end of the 1990s, networks were considered to be a way forward from the internal competition to collaborative working (Powell 1999). Managed clinical networks are characterised by an ethos of trust, reciprocity, understanding and loyalty. They operate as a form of clinical governance. By mapping current service provision and sharing knowledge, resources and information, better use can be made of scarce resources and they can reduce inequities and improve access to care.

SCOTTISH PERSPECTIVE

Health became a devolved issue in Scotland with the establishment of a Scottish Parliament. In many ways, Scotland has therefore been able to take a lead within the UK on health issues. The Scottish Diabetes Framework (SDF) established building-blocks for diabetes care (Scottish Executive 2002). These blocks were prioritised to ensure they would attract new government funding. One such example was a national retinal screening programme. This was set in motion with pump-primed funding for establishing managed diabetes clinical networks in each of the

15 area health boards. Hence, within Scotland, eye screening is undertaken on a national basis as opposed to local initiatives.

The Scottish Executive thereafter established the Scottish Diabetes Group (SDG) with the remit of implementing the SDF and monitoring the same. The SDG has established a variety of subgroups that address education, research and monitoring of the SDF implementation plan for example (www.diabetesinscotland.org/diabetes). This latter subgroup is the Scottish Diabetes Survey Monitoring Group.

The Scottish Diabetes Survey Monitoring Group provides an annual report of clinical parameters of people with diabetes for all the health boards within Scotland (http://www.scotland.gov.uk/Publications/2004/10/20023/44194#1). The supply of this information is an obligation on the health boards and it is submitted anonymously to a central source. Initially, structures and processes were submitted but now outcomes of care are included. This allows the determinants of care to be monitored and assessed.

As stated earlier, there must be a political drive to change healthcare practice. The Scottish Parliament has recently set up a cross-party group in diabetes. This group aims to provide a platform for politicians regardless of their party affiliations, people with diabetes, organisations with an interest in diabetes and professionals to discuss and promote good practice. It is also a forum where issues can be raised that can directly influence policy debates within the Scottish Parliament (www.scottish.parliament.uk/msp/crossPartyGroups/groups/cpg-diabetes.htm).

QUALITY CONTROL

The Audit Commission is an independent body within the UK that is responsible for ensuring that public money is spent economically, efficiently and effectively. It aims to promote good practice and to focus resources on those people who need public services most. The Audit Commission applies to England and Wales and information on its outcomes can be found on its website (www.audit-commission.gov.uk)

The NHS Quality Improvement Scotland (NHSQIS) is a special health board in Scotland with the remit of improving care for people in Scotland (www.nhshealthquality.org). It aims to:

- provide clear advice and guidance on effective clinical practice based on a review of available evidence
- set clinical and non-clinical standards of care
- review and monitor performance of the NHS in Scotland
- run development programmes for staff
- promote clinical risk management.

Under the auspices of NHSQIS, a standards development unit has been established. Its remit is to develop and monitor standards on a national basis. Crucially, people with diabetes are involved in this process and each team reviewing the standards has lay members. Under the auspices of NHSQIS, there are clinical standards in diabetes.

The individual who has diabetes within the UK should enjoy the standard of care set out in the above documents. However, although standards are set and care is delivered in a variety of ways and in different settings, individuals also have their own unique care needs. The right care for an individual with diabetes must take into account that person's own cultural and religious perspective of life and attempt to balance this with current clinical guidelines.

IMPACT OF RESEARCH ON ORGANISATIONAL ISSUES

Research plays an important role in the delivery of care. The Diabetes Control and Complications Trial (DCCT) Research Group (1993) and the UK Prospective Diabetes Study (UKPDS) (1998) are two large studies that have had a major impact on the delivery of care. Both these clinical studies show that the goal of all care is to work with the individual to reduce both blood glucose to near normal levels and, blood pressure. Research leads to the development of clinical standards and an emerging evidence base. The Diabetes Trial Unit based in Oxford University (www.dtu.ox.ac.uk) is a centre for diabetes research and its website informs readers of ongoing research and outcome summaries for practical use.

Within Scotland, the Scottish Intercollegiate Guidelines Network (SIGN; www.sign.ac.uk) was set up by the Royal Colleges of Medicine to develop research evidence based guidelines for the NHS in Scotland, not specifically for diabetes. SIGN first produced a series of diabetes guidelines in 1996; these were updated in 2001 (SIGN 2001) and can be accessed from the website. More recently, SIGN has become part of NHS Quality Improvement Scotland (www.nhshealthquality.org).

SIGN was Scotland's response to the St Vincent Declaration (Krans et al 1995). This was a WHO response to the mortality and morbidity of diabetes; the member countries agreed to take positive action to reduce the complications of diabetes. To commence this process, it was important to establish a research evidence base of interventions that are known to affect clinical outcomes. This was established under the auspices of SIGN and is maintained and updated every 5 years.

The National Institute for Health and Clinical Excellence (NICE) in the UK is an independent organisation that is responsible for providing national guidance on the promotion of good health and the prevention and treatment of ill health. The NICE develop and update various guidelines for diabetes care that can be accessed from their website (www.nice.org.uk). NICE also has the function of determining the cost effectiveness of treatments.

The right care is continually evolving in a cyclical manner. It requires the setting up of structures and processes to support it. Figure 12.1 shows the integration between research and audit using exemplars detailed above.

Fig. 12.1
Development of
diabetes

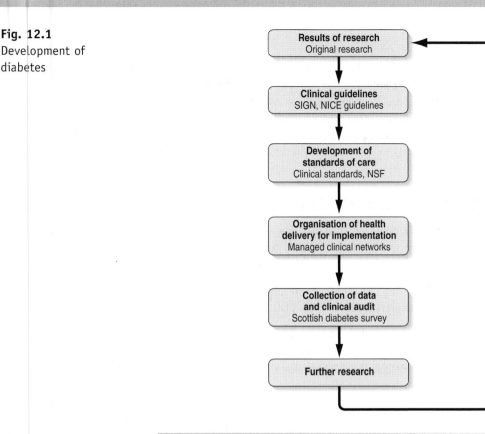

CONCLUSION

Several tiers of support are required if the appropriate treatment is to reach the individual with diabetes. People with diabetes are the experts in their own care. Their family, friends and support networks are their informal carers who are travelling with them on their journey through life. However, the actual living with diabetes can only be undertaken by individuals themselves.

Any organisation of health care must ensure that the needs of people living with diabetes are central and at the core of all health service delivery. Hence, it can be seen that the organisation of diabetes care has to consider who the right person is to deliver the care. This might be the individual with diabetes, his or her family and friends or healthcare professionals.

The timing of care is crucial to support individuals in managing their own diabetes. It is vital that specialist services are available when required. Likewise, it is also vital that when a person is ready to make a change in their diet or exercise, that the right support is offered at this time as well. As people travel through life and face many different challenges, it is important that they are equipped with the right care to manage their diabetes, on an ongoing basis.

The right place is that place that best meets the needs of individuals. This might be in their home, a GP's surgery or a hospital environment. The right care is emerging continually through research and evidence-based practice. This is an evolving field of care that is constantly being updated and reviewed. Underpinning all healthcare organisations is the political will to ensure that the above parameters are met.

REFERENCES

Bakker K, Bilo HJG 2004 Diabetes care in the Netherlands: now and in the future. Practical Diabetes International 21(2):88–91

Balance 2005 Prisoner cell block D. March–April:28–32

Benbow SJ, Walsh A, Gill GV 1997 Diabetes in institutionalised elderly people: a forgotten population? British Medical Journal 314:1868–1869

Department of Health (DH) 2002 National service framework for diabetes standards in Wales. DH, Wales

Department of Health (DH) 2003 National service framework for diabetes delivery strategy. DH, London

Diabetes Control and Complications Trial (DCCT) Research Group 1993 The effect of intensive treatment of diabetes on the development and progression of long-term complications in insulin-dependent diabetes mellitus. New England Journal of Medicine 329:977–986

Diabetes UK and Clinical Resource Efficiency Support Team (CREST) 2001 Northern Ireland task force on diabetes. CREST, Northern Ireland

Diabetes Update 2004 A framework for diabetes in Europe. Diabetes Update, Winter:7

Forbes A, Berry J, While A et al 2002 Issues and methodological challenges in developing and evaluating health-care interventions for older people with diabetes mellitus, part 1. Practical Diabetes International 19(2):55–59

Gordon D, McDowell J 1996 The organisation of diabetes care In McDowell JRS, Gordon D (eds) Diabetes: caring for patients in the community 249-261. Churchill Livingstone, Edinburgh

Greenfield S, Nicolucci A, Mattke S 2004 Selecting indicators for the quality of diabetes care at the health systems level in OECD countries. OECD health technical papers no 15. Online. Available: www.oecd.org/dataoecd/28/34/33865546.pdf

Griffin S, Kinmonth AL 2005 Systems for routine surveillance for people with diabetes mellitus. The Cochrane database of systematic reviews issue 4. Online. Available: www.cochrane.org/reviews/en/ab000541.html

Harris G 2005 Diabetic yearly reviews: the role of DNs. Journal of Community Nursing 19(7):12–17

Kenny C 2004 Primary diabetes care: yesterday, today and tomorrow. Practical Diabetes International 21(2):65–68

Krans HMJ, Porta M, Keen H, Staehr Johansen K 1995 Diabetes care and research in Europe: the St Vincent Declaration action programme. Implementation document. World Health Organization, Rome

Meakin J 2004 Diabetes behind the bars. Diabetes Update Winter:18–20. Online. Available: www.diabetes.org.uk/update/winter04/downloads/Prinsoners.pdf

Pedrosa HC 2004 Diabetes care in Brazil: now and in the future. Practical Diabetes International 21(2):86–87

Pender S 2005 Planning and information day for people with diabetes. Nursing Times 101(31):35–37

Powell M 1999 New Labour and the 'third way' in the British NHS. International Journal of Health Services 29:353–370

Renders CM, Valk GD, Griffin S et al 2005 Interventions to improve the management of diabetes mellitus in primary care, outpatient and community settings. The Cochrane database of systematic reviews issue 4. Art. No. CD001481. DOI: 10.1002/14651858. CD001481. Online. Available: www.cochrane.org/reviews/en/ab001481.html

Scottish Executive 2002 Scottish diabetes framework. Scottish Executive, Edinburgh

Scottish Intercollegiate Guidelines Network (SIGN) 2001 SIGN 55: management of diabetes. SIGN, Edinburgh

UK Prospective Diabetes Study (UKPDS) Group 1998 Intensive blood-glucose control with sulphonylureas or insulin compared with conventional treatment and risk of complications in patients with type 2 diabetes (UKPDS 33). Lancet 352:837–853

Urbancic V, Koselj M 2004 Diabetes care in Slovenia: now and in the future. Practical Diabetes International 21(2):92–94

USEFUL WEBSITE ADDRESSES

www.audit-commission.gov.uk: the Audit Commission in the UK.

www.childrenwithdiabetes.com: a support site drawing largely from the US. It is aimed at parents and children with diabetes.

www.diabetes.org.uk: Diabetes UK is an organisation that functions to meet the needs of people with diabetes and healthcare professionals caring for people with diabetes.

www.diabetes.org: American Diabetes Association.

www.diabetes-healthnet.ac.uk: the Tayside Diabetes Network, which contains several links to other relevant sites, including Scottish Care Information Diabetes Collaboration (SCI-DC).

www.diabetesinscotland.org: website for the Scottish Diabetes Group, with several excellent links.

www.dtu.ox.ac.uk: the UK Diabetes Trial Unit based at the University of Oxford.

www.easd.org: the European Association for the Study of Diabetes.

www.elib.scot.nhs.uk: the NHS Scotland e-library, which contains a diabetes portal.

www.fend.org: Federation of European Nurses in Diabetes.

www.idf.org: International Diabetes Federation.

www.jrdf.org: Juvenile Diabetes Research Foundation International.

www.nhshealthquality.org: NHS Quality Improvement Scotland.

www.nice.org.uk: the National Institute for Health and Clinical Excellence, which works on behalf of the National Health Service in the UK.

www.paho.org: the Pan American Health Organization, which includes diabetes within its topic area of non-communicable diseases.

www.scotland.gov.uk: the Scottish Executive.

www.scottish.parliament.uk: the Scottish parliament.

www.show.scot.nhs.uk: NHS Scotland.

www.sign.ac.uk: the Scottish Intercollegiate Guidelines Network (SIGN), which develops and disseminates national clinical guidelines with recommendations for effective practice based on current evidence.

www.who.int/topics/diabetes_mellitus/en: the World Health Organization.

Index